Essentials of Sonography and Patient Care

Essentials of
Sonography
and
Patient Care

Second Edition

Marveen Craig, RDMS

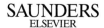

SAUNDERS
ELSEVIER

11830 Westline Industrial Drive
St. Louis, Missouri 63146

Notice

Knowledge and best practice in this field are constantly changing. As new research and experience broaden our knowledge, changes in practice, treatment and drug therapy may become necessary or appropriate. Readers are advised to check the most current information provided (i) on procedures featured or (ii) by the manufacturer of each product to be administered, to verify the recommended dose or formula, the method and duration of administration, and contraindications. It is the responsibility of the practitioner, relying on their own experience and knowledge of the patient, to make diagnoses, to determine dosages and the best treatment for each individual patient, and to take all appropriate safety precautions. To the fullest extent of the law, neither the Publisher nor the Author assumes any liability for any injury and/or damage to persons or property arising out or related to any use of the material contained in this book.

Previous edition copyrighted 1993

ISBN-13: 978-1-4160-0170-6
ISBN-10: 1-4160-0170-0

Acquisitions Editor: Jeanne Wilke
Developmental Editors: Christina Pryor and Linda Woodard
Publishing Services Manager: Pat Joiner
Project Manager: Jennifer Clark
Designers: Kathi Gosche and Andrea Lutes

Printed in the United States of America

Last digit is the print number: 9   8   7   6   5

To
ELIZABETH DIENES,
who nurtured the seed from which this book has grown.

Reviewers

Gina M. Augustine, MLS; RT(R)
Director
School of Radiography and Specialty Programs
Jameson School of Radiography
New Castle, Pennsylvania

Kevin P. Barry, M Ed; RDMS; RDCS; RT (R)
Department Head
Diagnostic Medical Imaging
New Hampshire Technical Institute
Concord, New Hampshire

Joan M. Clasby, BvE; RDMS; RT
Professor and Program Director
Diagnostic Medical Sonography
Orange Coast College
Costa Mesa, California

Janice D. Dolk, RT(R); RDMS; MA
Consultant to Sonography Projects
Performance Improvement Coordinator
Owings Mills, Maryland

Kathleen Murphy, MBA; RDMS; RT
Program Director Diagnostic Ultrasound
GateWay Community College
Phoenix, Arizona

Susanna L. Ovel, RDMS; RVT
Senior Sonographer and Instructor
RAS
Sacramento, California

Craig F. Peneff, BSAS; RDMS; RVT
Program Director and Assistant Professor
Lorain County Community College
Elyria, Ohio

Cheryl L. Zelinsky, MM; RT(R); RDMS
Associate Professor and Director
Diagnostic Medical Sonography
Oregon Institute of Technology
Klamath Falls, Oregon

Preface

In the 10 years since *Introduction to Ultrasonography and Patient Care* was first published, sweeping changes in ultrasound technology, the delivery of health care, and the practice of diagnostic ultrasound have occurred. To respond to this changing world, change has come to sonography education as well.

This second edition reflects a significant makeover in response to those needs. In addition to a new look on the cover is a new title. Inside are updated and expanded chapters on sonographer safety; legal, ethical, and legislative issues; current sonographic protocols; and basic patient care. Each chapter begins with a list of general objectives and key terms designed to help readers best understand the material. At the end of each chapter, bibliographic references offer direction to those seeking a more in-depth exploration of a given topic.

To help ease students into the working profession, new information on applying and interviewing for positions and understanding the hospital and nonhospital opportunities available to them have been added. The appendices contain an updated glossary, an abbreviated list of Spanish phrases useful in communicating with imaging patients, a list of laboratory tests specific to various clinical ultrasound specialties, and important regulatory practices regarding patient care and safety.

One sad note among all of this exciting change and promise for the future is the realization that the gains of the past extracted a severe toll on the health of many veteran sonographers. Their bittersweet legacy is already paving the way for current and future sonographers to enjoy their chosen profession without fear of career-ending injuries. We are all deeply indebted to them.

It is my hope that those who use this book find it helpful in enjoying safe, successful, and rewarding careers as diagnostic medical sonographers.

EVOLVE RESOURCES

Completely new Evolve resources have been created. They consist of an instructor's manual, focused teaching outlines, an expanded test bank, and an electronic image collection. The material is designed to help instructors develop class presentations, test student comprehension of the material, and create student interest and enthusiasm with interactive assignments. The resources for *Essentials of Sonography and Patient Care* are located on Evolve, an interactive learning environment.

Evolve works in coordination with *Essentials of Sonography and Patient Care*. Instructors may use Evolve to provide an Internet-based course component that reinforces and expands the concepts presented in class. Evolve may be used to publish the class syllabus, outlines, and lecture notes; set up "virtual office hours" and e-mail communication; share important dates and information through the online class calendar; and encourage student participation through chat rooms and discussion boards. Evolve allows instructors to post examinations and manage their grade books online. For more information, readers can contact an Elsevier sales representative.

Marveen Craig

Acknowledgments

In completing this book, many thanks are in order, and I hesitate for fear of omitting anyone. I am especially indebted to Joan Baker; Phil Bendick, PhD; Eric Blackwell, MD; Terry DuBose; Don Milburn; and Joseph Woo, MD, who supplied photographs—both elusive to obtain and difficult to reproduce. They helped to illustrate the old and the new, as well as just how far diagnostic ultrasound has come in 5 decades.

The final product would not have been possible without the valuable constructive criticisms and much appreciated encouragement of those who reviewed both manuscripts and of my editors at Elsevier Science: Jeanne Wilke, Linda Woodard, and the indefatigable Christina Pryor.

My heartfelt thanks go to my husband, Walter, and my family and friends for their emotional support and for allowing me to put the book first, when necessary.

My thanks also go to the following sonographers, who generously shared the scanning protocols used in Chapter 7:

Abdominal Protocols
M. Robert de Jong, RDMS, RDCS, RVT
Radiology Technical Manager
The Johns Hopkins Hospital
Baltimore, Maryland

OB/GYN Protocols
Pamela Foy, BS, RDMS
Clinical Coordinator of OB Ultrasound
The Ohio State University Medical Center
Columbus, Ohio

Echocardiography Protocols
Ann Dempsey, RDCS, RDMS, RVT, FASE
AcuNav Product Specialist
Siemens Medical Solutions
Mountain View, California

Marveen Craig

Contents

Chapter 1

The Origins and Evolution of Diagnostic Medical Sonography

Learning Objectives

Students who successfully complete this chapter will be able to do the following:

- Describe the evolutionary history of diagnostic ultrasound.
- Identify at least four of the leading pioneers who shaped the new technology of ultrasound.
- Define related imaging modality terms.
- Compare and contrast imaging modalities.

Key Terms

A-Mode	Doppler effect	real-time imaging
analog scan converter	gray-scale imaging	therapeutic ultrasound
B-Mode	harmonic imaging	3-D imaging
bistable	M-Mode	4-D imaging
cavitation	piezoelectric effect	ultrasound
digital scan converters		

The taproots of diagnostic ultrasound can be traced to one of the oldest sciences—that of sound, or acoustics—which dates back to the ancient Greeks. However, the goal of this chapter is to acquaint the student with some of the developmental milestones and contributing pioneers who shaped this new science, rather than to provide a detailed history of ultrasound.

The systematic study of sound began in 500 BC with the Greek mathematician Pythagoras, who observed the relationship between sound pitch and frequency. But much earlier cultures such as those of the Egyptians, the Persians, and the Chinese had developed musical instruments and become interested in the propagation of sound. Pythagoras is said to have invented the sonometer, an instrument used to study musical sounds.

A hundred years later, the Greek scholar Archytas of Tarentum defined the nature of sound, deducing that sound is produced by the motion of one object striking another, with swift motion producing a high pitch and slow motion producing a low pitch. It was not until 350 BC that Aristotle developed the theory of sound propagation (i.e., sound is carried to the ears by the movement of air).

A familiar sound analogy, which is still used by contemporary physics teachers, can be attributed to the Roman philosopher Boethius, who was the first to compare sound waves with the waves produced by dropping a pebble into a calm body of water.

From then until 1300 AD, little scientific investigation occurred in Europe, although scientists in the Middle East and India were developing new ideas about sound by studying music and working out systems of music theory.

The study of sound remained relatively dormant during the Middle Ages but experienced a revival in the upsurge of scientific interest after the Renaissance.

In 1500 the illustrious Leonardo da Vinci became intrigued with the physical properties of sound, and he is thought to have originated the idea that sound travels in waves. He is also credited with discovering that the angle of reflection is equal to the angle of incidence.

Europeans did not begin extensive experiments on the nature of sound until 1638, when Galileo demonstrated that the frequency of sound waves determines pitch. In the late 1600s, Sir Isaac Newton announced the derivation of the theory of velocity, and the English chemist Robert Boyle popularized the theory of the elasticity of air.

Over the next two and a half centuries, experiments would be performed and mathematic calculations developed that would lead to the current understanding of the fundamentals of acoustics. The end of the nineteenth century marked the beginning of the modern study of acoustics, with the publication of *Theory of Sound* (1877) by the British scientist Lord Rayleigh. In his remarkable book, Rayleigh gathered, clarified, and expanded the current knowledge of acoustics.

THE NATURE OF ULTRASOUND

One of the first experiments dealing with **ultrasound** (sound with frequencies above the limits of human hearing) occurred in 1793, when Lazzaro Spallanzani, an Italian priest-scientist, studied the activities of bats. Observing that bats could function effectively in the dark even if blinded—but not if deafened—Spallanzani theorized that the bats were listening to something he could not hear. Exactly what it was eluded him.

During the scientifically rich nineteenth century, theories, investigations, and discoveries about sound abounded. Among them were the theory of wave diffraction proposed by the

French physicist Augustin Fresnel, the invention of the ultrasonic whistle by Sir Francis Galton, and the description of the ferromagnetic effect by James Joule.

The effect of motion on the pitch of sounds was first postulated by Austrian scientist Christian Johann Doppler and named the Doppler effect in his honor. In 1845 Doppler formulated his principle that when a source of wave motion itself moves, the apparent frequency of the emitted wave changes.

Even Wilhelm Roentgen was involved in studying sound before radiographs captured his attention. The field of ultrasound was made accessible, however, in 1880, with the discovery by the Curie brothers (Jacques and Pierre) of the phenomenon of piezoelectricity. These researchers established the presence of the **piezoelectric effect** when they observed that certain crystals would expand and contract slightly when placed in an alternating electrical field. Reverse piezoelectricity permitted the same crystal to create an electric potential, or voltage, making the crystals useful as both receivers and sources of sound waves, from audible to ultrasonic frequencies. Their accomplishments ultimately led to development of the modern ultrasound transducer.

Not until the twentieth century did scientists learn how to produce ultrasound and put it to work. Until then, ultrasonic waves were little more than a scientific curiosity.

During World War I, French physicist Paul Langevin and Constantin Chilowsky studied controlled sound frequency and intensity and discovered a way to use the property of echoing sound waves to detect underwater objects. Their device, the hydrophone, was used extensively in the surveillance of German submarines. It was in 1916, during World War I, that the first submarine detected by the hydrophone was sunk. Even more important was the fact that their studies laid the groundwork for the development of sonar in the next great war.

Langevin also discovered the harmful effects of ultrasound on marine life when he observed that small fish swimming through ultrasound beams were killed instantly. He realized the potential power of the energy with which he was dealing when one of his assistants, holding his hand briefly in the path of the sound wave, experienced agonizing pain—as if the very bones were being heated!

The answer to Spallanzani's eighteenth century questions had to wait until 1938, when G. W. Pierce invented a sonic detector. This instrument was able to pick up the high-frequency vibrations of bats and convert them into audible sounds.

Science and industry are jointly responsible for the great strides made in the understanding and refinement of ultrasonic energy. Industrialists such as Floyd Firestone, with his ultrasonic invention called the *reflectoscope,* harnessed its awesome power and found many uses for it such as metallic flaw detection and cleansing.

MEDICAL APPLICATIONS

In 1927, Robert Williams Wood and Alfred Lee Loomis first discussed the destructive nature of ultrasound on biologic organisms and living tissues. The effect of high doses of ultrasonic energy on the body is as injurious as radiographs and atomic radiation. In lower doses, however, ultrasonic energy can be a therapeutic agent. The effects produced by high-energy ultrasonic waves normally are irreversible and arise from cavitation, intense mechanical stresses, or intense localized heating. Focused high-energy ultrasound waves are used as **therapeutic ultrasound** to remove unwanted tissue. The minimum-damaging ultrasound

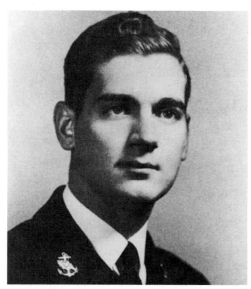

A

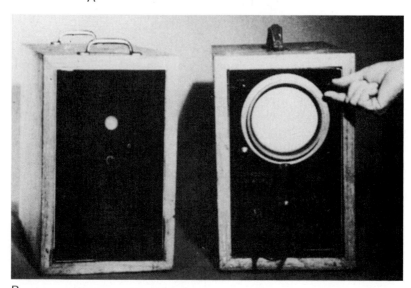

B

FIGURE **1-1 A,** Dr. George D. Ludwig conducted A-mode experiments for the U.S. Navy to detect the presence of gallstones and other foreign bodies embedded in animal tissues. One of his primary concerns was establishing the physical and physiologic standards of the velocity of ultrasonic transmission through gallstones versus tissue. **B,** Scanning apparatus used by Dr. Ludwig to investigate sound transmission and the acoustic properties of tissue.

dose is not easily defined at present, nor is it possible to correlate a definite type of tissue damage with a universally standardized dosage.

In contrast, low-intensity ultrasonic waves can be used to visualize the interior of the body. An ultrasonic examination is noninvasive, and since the late 1960s, scientists have been painlessly probing the soft tissues of the human body, seeing with sound.

In 1942 Austrian Karl Dussik was one of the first physicians to use ultrasound for diagnostic purposes. Using **A-Mode**, the 1-D representation of reflected sound waves, he claimed that tumors of the brain could be detected ultrasonically. He referred to these images of the brain as *hyperphonograms.*

The development of metal flaw detectors and naval sonar also made possible the work of three independent American investigators: George Ludwig, John Wild, and Douglass Howry.

From 1947 to 1949, Ludwig, a Pennsylvania surgeon, working first at the Naval Medical Research Institute and then with colleagues at the Massachusetts Institute of Technology, successfully used ultrasound to detect gallstones embedded in animal tissues (Fig. 1-1).

Wild, a surgeon who emigrated from England to America, first thought of using ultrasound to detect tissue thickness. In his work at the University of Minnesota, he realized that cancerous tissues differed greatly from normal tissues. Along with engineer John Reid, he constructed an early prototype breast scanner that employed the use of an externally placed water path. Their **B-Mode** techniques used 2-D presentations of echo-producing interfaces (Fig. 1-2). Wild also pioneered in the development of early internal scanners, devising a rectal transducer to obtain images of the large bowel.

In Denver, radiologist Douglass Howry worked independently of the other groups. Howry had pursued an interest in diagnostic ultrasound since 1948; however, it was not

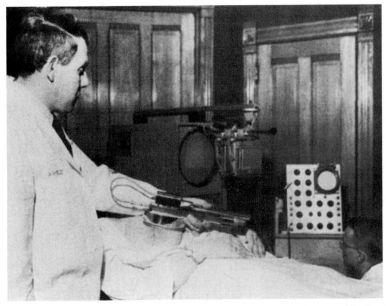

FIGURE **1-2** Dr. John A. Wild (*left*) applying a B-mode scanner to a patient's breast, while Dr. John M. Reid operates the system controls (*lower right*).

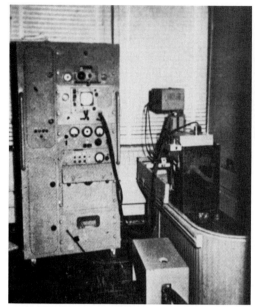

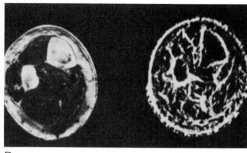

A

FIGURE **1-3 A,** The "cattle-tank" immersion scanning system. The transducer assembly is mounted on the wooden track running along the outside edge of the tank. The actual transducer was submerged within the water-filled tank. **B,** Horizontal ultrasonic scan of a human leg produced by the cattle-tank scanner.

until 1951, using war surplus electronic components, that he constructed a "water-path" scanner. He used a laundry tub and later a cattle tank for his first prototypes, in which the subject or the body part to be imaged was submersed in water (Fig. 1-3). However, the resulting 1-D images were disappointingly incomplete. Joining forces with his friend and mentor Joseph Holmes, a University of Colorado physician, resulted in the development of a compound scanner. Howry and Holmes discovered that by simultaneously moving the transducer in two different motion patterns, a more complete anatomic picture could be formed. The cattle tank eventually was replaced by an upturned B-29 gun turret in which the subject was not only immersed but also weighted down to avoid floating or introducing motion artifacts as the mechanically circling transducer cut a path through the water (Fig. 1-4).

The impracticality of using this method on sick patients spurred these scientists to simplify the procedure and to successfully develop a "pan" scanner (1957) that permitted the patient to sit next to, but outside, a small pan of water through which the transducer moved.

The experience Howry and Holmes gained eventually led to the development of a compound contact scanner, which permitted direct scanning of the body with the use of a light film of oil or lubricating gel to replace the cumbersome water path (Fig. 1-5). These early **bistable** images registered echoes on a phosphorus-coated oscilloscope screen as dots of light, using a *storage* or *bistable* cathode ray tube. All echoes greater than predetermined specific amplitudes were displayed as constant-intensity dots of light.

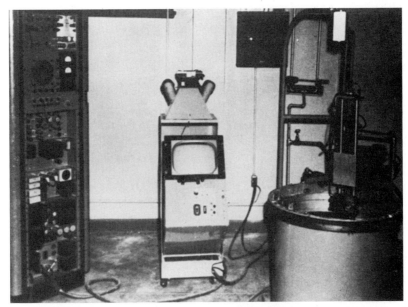

FIGURE **1-4** Douglass Howry and Joseph Holmes' B-29 gun turret water-bath scanner (c. 1953-1954). The transducer assembly is mounted on a ring encircling the tank. This arrangement provided a complete 360-degree scan path around the immersed patient. The transducer could be raised and lowered to a desired level within the tank. A second motor moved the transducer in a 4-inch back-and-forth-sectoring motion. *Left*, the tall console contained the electronic system; *center*, the display console; *right*, the gun turret and transducer carriage assembly.

A major limitation of the bistable imaging technique (existing in either black or white) was that the storage phosphor was either "off" or "on." This resulted in a white dot from an echo, at or above threshold strength, appearing on the screen. If the echo reflection was below the established threshold strength, no echo dot would be visible on the screen.

After Howry left Denver to work at the Massachusetts Institute of Technology, Holmes worked closely with William Wright, an electronic engineer. The fruits of their labors were realized in 1962 with the introduction of the first commercially available portable ultrasonic system, a compound contact scanner known as the *Physionics Engineering Porta-Arm* (Fig. 1-6). This system gained worldwide acceptance and use. The work of the Denver group is considered one of the most seminal pioneering contributions in B-mode imaging and contact scanning. The Porta-Arm scanner was the direct precursor to the imaging systems in use today.

In the mid-1950s, Ian Donald, aware of Howry's work and that of the Japanese, began his study of diagnostic ultrasonography in Scotland. His interest developed from World War II experiences with the Royal Air Force, during which he witnessed the ultrasonic testing of aircraft to detect metal stress and fatigue. Donald vowed to pursue his notion that ultrasound might be used in a similar fashion on patients.

By means of comparative examinations of an excised tumor and a beefsteak (from the local butcher shop), Donald proved that tumors possessed echo patterns different from those of normal tissue. This work was conducted in an atomic boiler plant outside Glasgow with

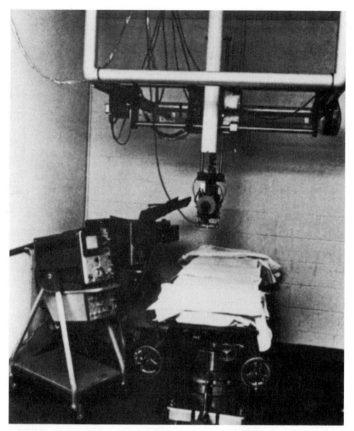

FIGURE **1-5** The University of Colorado's first compound contact scanner as constructed by consulting engineers William Wright and Ed Meyer for Dr. Joseph Holmes. The system required one individual to manually guide the ceiling-mounted transducer carriage across the patient's body, as the transducer mechanically sectored 30 degrees to either side of the perpendicular. A second individual operated the controls and the camera (*left*). This system was used during the 1960s to develop many of the scanning protocols still practiced today.

use of a borrowed flaw detector. Later, again using borrowed equipment and A-mode technique, he began detecting ovarian cysts, ascites, and polyhydramnios in his patients. Donald is credited with perfecting the A-mode measurement of the fetal biparietal diameter (1959), making it possible to ultrasonically estimate fetal age, weight, and growth rate.

In 1957 Donald collaborated with industrial engineer Tom Brown to develop a contact compound scanner. They mounted it on a bedside table and suspended it over the patient. Manipulating the transducer by hand underneath the table, Donald, using brightness modulation (B-mode) technique, produced the first crude fetal scans. By 1960 Donald and Brown had developed a mechanical sector scanner and later a hand-held scanner called the *diasonograph,* suitable for commercial distribution (Fig. 1-7).

Despite Donald's involvement in the research and development of ultrasound equipment, his primary interest was in applying diagnostic ultrasonography to his specialty of obstetrics

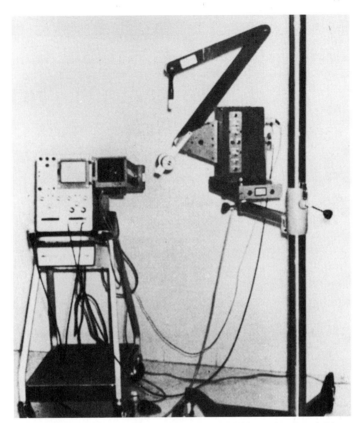

FIGURE **1-6** Porta-Arm scanner. Engineers William Wright and Ed Meyer developed this portable compound contact scanner after forming their own company, Physionics Engineering. Freed from the ceiling mount and positioned on a wheeled tripod, the transducer mechanism, a three-jointed scanning arm, and a mechanical and electronic "box" could be moved along a calibrated metal track. Horizontal or longitudinal positioning of the "arm" permitted scans in two planes. A single operator could now operate the scanner, controls, and camera.

and gynecology (Fig. 1-8). He is credited with contributing to the diagnosis of multiple pregnancies, hydramnios, and hydatidiform mole, and the introduction of the fluid-filled bladder technique used in early pregnancy and gynecologic studies. His crowning achievement occurred in 1954 when he was the first to demonstrate a fetal gestational sac, which earned him the title "father of obstetric ultrasound."

The year 1954 witnessed another exciting discovery. In Sweden, physicist Carl Hellmuth Hertz and Dr. Inge Edler, using a flaw detector borrowed from the Malmo shipyards, demonstrated a motion display of the heart and intracardiac structures called **M-mode**. Employing both A- and B-mode techniques, they added a continuously moving display of the returning cardiac echoes (Fig. 1-9). At first they were stymied by an inability to identify the various motion patterns, until Edler realized that he was seeing the characteristic motion patterns of the anterior leaflet of the mitral valve. Dr. Sven Effert, placing a transducer directly on the heart, verified all of Edler's previous identification and motion patterns,

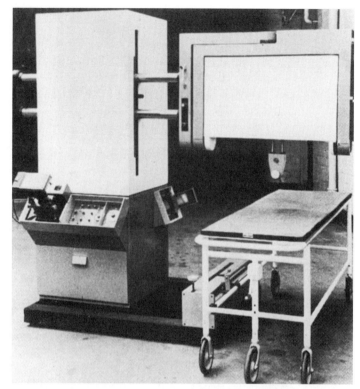

FIGURE **1-7** Developed from prototypes designed by Ian Donald and Tom Brown, the Diasonograph was introduced commercially by Nuclear Enterprises, Ltd., Edinburgh, in 1964.

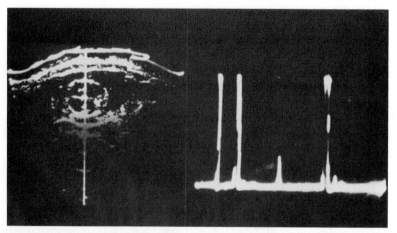

FIGURE **1-8** Fetal head and biparietal measurement. *Left,* A cross-sectional scan of the fetal head outlined in B-mode presentation. *Right,* An A-mode presentation of the midline echo. This scan (c. 1964) is thought to have been produced with the diasonograph.

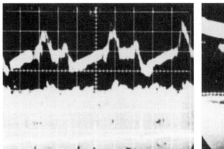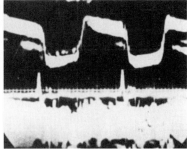

FIGURE **1-9** Early M-mode scans of the mitral valve. Carl Hellmuth Hertz and Inge Edler developed an ultrasonic technique to display graphic cardiac motion. Reflected echo information appeared as a bright dot moving along the screen as the structure being imaged moved or shifted position. A special camera and continuous moving film displayed the wave form motion of the echo dot reflected from the intracardiac structures. *Left*, Normal mitral valve patterns. *Right*, An abnormal, flat-topped stenotic mitral valve pattern.

validating Edler's observations. With this achievement, the diagnostic potential of echocardiography became apparent. Construction of echocardiography equipment would not occur, however, until cardiologist Claude Joyner and Reid at the University of Pennsylvania collaborated with Howry and Holmes at the University of Colorado.

Arvo Oksala (Finland) and Gilbert Baum (United States) each pioneered early ophthalmologic ultrasound applications during the 1950s. Oksala was the first to adapt A-mode technique for use in the eye and to correctly interpret the resulting ophthalmic echo data. Baum initially worked with the A-mode presentation but, dissatisfied with its lack of precision, turned his efforts to applying B-mode techniques to ophthalmology. He and his colleagues were the first to employ ultrasonic frequencies of 10 to 15 MHz, which produced significantly higher resolution. Baum also was successful in producing a 3-D image of the eyes with what he called "third-generation" B-mode ultrasound equipment. The system employed successive scans at each millimeter of eye depth.

The early 1960s also found J. Stauffer Lehman (United States) involved in the early investigation of ultrasound technology. His association with Smith-Kline Instruments resulted in the development and production of a water-bag and contact B-mode scanners, as well as A- and M-mode echocardiography systems. Lehman was later joined by Barry Goldberg, who was published extensively on wide-ranging clinical ultrasound subjects and was the first investigator outside Europe to detail the methods and advantages of fetal cephalometry (1965).

In New York City Lajos von Micsky focused attention on abdominal and endoscopic ultrasound instruments and produced some of the earliest abdominal, transvesical, rectal, and transvaginal systems.

A dramatic application of ultrasonography in ophthalmic medicine took place in the late 1960s, when Dr. Nathaniel Bronson, working in New York City, combined two new medical developments. The first was a tiny forceps that could grasp small objects easily and accurately. The other discovery was spurred by a suggestion of the aforementioned Finnish scientist, Arvo Oksala, to use a sonar beam to "see" inside the eye.

Using war surplus electronic components, Bronson assembled a sonar device that could explore the eye from the outside. Then he devised a hand-held, combination sonar transducer-probe, small enough to operate inside the minuscule incisions used in eye surgery.

Hooking the probe up to a small oscilloscope screen to display the echoes, Bronson tested the probe on every bit of foreign matter that could conceivably lodge in the human eye. In September 1964 at Walter Reed Hospital, outside Washington, D.C., Bronson's device was used successfully on a human being for the first time to remove a ¼-inch brass sliver from the eye of an 11-year-old boy.

The bistable years

From the mid-1960s, how bistable ultrasound imaging might enhance clinical diagnosis was studied around the world. In Denver Joseph Holmes and obstetric colleagues Ken Gottesfeld and Horace Thompson were awarded grants to investigate such diverse areas as adult polycystic kidney disease, liver transplantation, visualization of the placenta, diagnosis of fetal death in utero, midline brain shifts in workers exposed to industrial toxins, and A-mode investigations of the heart. Interested in education as well, Holmes extended an open-door policy to any individuals interested in ultrasound so that they could learn by observing the daily operation of his research and clinical laboratories. The visitor's logbook filled rapidly with the names of many early ultrasound pioneers and individuals who were—or would soon become—luminaries in the field. In addition to the ongoing "show-and-tell" sessions, the Denver group was active in publishing research, organizing numerous ultrasound seminars and conferences, and lecturing nationally and internationally.

Biophysical and bioeffects research

The biophysical and therapeutic applications of ultrasound have a longer history than the diagnostic ultrasound applications. Among the major contributors to the understanding of ultrasound applications in biology and medicine were William Fry, a physicist at the University of Illinois, and his brother, Francis Fry, founder of the Bioacoustics Research Laboratory. William, aided by a Navy research grant, explored the possibilities that high-intensity ultrasound eventually could provide a noninvasive, lower-risk surgical technique, as compared with standard invasive surgery. He was to find that it also offered unique advantages in the investigation of how the brain functioned. William designed a sophisticated system employing a multiple transducer system of focused, high-intensity sound beams that could produce a pinpoint lesion without damaging to surrounding tissue.

Francis later became interested in developing a computer-based, low-intensity ultrasound instrument for soft tissue visualization. With his coworker Elizabeth Kelly, he embarked on the study of using ultrasound to detect breast cancer. Elizabeth Kelly Fry is recognized today as one of the leading authorities on ultrasonic breast scanning.

From its inception, the safety of ultrasound has been continuously studied. As early as 1967, Donald conducted extensive experiments that demonstrated no harmful effects from the ultrasonic insonation of human cells. His work agreed with previous Japanese studies (1963) on pregnant rats that found no ill effects from ultrasound exposure at low power levels. Early research carried out at various American universities by Wesley Nyborg, Paul Carson, Raymond Gramiak, William and Francis Fry, William O'Brien, and Marvin Ziskin focused on the in vitro effects of ultrasonic insonation in producing heating, **cavitation** (the formation of gas- or vapor-filled cavities), and bubbling in tissue. As a result of these efforts, a document entitled *Guidelines on Biological Safety* was published.

Twenty years later, it would be possible to study the long-term effects on children who had been exposed prenatally to ultrasound. Again, even in these longitudinal studies, no adverse effects were demonstrated. As a result of these and ongoing research studies, safety statements have been issued. These statements support the widely held belief that clinical use of diagnostic ultrasound has not been found to cause any adverse effects in humans.

The gray-scale revolution

The 1950s and 1960s were to become the golden age of diagnostic ultrasonography. The problem with the current bistable images was their failure to show the subtle amplitudes of soft tissue. The solution came in the form of an **analog scan converter**, an advance that was primarily due to work started by George Kossoff and William Garrett in Australia in 1969. With the new analog scan converter systems, when reflected echoes were returned from the body, computer-processor technology was used to process them as signals, which allowed them to be "scaled." Clinically relevant echoes reflecting from the internal texture of soft tissues could now be displayed in varying shades of gray on and recorded from a television monitor. This advance was called **gray-scale imaging**. As an added bonus, calipers could now be applied directly on the screen. Image recording of the time used videotape, emulsion films, and thermal printing devices. With the help of Garrett, Kossoff designed and constructed a compound water-path scanner for obstetric use. Their pioneering achievements resulted in the development of gray-scale imaging, dramatically increasing the information content of images and revolutionizing diagnostic ultrasonographic equipment design and acceptance (Fig. 1-10). In 1975, Kossoff and his colleagues created the Ultrasonic Institute Octoson, a rapid multitransducer water-bath scanner. Using the latest scan converter technology, the Octoson produced high-resolution compound scans at an astonishing rate of one scan per second.

The continued quest to improve the resolution and display of echo information eventually resulted in analog scan converters being replaced with **digital scan converters**, which stored echoes in a digital format. One of the earliest digital scan converters was produced in 1976 (Searle Ultrasound) and was capable of producing 64 shades of "gray."

Japanese work in diagnostic ultrasonography, which began in 1950, roughly paralleled the developments taking place in Europe and the United States. The Japanese placed considerably more emphasis on Doppler and echocardiography than scientists in any other country. At the same time that Kossoff and Garrett were perfecting their water-path scanner, physicist Rokuru Uchida and Dr. S. Oka were building a special apparatus for the new ultrasound application of shattering renal stones.

The Doppler revolution

In the United States, serious Doppler ultrasound research was not undertaken until the late 1950s. Medical ultrasound uses the **Doppler effect**, in which the frequency of sound increases or decreases as the source moves toward or away from the transducer to recognize echo signals from moving reflectors. In 1958 Donald Baker, who designed several sophisticated, implantable flowmeters, joined Robert Rushmer and Dean Franklin. This University of Washington group is credited with the development of a small, hand-held, portable, continuous-wave Doppler device for transcutaneous use. In 1964 Eugene Strandness, a vascular surgery resident, joined the group to conduct clinical trials. His involvement with the project inspired him to devote his career to the study and development of noninvasive measuring of the peripheral vascular systems. A giant step

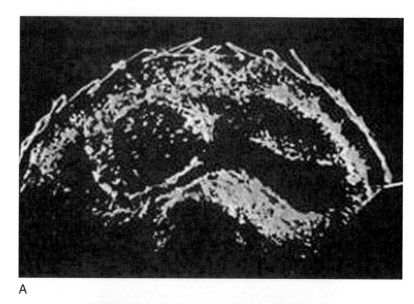

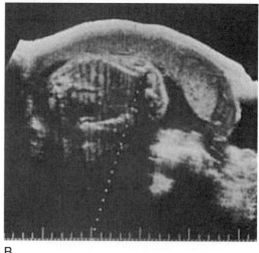

FIGURE **1-10** Comparison scans of early bistable and gray-scale images. **A,** Bistable, compound-contact B-scan of a pregnant abdomen made with the diasonograph (c. 1960s). **B,** Gray-scale scan of the fetal trunk and placenta made with a Picker 80L static scanner (c. early 1980s).

forward came with his 1967 publication on assigning particular waveforms to specific disease conditions.

Work on pulsed Doppler applications began in 1966 and in 1970 culminated in the development of the first pulsed Doppler system by Baker and his coworker Dennis Watkins (with guidance from Reid) (Fig. 1-11). Baker also worked on a technique for determining blood flow volume from Doppler velocimetry measurements. In 1974 the Seattle group

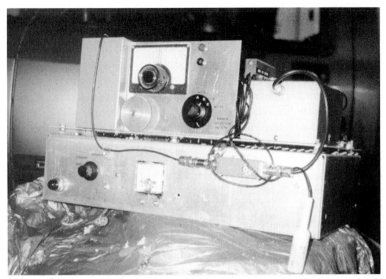

FIGURE **1-11** The first pulsed-Doppler system developed by Donald Baker at the University of Washington in 1966.

designed the first pulsed-Doppler scanner capable of combining with 2-D gray-scale imaging. It was now possible to use gray-scale imaging to guide the placement of the ultrasound beam for Doppler signal acquisition. Additional early work in pulsed Doppler was carried out in England, France, Japan, Norway, Finland, and Australia as well.

The next Doppler breakthrough provided color-coded velocity waveforms and flow images superimposed on M-mode and 2-D gray-scale images (1975). Early color-flow Doppler systems were limited by processing power, lack of good duplex arrays, and inadequate algorithms and techniques for estimating Doppler frequency. It would take Japanese investigators (Chihiro, Kasai, Koroku, Damekawa, and Omoto) to demonstrate that real-time color-flow imaging was possible with the use of a phased detector. Their approach to color-flow mapping continues to be used today and contributed indirectly to supplying an intricate piece to the puzzle of medical diagnosis, by demonstrating that tissue vascularity increases in the presence of malignant conditions.

Early cardiac investigation

The field of echocardiography found a passionate proponent in Harvey Feigenbaum (United States), whose work on the ultrasound detection of pericardial effusion was published in 1965. Feigenbaum was captivated by the technique and became a tireless apostle and mentor. He established and conducted some of the first echocardiography courses and wrote *the* definitive text on echocardiography (1972), which, after many updates and printings, is still revered today.

Gramiak and Shah, at the University of Rochester, introduced the concept of contrast echocardiography in 1969, thereby greatly advancing cardiac ultrasonography.

The 1970s and 1980s were a rich period, as publications by Goldberg, Shane, Seaward, Popp, Nana, De Maria, and Chisels advanced the acceptance of echocardiography in the exploration of all forms of cardiac disease. The search for better echocardiographic windows into the heart resulted in the development of transesophageal transducers during the 1980s. Within the next decade, biplane and omniplane transducers with color-flow and Doppler capabilities also were introduced, quickly becoming indispensable to the practice of cardiology.

The 1980s also saw the formation of many companies and commercial divisions of major corporations devoted to the manufacture of ultrasound equipment. Picker, Toshiba, Aloka, KretzTechnic, Johnson & Johnson, Siemens, Unirad, Acuson, Diasonics, Philips, and ATL were among the largest and most successful in worldwide sales.

The real-time revolution

Real-time imaging refers to images produced by automated scanners with sufficient speed to visualize and record moving structures, as well as stationary echo reflectors. The first moving ultrasound images were achieved with an instrument called a fast B-scanner that was developed by German scientists Krause and Soldner.

Siemens Medical Systems eventually marketed this machine as the Vidoson system in 1965. The Vidoson used rotating transducers housed in front of a parabolic mirror in a water coupling system and produced 15 images per second. The resulting 120 line images were of good resolution and were displayed in basic gray-scale format. The system was relatively large, however, because the transducer housing was mounted on a mobile gantry and rigidly connected to a main console. The Vidoson enjoyed 10 years of European popularity because of its ability to display and study movement, especially fetal cardiac motion, fetal breathing, and gross fetal body movements. Radiologist Fred Winsberg (Canada) was one of the Vidoson's earliest North American proponents and published many of the earliest papers concerning real-time imaging.

In 1973 Griffith and Henry, at the U.S. National Institutes of Health, produced a mechanical oscillating real-time scanner. Because it was capable of producing a clear, 30-degree sector, real-time image, it significantly advanced the development of echocardiography.

The first multielement linear electronic array transducer was produced in 1964 by Werner Buschman (East Germany). However, it was Martin Wilcox, founder of the Advanced Diagnostic Research (ADR) Corporation, who designed one of the most popular commercially available, linear-array, real-time scanners in 1973 (Fig. 1-12). The ADR scanner would set the standard for many subsequent designs by being smaller and more compact than the current static imagers. In 1975 the newest ADR unit used focusing techniques, which were so popular that an unprecedented 5000 units were ordered worldwide. A 3-MHz variable focus transducer was added in 1980. It boasted both mechanical and phased focusing, improved gain, reduced noise, switchable focal zones, and a much *quieter* transducer.

Initially, the intent was to use the smaller real-time scanners only to complement static scanners. The poorer resolution, smaller field of view, and less accurate measuring systems of the fledgling real-time scanners created a reluctance to switch from static scanners exclusively to real-time systems. Eventually, as those areas were remedied, the large, bulky, static scanners were rapidly phased out or replaced as the advantages of the much improved real-time scanners became apparent. The new systems were more mobile and flexible, and the only remaining drawback that critics could find was the systems' limited field of view. Mass conversion from static to real-time scanners, however, would not happen until 1985.

One early ultrasound application that eventually gained wide acceptance was its use in amniocentesis. Initially, patients were scanned in the ultrasound laboratory and the optimum

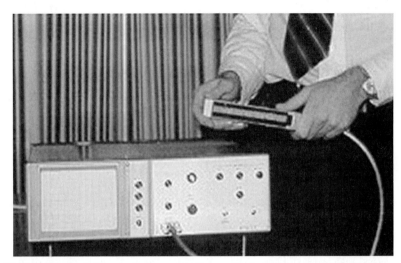

FIGURE **1-12** The Advanced Diagnostic Research Corporation's linear-array real-time ultrasound system. Designed by Martin Wilcox, the scanner made its debut in 1974, setting an industry standard for abdominal and obstetric imaging.

site for amniocentesis was determined. Then patients returned to their obstetricians for performance of the procedure. It was not until the late 1970s that Jason Birnholz, at Harvard, pioneered the concept of using a real-time phased array not only to localize the best fluid pocket but also to identify the needle tip. This permitted a safer and more convenient procedure to be performed in the ultrasound setting. Manufacturers quickly developed needle guide adapters to be used not only for amniocentesis but also for the aspiration of cysts within the abdominal organs and cavities. Performing invasive procedures with the use of real-time ultrasound gained wide acceptance; however, the use of needle adapters was eventually discarded because their configuration often limited the areas of needle placement. In addition, the need to sterilize needle adapters between procedures meant they were not always readily available.

The era of transducer technology

The 1980s ushered in an era devoted to improving image resolution by means of innovative and sophisticated transducer designs. Real-time scanners now offered curvilinear (convex) transducers, which virtually replaced the larger linear arrays. Transducer crystal technology blossomed, yielding broadband capabilities, increased arrays, faster computation times, increased numbers of focal zones, and automatic time-gain controls. Outmoded analog functions were replaced with high-speed digital electronics. These breakthroughs were made in large part because of technology advances in the nonmedical areas of telecommunications, radar, and consumer electronics.

The advent of real-time imaging had its greatest impact on the field of obstetrics. The ability to visualize such structures as the fetal yolk sac, measure crown rump lengths, and visualize fetal heart activity early in the first trimester of pregnancy pushed the boundaries of reproductive knowledge farther and faster than ever before. Observing fetal activity and fetal breathing spurred interest in the early diagnosis of intrauterine fetal growth restriction.

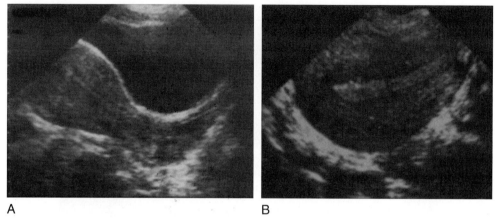

A   B

FIGURE **1-13 A** and **B,** Comparison of transabdominal and endovaginal imaging. **A,** This sagittal transab-dominal scan uses the full-bladder technique to demonstrate early fibroid development in a uterus. **B,** An endovaginal sagittal scan showing a normal adult uterus and high-resolution imaging of normal proliferative phase, thickened endometrium.

Manning and Platt (United States) introduced the concept of the fetal biophysical profile, the ultrasound equivalent of an intrauterine American Pediatric Gross Assessment Record (APGAR), to evaluate fetal well-being. High-risk pregnancy conditions such as twin transfusion syndrome, RH incompatibility, and diabetic effect were monitored by ultrasound, and the resulting information contributed greatly to the management and outcomes of such pregnancies.

Reintroduction of endocorporeal transducers in the mid-1980s was a boon to obstetrical, gynecologic, and urologic diagnosis. The improved higher-resolution transducers made possible earlier diagnosis of pregnancy and complications, as well as the earlier diagnosis of benign and malignant masses (Fig. 1-13). The ability to visualize subtle fetal malformations, especially before the third trimester, opened new avenues to prenatal diagnosis. In 1985 Greg De Vore (United States) demonstrated the value of combining Doppler color-flow mapping with the investigation of fetal cardiac malformations.

The application of real-time ultrasound spread to multiple medical specialties, and its popularity continued to expand rapidly. At a time when many of the early pioneers were retiring from the field, the individuals that they had mentored were stepping forward to continue further investigating the potential of ultrasound. Additionally, they assumed the extra responsibilities of creating education and training programs throughout the world. An incredible body of work was produced by luminaries such as Stuart Campbell (England); William Garrett (Australia); Lyons, Sauerbrei, and Cooperberg (Canada); and Goldberg, Feigenbaum, Leopold, Taylor, Hobbins, and Grannum (United States). Landmark articles by Fleischer, Sanders, Callen, and Rumack laid the groundwork for the first of many textbooks devoted exclusively to the study of diagnostic medical ultrasound.

Vascular sonography became a standard diagnostic tool by 1987, providing rapid and noninvasive imaging of the peripheral vasculature. By the mid-1990s Doppler instrumentation had been incorporated into most ultrasound systems, and vascular ultrasound quickly became the modality of choice for diagnosing lower-extremity deep venous thrombosis (Fig. 1-14).

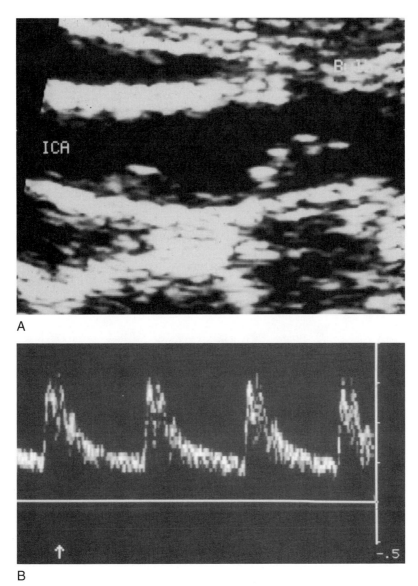

FIGURE **1-14** Early Doppler studies. **A,** An ulcerated carotid plaque obtained using a 7.5-MHz mechanical sector scanner (Diasonics 400). **B,** A normal Doppler spectrum (Diasonics 400).   (*Continued*)

In the late 1990s **harmonic imaging**, a quantitative method of characterizing/recognizing various tissue types, revived the old quest for tissue characterization. In specific patients, the new approach could dramatically improve resolution by reducing artifacts, achieving better penetration, and selectively processing returning echoes.

Twenty-first century ultrasound

Twenty-first century ultrasound is already off to an exciting start with the introduction of 3-D and 4-D ultrasound imaging. The results represent the difference between a video and

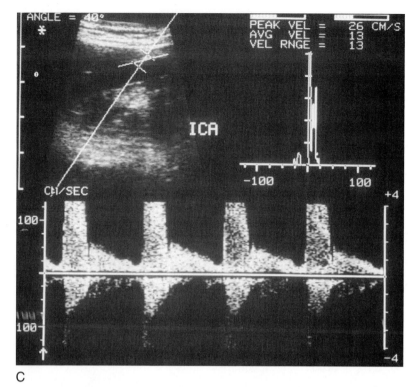

C

FIGURE **1-14, cont'd C,** An aliased Doppler spectrum (also using the Diasonics 400).

still photography because **3-D imaging** produces a volume, rather than a single-angle approach (Fig. 1-15). The displayed volume image offers a software rendering of all of the detected soft tissue that can be produced in a still image. By adding another dimension, **4-D imaging**, numerous images are captured in rapid succession, creating a motion video of the target.

Hand-held compact ultrasound systems weighing less than 10 lb are making it easier to perform ultrasound wherever and whenever it is needed (Fig. 1-16). This is made possible by the integration of millions of transistors on a single chip enabling lightweight mobile systems to provide high-performance studies. Already tested and in regular use in the space program and on battlefields, these tiny giants are bringing ultrasound diagnosis for the first time to many of the most remote and harshest settings in Third World countries.

The versatility of diagnostic ultrasound guidance is valuable in many invasive procedures. Its use in radiofrequency ablation is having a profound effect on medicine and the treatment of tumors, especially for patients who are not candidates for surgery or chemotherapy. Ultrasound is used to guide the placement of the radiofrequency probe into the tumor and monitor the lesion's size and position while it is being destroyed. Doppler ultrasound is used to observe blood flow in the tumor before and after the procedure.

Image quality has been further enhanced with the latest adaptive, digitally encoded real-time software. The new feature dynamically suppresses the granular speckled appearance of a standard ultrasound image to enhance features such as vascular borders and tissue boundaries that may be obscured with conventional imaging approaches.

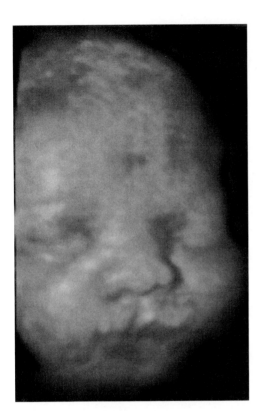

FIGURE **1-15** 3-D fetal ultrasound scanning. To create 3-D images, the ultrasound system determines the volume of the fetus and then reconstructs the image in three dimensions.

Ultrasound has gone wireless, as well as digital. Voice-activated technology now allows physicians and sonographers to control more than 100 system functions using only their voice. This is a boon when working with difficult patients and children or doing portable examinations in critical care settings. By freeing sonographers from the ultrasound console and keyboard, it is anticipated that voice-activated systems will help reduce the number of sonographer upper arm musculoskeletal injuries (Fig. 1-17).

A promising new hand-held device, the Sonic Flashlight, was developed by researchers at Carnegie Mellon Institute and is currently undergoing clinical trials. The instrument positions a real-time ultrasound scanner and monitor on opposite sides of a see-through mirror. When the device is placed against the patient's body, the monitor projects the ultrasound image onto the mirror. Viewing the image directly eliminates the need to look away from the patient to view a traditional real-time display in order to place biopsy needles and catheters. The new system is expected to make it easier to access vessels and fluid collections, as well as assist in the placement of needles and catheters.

What the future holds

Along with the computer and electronic developments that have extended ultrasound's vision, expect to see considerable diagnostic advancement with the expanding use of contrast ultrasound techniques, to the level of molecular imaging and therapy.

The potential of diagnostic ultrasound seems limitless, and the future of ultrasonography in medicine is secure as it continues playing vital roles not only in diagnosis but also in the treatment of many medical conditions and diseases.

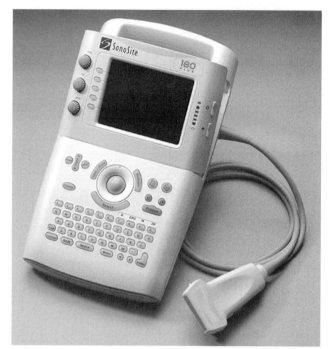

A

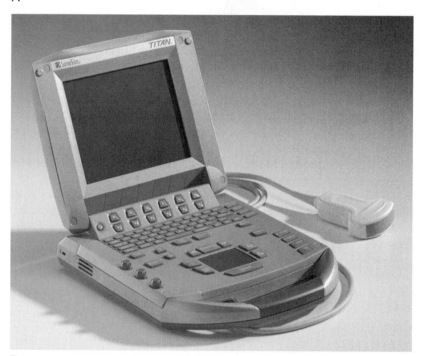

B

FIGURE **1-16** The SonoSite hand-carried portable ultrasound unit. **A,** The SonoSite 180Plus hand-carried ultrasound unit was designed for point-of-care ultrasound scanning. This unit took ultrasound out of the hospital and into developing countries and distant battlefields. **B,** The Titan laptop-sized ultrasound system's advanced features and size made it ideal for use in the NASA space and underwater programs, as well as in imaging centers and office practices.

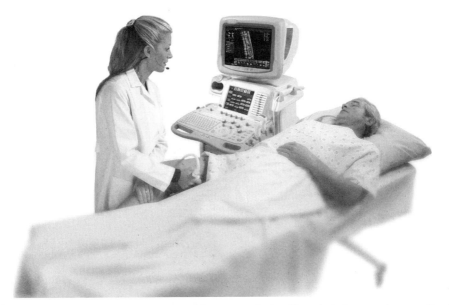

FIGURE **1-17** Voice-activated ultrasound system. The system depicted here includes speech recognition technology. The operator controls the system by voice via a head set, thus freeing both hands throughout the study and eliminating the need to keep one hand on the control panel.

Ultrasound technology, like progress, is ever changing. As with any new technology, sonographers must learn how to use it to their advantage and to avoid abusing or misusing this marvelous technology. Now that the importance of ergonomics has been revealed, the future should hold no more large-scale, job-related sonographer injuries. Equipment manufacturers have already responded with improved equipment design. With the support of the Occupational Safety and Health Administration (OSHA), hospital, clinic, and office practice managers are aware of the need to create an ergonomically safe workplace.

Diagnostic ultrasound has continued to advance because of the early and ongoing unique partnerships among engineers, physicists, physicians, sonographers, and commercial entrepreneurs. From the 1940s to the present, the field continues to grow and improve through innovative technologic breakthroughs. The availability of extended view equipment; the merging of old with new technology in the case of 3-D and 4-D imaging; the growing popularity of contrast agents; the expansion of Doppler applications to all the specialty areas of sonography; and the rise of transcranial ultrasound have all contributed to the continuing excitement, acknowledgment, and respect for this profession.

The infant is still coming of age. What will tomorrow bring? The results remain to be seen, but judging by past history and performance, the extraordinarily exciting prospects promise to be not only evolutionary, but also revolutionary.

Summary

From the ancient Greeks and Romans to present day scientists, practitioners and engineers, diagnostic ultrasound has captivated the imagination. The work of scores from ultrasound pioneers such as Langevin, Dussik, Donald, Howry, Edler, Wilcox,

Kossoff and Baker has earned sonography a secure place in diagnostic imaging arenas throughout the world.

Who would have dreamed that the static imaging devices that were so lauded in the 50s and 60s would lead to real-time imaging that would revolutionize what is understood about developing fetuses and cardiovascular performance today?

Who could have imagined ultrasound systems so small and portable that they would be found bringing help and hope to patients in underprivileged countries, in refugee camps, and on battlefields?

Though relatively new by medical standards, what established diagnostic ultrasound as one of the most useful and popular diagnostic tools is its noninvasiveness, multidisciplinary applications, mobility, and affordability. There is no doubt that it will remain a preferred and viable diagnostic choice far into the future.

The 21st century has brought 3D and 4D imaging, contrast agents, and harmonic imaging. Amazing technological breakthroughs and previously unthought-of applications have become the expected, rather than the rare exception, in the history of sonography.

What a privilege it was to work alongside many of the men and women mentioned earlier, observing talented and visionary individuals build the foundations of diagnostic ultrasound. They set the bar of excellence very high; it is up to the sonographers and sonologists of today and of the future to carry on those ideals.

BIBLIOGRAPHY

Cronan JJ: History of venous ultrasound, *J Ultrasound Med* 22:1143-1146, 2003.

Fleischer AC: Gynecologic sonography. Past, present, and future, *J Ultrasound Med* 22:759-763, 2003.

Goldberg BB: *Medical diagnostic ultrasound: a retrospective on its 40th anniversary,* Bethesda, Md, 1988, American Institute of Ultrasound in Medicine.

Holmes JH: Diagnostic ultrasound during the early years of A.I.U.M, *J Clin Ultrasound* 8:299-308, 1980.

Meyer RA: History of ultrasound in cardiology, *J Ultrasound Med* 23:1-11, 2004.

Nelson LH: Echoes from the past: history of obstetrical ultrasound, *J Ultrasound Med* 22:667-671, 2003.

Woo J: A short history of the developing of ultrasound in obstetrics and gynecology. Available at: *http://www.ob-ultrasound.net/history.html*

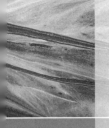

Chapter 2

Sonographer Development

Learning Objectives

Students who successfully complete this chapter will be able to do the following:

- Define the role of the sonographer.
- List the specific aptitudes, abilities, and skills desirable in sonographer candidates.
- Compare and contrast the advantages and disadvantages of a sonography career.
- Describe the benefits of membership in a professional society.
- Explain the difference among accreditation, certification, and registration.

Key Terms

accreditation   certification   registration

The past 2 decades have produced a marked growth in the field of allied health careers. This growth has occurred partly because the proliferation of medical technologic advances that occurred during that time created a critical need for professionals adept at using new and complex instruments.

The "high-tech" era has also added new dimensions to the practice of medicine, as advanced research techniques promote the discovery of new causes and cures for diseases. It has encouraged the concept of physician specialization, and in so doing, has provided room for expanding the role of allied health professional to one of physician assistant.

At first glance, the daily practice of sonography appears deceptively simple. On closer inspection and exposure to the process, it is apparent that sonographers face a workday filled with complex challenges. Such exposure also makes it apparent that the transducer-wielding sonographer has a profound effect on the quality of an examination and that in-depth education and training are required to achieve the greatest possible diagnostic benefits.

With each advance in technology, sonographers are expected to develop skills that might not have been part of their training programs even 5 years ago. Learning such skills as increased expertise in patient care, pathophysiology, and computer literacy, added to rapid and ongoing instrumentation changes, can be both exciting and frustrating.

Truly committed sonographers will want to obtain peer recognition of their sonographic competence and work toward earning **certification** and the credentials that verify their proficiency in one or more ultrasound specialty areas.

THE ROLE OF SONOGRAPHER

Role is a specific behavior that an individual demonstrates to others; function, on the other hand, involves the tasks or duties one is obligated to perform in carrying out a role.

The term *sonographer* literally means one who graphs or draws with sound. A sonographer performs ultrasound studies and gathers diagnostic data under the direct or indirect supervision of a physician. The sonographer's role, however, is more than tasks delegated by physicians. Sonography is a unique profession with its own theoretic basis. Sonographers provide both physical and emotional care by using the most advanced equipment available and by relying on their hearts for a nurturing approach to patients. To be a good sonographer today, it is necessary not only to possess strong scientific knowledge and skills but also to work diligently to keep abreast of the field and to cultivate tender care and concern for one's patients.

Qualities of a sonographer

What specific aptitudes, abilities, and skills are indicative of a good sonographer? To answer that question, it is important to realize that aptitudes are not skills or abilities but rather undeveloped and untrained talents. The possession of an aptitude produces a natural tendency to do well. The following categories list some of the most desirable sonographer qualities.

INTELLECTUAL CURIOSITY

Sonographers should be intrigued by science and challenged by the thought of putting it to work to help people. A paramedical background or clinical expertise is a requirement for entering the field. Eventually, many sonographers become interested in teaching or research, or both.

EAGERNESS AND PERSEVERANCE

Candidates for sonography training must be willing to attend an academic program beyond high school level and be ready to spend untold hours studying. Sonographers are required to take mathematics and scientific courses and be able to integrate that knowledge in their clinical activities to produce better scans. These qualities remain important after graduation as well, because sonographers are expected to constantly strive to improve their scanning abilities, learn new specialty areas, further their education, and move into supervisory or management positions.

CRITICAL-THINKING AND ANALYTIC CAPABILITIES

Sonographers must be capable of making accurate, independent judgments because patients' lives may depend on those judgments. The abilities to plan and organize time and resources are important traits, inasmuch as sonographers are expected to adapt the pace of an examination to fit prevailing needs.

TECHNICAL ORIENTATION

Two of the most critical needs are the ability to conceptualize images in 3-D form and to possess good psychomotor skills. Sonographer candidates should be interested in working with their hands and with equipment and be constantly willing to learn new technical skills. In addition to adeptness at using many sophisticated machines and devices, sonographers must be adaptable and creative in those instances when equipment malfunctions.

DEXTERITY

Possessing good hand coordination is critical when manipulating the transducer in minute angles or tilts to achieve the best sound transmission. Dexterity is also required when the nonscanning hand must simultaneously change control settings and monitor display and recording devices.

PHYSICAL HEALTH

Good health is important because physical stamina is required for the hard work involved: long periods on one's feet, moving about, lifting and positioning patients, and performing other physically demanding tasks. Sonographers should be able to handle stress and be skilled in helping others cope with it.

SELF-DIRECTION

Because sonography is never dull or routine, sonographers must be creative; i.e., able to "roll with the punches" and make independent decisions. They should be capable of remaining unfrustrated by disruption of routine and be able to function autonomously.

EMOTIONAL STABILITY

Sonographer candidates should be stimulated by the prospect of daily involvement in life and death situations. Not all examinations have happy endings, and often sonographers find themselves working with patients under great stress. It takes an emotionally stable person to be nurturing and compassionate in such situations.

COMMUNICATION SKILLS

Sonographers must be effective communicators, as well as good listeners, because they are frequently required to teach patients and family members, medical students, interns, and other sonographers. The abilities to interact effectively with patients and medical personnel and to work as part of a team are critically important.

Strong verbal communication skills and the competence to develop written reports also are necessary. A sonographer must feel comfortable in delegating tasks to coworkers and interacting with physicians and other health care personnel. As they move up through the ranks of the profession and take on more responsibilities, sonographers also need persuasive negotiating, leadership, and management skills.

DEDICATION

Sonographers should find satisfaction in working with all types of patients including children, expectant mothers, and elderly persons. They should be sensitive and giving, as well as tenacious and flexible, as they seek the best results for their patients. Above all, they must be dedicated to their profession and willing to continue their studies in order to advance their knowledge, often after working a busy day. Graduate sonographers display dedication by performing on-call services and returning the following day for their regular shift, sometimes with only limited time to sleep or rest.

CAREER ADVANTAGES

Why become a sonographer? The greatest reward in sonography is the satisfaction of helping a patient—knowing that one's skills and abilities made a difference. Another strong attraction of the field is respect. A good sonographer is treated as a competent resource person, even as a colleague, and is held in high esteem.

Being a member of a unique profession is a definite plus, as is the freedom to express creativity, authority, and judgment. It is highly satisfying to work one-on-one with patients, to tailor a study to the individual patient, and to deliver personalized patient care.

The diversity of career options offered in sonography also exerts a magnetic effect. The variety of specialties to choose from, the fact that daily work is so vastly different, and the opportunity to obtain employment anywhere in the world are strong attractions. Attractive salaries and the flexibility of designing work hours to fit personal requirements (e.g., part-time vs. full-time work and shared jobs) are other benefits.

The field of sonography offers rich human experiences and is never dull. Although it is often stressful and demanding, the opportunities to solve problems and to meet professional challenges are personally rewarding.

What makes medicine appealing is its reverence for life—its power and sacredness. The integration of science into this mystery is exciting. Searching for pieces of a puzzle that do not fit perfectly and then working to restore the balance bring a great sense of accomplishment. Although individual situations may require only a one-time use of their medical skill, sonographers require an understanding of many facets of disease to make good decisions. Thus the field allows them to satisfy their intellectual curiosity while serving humanity.

In addition to considering a profession's advantages, it is equally important to evaluate its challenges. Accepting the challenge of professionalism often means accepting that there may be no cure for a particular disease and that some patients will die. The only consolation in this case is the knowledge that a sonographer's concern and skill have improved the patient's quality of life and ultimately will influence the care of future patients.

Career sonography cannot be compared with traditional 9-to-5 jobs, as evidenced by the following:

- Frustration can occur when patients have not been properly prepared for their studies or when having to reschedule a patient whose ultrasound study was ordered out of sequence (after other diagnostic tests that might prevent obtaining a diagnostic ultrasound study). Frustration levels are also high when better equipment is not provided.
- Fatigue can occur when scanning in an environment that is not ergonomically sound or when emergency and add-on patients must fit into an already full schedule. Fatigue is common when a sonographer is on call and must report for duty the next day without adequate time to rest or sleep.
- Depression can occur whenever emotional distances are not properly maintained or when sonographers try to do too much for patients and coworkers at the expense of neglecting themselves.

However, for each of these challenges the sonographer has a small triumph in knowing that he or she has done the job well and patients have benefited. The profession does not appeal to everyone. Only the individual can decide whether he or she is up for the challenge and whether the benefits outweigh the challenges.

BENEFITS OF MEMBERSHIP IN A PROFESSIONAL ORGANIZATION

The evolution of sonography as a career has been almost as colorful as the field of diagnostic medical sonography itself. Early operators of ultrasonic equipment in the United States were medical students; interns; residents; and "research assistants" plucked from such unlikely occupations as receptionists, secretaries, orderlies, teachers, and housewives, as well as from the fields of nursing and radiology.

Interest in ultrasound grew quickly and, to meet the demands for training, pioneering laboratories and commercial equipment manufacturers opened their doors to any interested observers. The transfer of technical knowledge occurred in a show-and-tell fashion as the number of "trained" technicians slowly increased. The allied health profession of sonography could not have developed without the aid of those early workers and the important ultrasound organizations that continue to serve the sonography community today.

Some sonographers opt not to join professional organizations, citing the costs and their lack of time as primary reasons. Paying dues, especially when money is tight, is difficult. However, in reality, those dues are a veritable investment in the future if a member fully uses the organization by becoming involved and networking. The time devoted to membership involvement is another investment that places sonographers side by side with people who can advance their careers.

With the rapidly changing fields of sonography and health care, it is critical to be seen as someone who is moving forward, working on the cutting edge of what is happening in the profession. Modern sonographers including sonography students cannot afford to ignore

membership in a professional society because it adds both credibility and advancement. Membership benefits that should be considered follow:
- Continuing education opportunities
- Access to professional information
- Participation in volunteer leadership roles
- Professional development
- Advocates of federal and state regulatory issues
- Lobbying the government on behalf of the membership
- Aiding career advancement
- Staying current with the latest research through conferences, seminars, and annual meetings
- Publications (newsletters and professional journals)
- Networking
- Access to financial, insurance, and health programs

MEMBERSHIP ORGANIZATIONS

American Institute of Ultrasound in Medicine

In August 1951 an organization to promote the use of ultrasound in physical medicine was formed. One year later, the group, calling itself the American Institute of Ultrasound in Medicine (AIUM), conducted its first annual meeting in conjunction with the American Congress of Physical Medicine. Initially, membership was open only to physiatrists, but by 1964 the AIUM welcomed all physicians and bioengineers interested in the medical applications of ultrasound, particularly those in the field of diagnosis.

Over the years the number of physiatrists declined, leaving the diagnostically oriented members in the majority. The organization has continued to flourish, and today the AIUM remains the primary multidisciplinary, nonprofit society dedicated to advancing the art and science of ultrasound in medicine and research.

The AIUM has a global membership composed of physicians; scientists; engineers; sonographers; technicians; manufacturers and their representatives; and medical students working toward the professional, educational, research, and scientific needs of medical specialists practicing ultrasound in medicine. The AIUM offers a voluntary Diagnostic Ultrasound Accreditation program aimed at improving the quality of ultrasound examinations in the United States and Canada. Complying with the AIUM's minimum standards and guidelines enhances the quality of ultrasound practices and the end point of patient care.

Society of Diagnostic Medical Sonography

In 1965 the AIUM invited interested ultrasound technicians to attend its scientific sessions until such time that the technicians could found their own technical society. That event occurred in 1970, with the formation of the American Society of Ultrasound Technical Specialists (ASUTS), with a total membership of six. The society's goal was to promote, advance, and educate its members, as well as the medical community, in the science of diagnostic medical ultrasound and, as a consequence, to contribute to the enhancement of patient care. Within several years, membership had grown to several hundred technicians, and the ASUTS turned its efforts toward gaining recognition of ultrasound technology as a new health career.

On October 4, 1974, the American Medical Association (AMA) responded to a request by the ASUTS for the creation of a new and separate health occupation, as well as a new title: the diagnostic medical sonographer. Under the guidance of the AMA, the ASUTS and other collaborating organizations developed a *Document of Essentials,* which set forth the minimum educational requirements for sonography training and served as a guide to curriculum development in formal ultrasound educational programs.

For consistency with the new terminology, the name of the ASUTS was formally changed in 1978 to the Society of Diagnostic Medical Sonographers (SDMS) and again in 2001 to the Society of Diagnostic Medical Sonography. In 2002, through the efforts of the SDMS, the U.S. Department of Labor *(Occupational Outlook Handbook)* recognized diagnostic medical sonographer as an independent profession, marking a major turning point for the profession. This classification is important because of its impacts on sonographer job descriptions, classifications, and pay scales.

With a membership in the tens of thousands, the SDMS continues to set high educational standards, monitor the socioeconomic concerns of its membership, and promote excellence in the field. Through the efforts of its Professional Status Committee, a code of conduct, scope of practice statement, and job description have been adopted.

American Society of Echocardiography

Dedicated to the field of echocardiology, the American Society of Echocardiography (ASE) meets the needs of physicians and sonographers. With more than 8000 members, the society offers student membership, as well as online continuing medical education, a professional journal and newsletter, and job and resumé postings.

Society of Vascular Ultrasound

Dedicated to the field of vascular sonography, the Society of Vascular Ultrasound (SVU) provides members with an online journal and newsletter, continuing medical education via seminars and annual meetings, professional performance guidelines, a job center and awards program, and student membership.

American Society of Radiologic Technologists

The mission of the American Society of Radiologic Technologists (ASRT) is "to lead and serve its members, the profession, other health care providers and the public on all issues that affect the radiologic sciences." For some sonographers, ultrasound is a subspecialty to their primary careers as x-ray technologists. The ASRT keeps them apprised of technologic advances, trends, and pertinent legislation in addition to providing continuing education opportunities for them in publications and meetings.

CERTIFYING/ACCREDITING ORGANIZATIONS

American Registry for Diagnostic Medical Sonographers

Recognizing that the new profession needed some way to evaluate and certify the proficiency of sonographers, the American Registry for Diagnostic Medical Sonographers (ARDMS) formed an examination committee to explore the possibility of measuring the levels of competency of persons who perform various diagnostic ultrasound studies. Its goal was achieved in 1975, with the formation of the American Registry for Diagnostic Medical Sonography (ARDMS). This organization conducts certifying examinations for qualified sonographers in each specialty area of diagnostic ultrasound and maintains a list of those sonographers who have successfully passed their registry examinations. Box 2-1 lists the

BOX **2-1** American Registry for Diagnostic Medical Sonography Roster of Specialty Credentials

Registered Diagnostic Medical Sonographer (RDMS):
Abdominal, OB/GYN, Fetal Echocardiography,* Neurosonology, Breast
Registered Diagnostic Cardiac Sonographer (RDCS):
Adult and Pediatric Echocardiography, Fetal Echocardiography*
Registered Vascular Technologist (RVT):
Noninvasive Vascular Sonography

*The fetal echocardiography specialty can be acquired under either the RDMS or the RCDS credential.

credentials awarded to candidates who successfully complete the examinations in major specialty areas.

Although **registration** is a voluntary activity in all but a few states, registered sonographers must provide proof of 30 hours of continuing education each triennium to maintain their registry status. As of this writing, the ARDMS has certified more than 44,000 individuals and is considered the premier certifying agency for the sonography community.

American Registry of Radiologic Technologists

The American Registry of Radiologic Technologists' (ARRT) "Sonography Suite" includes three separate certification programs covering the gamut of procedures from general to vascular to breast. Along with Radiography, Nuclear Medicine Technology, and Radiation Therapy, ARRT's general Sonography certification is a primary category open to recent graduates of approved educational programs who can demonstrate the appropriate education, ethics, and examination qualifications.

Cardiovascular Credentialing International

Offering testing that provides an accurately measured index of performance, Cardiovascular Credentialing International (CCI) has credentialed more than 3000 individuals in the fields of noninvasive cardiovascular technology and echocardiography.

Joint Commission of Allied Health Professionals in Ophthalmology

Since 1969, the Joint Commission of Allied Health Professionals in Ophthalmology (JCAHPO) has provided certification and continuing education opportunities to ophthalmic allied health professionals. JCAHPO's mission is to enhance the quality and availability of ophthalmic patient care by promoting the value of qualified allied health personnel and by providing certification and continuing education. In pursuit of its mission, JCAHPO became the credentialing program for the Registered Ophthalmologic Ultrasound Biometrist (ROUB) in 2004.

Joint Review Commission–Diagnostic Medical Sonography

The mission of the Joint Review Commission–Diagnostic Medical Sonography (JRC-DMS) and its sponsoring organizations is to cooperate to establish, maintain, and promote appropriate standards of quality for educational programs in diagnostic medical sonography and to provide recognition through **accreditation** for educational programs that meet or exceed the standards.

Summary

The term *sonographer*, like the discipline, is deceptively simple; no matter how sophisticated instrumentation becomes, without the expertise of the sonographer, the bright dots on the TV monitor are simply electrical impulses being converted to light. Just as a sculptor can envision a form within raw material, so too do sonographers see valuable and critical information in the dancing electronic displays before them. Through their talents and intelligence, they know when and how to produce the images that will enable physicians to convert those same dots and dashes of light into healing answers.

It is impossible to categorize sonographers within other allied health care areas. They are unique, straddling many career fields as they care for their patients, assess both clinical and ultrasound problems, and work diligently to create high-quality diagnostic studies. "Versatile," "intellectually stimulated," "resilient," and "idealistic" are only a few of the adjectives that personify a sonographer.

Just as there are differences among physicians and nurses, there are differences among sonographers, other allied health technologists, and nurses. The government's official recognition of the diagnostic medical sonographer was an appropriate and long-awaited outcome for members of the profession willing to go beyond the basic requirements of the job. These sonographers take the initiative to join professional sonography organizations to stay current with continuing education and socioeconomic changes that may affect the profession.

BIBLIOGRAPHY

Abuhamad AZ et al: The accreditation of ultrasound practices. Impact on compliance with minimum performance guidelines, *J Ultrasound Med* 23:1023-1029, 2004.

American Institute of Ultrasound in Medicine. Available at: *htpp://www.aium.org*.

American Registry for Diagnostic Medical Sonographers. Available at: *http://www.ardms.org*.

American Registry of Radiologic Technologists. Available at: *http://www.arrt.org*.

American Society of Echocardiography. Available at: *http://asecho.org*.

Cardiovascular Credentialing International. Available at: *http://wwwcci-online.org/credentials.html*.

Joint Commission on Allied Health Personnel in Ophthalmology. Available at: *http://www.jcahpo.org*.

Joint Review Commission-Diagnostic Medical Sonography. Available at: *http://www.jrcdms.org*.

Society of Diagnostic Medical Sonography. Available at: *http://www.sdms.org*.

US Department of Labor Statistics: *Occupational outlook handbook, January 2002*. Available at *http://www.bls.gov*.

Chapter 3

The Sonographer as a Student

Learning Objectives

Students who successfully complete this chapter will be able to do the following:

- Identify the three types of memory and describe how each is used.
- Discuss the recommended methods of taking notes while reading or listening to tapes or lectures.
- Name the steps in the PQRST method of note taking.
- Discuss competencies commonly evaluated in clinical education.
- Discuss the various types of educational and training options available to sonographers.

Key Terms

association	memory	subjective test
clustering	mnemonics	visualization
didactic	objective tests	

As one of imaging's most accessible instruments, diagnostic ultrasound has also rapidly become a broad-based instrument. Its appeal to a wide spectrum of specialty physicians and their patients has resulted in increasing demands for competent sonologists and sonographers. Unfortunately, the current lack of nationally accepted and defined clinical and educational standards has permitted extreme variables in sonologist and sonographer education and training. Until training standards for both sonologists and sonographers are adopted in the United States, sonographers must be apprised of this situation and be made aware that pressures and unrealistic expectations may await them as they enter the workplace. Consequently, they must learn not only how to operate ultrasonic equipment but how to distinguish normal from abnormal sonographic anatomy; correlate pertinent clinical data; and fully recognize their own technical and educational limitations, as well as their strengths.

Regardless of their background in allied health education or the length of time since graduation, sonographer-students will learn many things besides sonographic technique. Some students will learn about hospital rules and regulations for the first time and about the many ways of getting along with patients, staff members, and fellow students. Even veteran allied health professionals may find themselves spending time struggling to understand new and unfamiliar medical terminology as they expand their knowledge of patient care and the need to correlate clinical information from patients' charts.

The goal of this chapter is to help sonographer-students get the most out of their experience by doing the following:
- Explaining the complex process of learning
- Offering suggestions on the art of studying to learn
- Explaining the various methods of testing
- Offering strategies for getting the most out of a clinical rotation
- Explaining how to choose a program of study
- Providing information on current educational options in the United States

LEARNING DYNAMICS

Critical thinking and action

For many years, the American educational model has been to "drill" students to memorize information rather than to understand it. Who can forget reciting the multiplication tables by rote, only to stumble through the concepts of long division?

Today, modern educators are calling for educational reform that will teach students how to think rather than to memorize and then possibly forget. Educational methods now focus less on simply imparting facts and theories and more on developing students' capacities for judgment, fact gathering, analysis, and synthesis to prepare them to meet the educational and employment challenges of the 1990s and the next century.

Educating sonographers should be no different. Old habits die hard, however, and some students begin their sonography education expecting to be handed a master list of facts to memorize. Such students are doomed to frustration until they realize that working in the field of diagnostic medicine is a problem-solving activity, comparable to working on a complex jigsaw puzzle. Simply taking an inventory of all the puzzle pieces will not provide the answers. The key to a solution lies in observing how the shapes of individual pieces might interconnect with other pieces in various areas of the puzzle. Only through trial and error and by blending experience (memory) and logic (reasoning) can difficult puzzles be solved correctly.

Memory

Every individual has three completely different types of **memory**: immediate memory, short-term memory, and long-term memory. Immediate memory is for instantaneous use, whereas short-term memory usually is reserved for the temporary storage of facts—only long enough to use them—because they quickly fade. In contrast, long-term memory allows the permanent storage of information that is to be used (often repeatedly) over lengthy periods of time.

IMMEDIATE MEMORY

Immediate memory is the least understood and most often overlooked of the three types. It is employed to remember things only long enough to respond to them. Reading this page is an example of immediate memory. Each word that is read remains just long enough in the individual's immediate memory to make the transition from one word or idea to the next. Many of the words just read were discarded immediately, but they had to be remembered long enough to make sense out of them.

The major problem with immediate memory is that it is extremely limited. That is, people can respond to only one thing at a time, and the amount of information retained is limited to approximately two to four items. Another problem with immediate memory is that it requires singular attention to determine which items require prompt response and which items require transfer from the immediate memory before they decay and are lost forever.

SHORT-TERM MEMORY

Short-term memory comes into play after the information has been sorted out as being important enough to remember. It sometimes is called "working memory" because it is the system used to remember information that must be recalled or responded to within seconds or minutes after receiving it. Short-term memory is what people use to look up a telephone number and remember it only long enough to dial. The basic difference between short-term and immediate memory is that short-term memory allows people to remember several things at once, for periods of time greater than 1 second. One negative aspect of short-term memory is that it is a rather limited system, capable of remembering only a maximum of seven items at a time. The short-term memory also is subject to rapid information loss, although not as rapid as that of the immediate memory. Because disturbances can cause memory loss, the short-term memory can even be overloaded, causing us to forget "everything" taken in at the time of the overload. This is why reasonable study schedules and study breaks are encouraged.

LONG-TERM MEMORY

Long-term memory is used for information that must be stored for long periods (days, months, years) before use. Retrieving information from the long-term memory collection requires a search. If the long-term memory is unorganized, a big load is placed on the short-term memory. For this reason, it is important to process incoming information correctly or it will be irretrievable. The major advantages of the long-term memory system are (1) its limitless capacity to store information and (2) the number of items it can retain. Long-term memory facilitates learning and memorization of new material, and it is believed that the more information in long-term memory, the easier it is to enter new information.

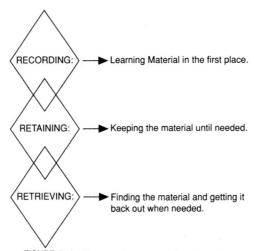

RECORDING: ⟶ Learning Material in the first place.

RETAINING: ⟶ Keeping the material until needed.

RETRIEVING: ⟶ Finding the material and getting it back out when needed.

FIGURE **3-1** Stages of memory: The three Rs.

To store information in long-term memory requires attention, organization, and association (Fig. 3-1). Attention can be defined as focusing on material one wants to remember and the ability to block any disturbing stimuli. The primary purpose of attention is to determine what is important enough to remember. Organization is the art of putting memory in order. The mind can be thought of as an expanding library of all previously acquired knowledge, stored by appropriate categories. Every time new knowledge is acquired, it is added to any associated facts that were previously stored and waiting to be checked out. If a particular category of facts is used or added to only infrequently, it is treated as inactive and displaced to make room for new or additional facts. This process is unfortunate because inactive information sometimes becomes difficult to locate or may even be lost.

One popular method of remembering things is called **association**, a technique that involves forming an association with a fact. Engaging in this activity leads one to learn and think more about that fact. As a result, the more facts that are associated with an item of memory, the more permanently those facts will be stored.

INACCURATE MEMORY

Humans have a tendency to alter and distort details. This tendency often occurs when some parts of a memory fail to fade in a uniform manner and are held together, but with missing or altered details. The motivation to distort the reality of events and experiences can be traced to a desire to make memories more appealing. By doing so, people support their beliefs and values, as well as their notions and hopes, and can defend their prejudices. Often people add details to their recollection of events to complete and make sense out of sketchy or incomplete memories. By filling in and rounding out missing details, they can create a memory that is satisfyingly whole or complete.

Although it is impossible to eliminate inaccurate remembering altogether, it is possible to decrease it to some extent. The key lies in remembering well and correctly. People can guard against inaccuracies by taking notes to ensure the precise remembrance of the information they want to recall. If people understand a subject clearly from the start, errors in thinking are not likely to occur. Their memories also improve if they prepare their bodies for the task.

By resting and getting sufficient sleep and by healthy eating habits (particularly eating breakfast), the brain's ability to function is improved.

FORGETTING

If one has ever failed to recall a name or a fact for a test, the frustration of forgetting is understandable. If one were unable to forget, however, the constant remembrance of pain, disappointment, and trauma would make life intolerable. Forgetting is a critical survival mechanism that allows the memory of painful experiences to lessen somewhat in intensity and eventually to fade. High pleasure and pain levels enhance remembering, making it possible to retain painful physical or emotional memories and to remember them as needed. When the rewards of remembering do not reach such highs, people have a tendency to forget. This characteristic explains the common failure to remember names, dates, places, and material that was not originally understood, and it illustrates the importance of interesting learning materials; otherwise, the individual must find artificial ways of remembering factual data.

MEMORIZATION

Memories can be stimulated in both conscious and subconscious fashions. Health care professionals often relate how the sensory triggers of sight, sound, touch, and smell are frequently associated with a particular patient or disease. Although these factors were not intentionally memorized, they still were registered in a subconscious fashion.

Conscious or intentional memorization occurs only when people deliberately and systematically devise ways to recall specific facts. As such, it relies heavily on both perception and attention.

Perceptions are greatly influenced by previous memories; therefore possessing a memory bank rich in similar information increases the accuracy of perceptions. The mind is not only a computer-like processor of information, but also a museum that stores past experiences and images. Thus when sonographers scan patients, the brief appearance of a partial shape or prominent echo-pattern often is sufficient to trigger recognition. Experience has shown that any increase in such memories is proportional to the sonographer's scanning activity. This occurrence can be explained by the fact that during a sonographic examination, each time information is displayed on the viewing monitor, it also is stored in the sonographer's memory. In addition, it has been demonstrated that sonographers who have logged many transducer hours reproduce their perceptions of patients' anatomy more rapidly and with greater detail and accuracy than do novice sonographers. Veteran sonographers subconsciously demonstrate their ability to retrieve data from a large body of organized and synthesized information.

As stated previously, attention requires concentration and a sharp focus on a specific fact or activity, whereas concentration requires discipline and vigilance to ignore interfering thoughts or distractions. An individual can improve the ability to concentrate by preparing to receive new information and to learn something about a subject in advance.

MEMORY TECHNIQUES

Whenever people are confronted with a large volume of new or unfamiliar information or an inadequate amount of time in which to learn that information, they commonly use memory aids. The memory techniques most commonly employed are clustering, relating (association), imagining (visualization), and mnemonics.

1. Baby's block bearing the letters A, B, and C.
2. A "plus" sign.
3. A bowl of soup.
4. An "equal" sign.
5. Alphabet Soup

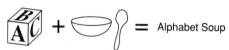

FIGURE **3-2** Visual associations.

Clustering is a method of memorizing long series of data by arranging them in segments. Usually it is easier to remember numbers grouped in segments of three to five. This is how people recall telephone numbers, Social Security numbers, and zip codes.

Rhyming can also make remembering easier. When facts or phrases are set to music, they are easier to recall. Examples are the songs used to master the alphabet (ABCD . . . EFG . . .) and numbers ("one, two, buckle my shoe . . .").

The use of visual or verbal associations enhances remembering by bridging memory gaps. Figure 3-2 shows some examples of association. The most successful associations are tied to prior knowledge. For instance, one might choose to remember the number of white and black keys on a piano (52 white keys and 36 black keys) by associating them with the facts that there are 52 weeks in a year and 36 inches in a yard. Sometimes, the similarities in spelling two different words can cause memory difficulties. For example, with the words *stationery* and *stationary,* it might be helpful to remember that the "e" in stationery stands for letters.

The use of acronyms, initialisms, and acrostics can make material meaningful by gathering information into mnemonic clusters so that one does not have as much to remember. For example, the names of the Great Lakes form the acronym HOMES, which stands for Huron, Ontario, Michigan, Erie, and Superior. Acronyms and initialisms are widely used to represent associations, organizations, government agencies, and military titles and terms (Box 3-1).

Another popular mnemonic technique involves creating a rhyme or story that contains the facts to be remembered. To remember when to begin and end the use of daylight savings time, people say:

Spring ahead in the spring; fall back in the fall.

Medical students have traditionally used an acrostic to remember the 12 cranial nerves (olfactory, optic, oculomotor, trochlear, trigeminal, abducens, facial, auditory vestibular,

BOX **3-1**   Using Initialisms and Acronyms as Memory Aids

EXAMPLES OF COMMON INITIALISMS AND ACRONYMS
SDMS: Society of Diagnostic Medical Sonographers
UN: United Nations
NCO: Noncommissioned officer
SNAFU: Situation normal, all fouled up!

glossopharyngeal, vagus, spinal accessory, hypoglossal) by assigning the first letter of each nerve to a word in a sentence:

On Old Olympus' Towering Top A Finn And German Viewed Some Hops.

First-letter **mnemonics** provide dual cues to help retrieve items and also indicate how many items are to be remembered so that one knows when they have all been recalled.

The memory technique that works best for concrete objects and actions such as remembering the items on our shopping lists is imagery, or **visualization**. The major drawback to this technique is that it works poorly on abstract concepts (such as justice and mercy). Whenever ultrasonic equipment controls are mentioned, most sonographers mentally visualize an instrument console and each control that is being discussed. Hearing a sonography term such as *increased gain* might trigger the memory of an ultrasound scan filled with predominantly bright echoes.

The obvious value of memory aids is that they make people organize, associate, and visualize meaningful information, forcing them to concentrate and pay attention. The painful truth is that the things people understand do not require memorization; people only memorize the things they do not understand.

Deductive reasoning

One of the greatest challenges in teaching sonography lies in getting students who are the product of American schools to develop the skill of deductive reasoning. This form of thinking involves drawing conclusions from facts and depends on the storage of facts in the individual's memory bank and on the ability to recover and logically manipulate that information to correlate with the clinical questions at hand. Logic represents an important creative thinking tool that is especially useful in the practical phases of the creative thinking process, when the individual is evaluating ideas and preparing to apply them.

Effective listening

The student who wants to learn must increase his or her reading rate and listening skills. Studies have shown that people rarely listen with maximum efficiency, and they consciously pay attention to only 25% of what they hear. The average speaking rate has been measured at approximately 100 words per minute, whereas the average listening and thinking rate is 400 to 500 words per minute. Such a great time lag encourages the mind to wander. Knowing this fact should prompt students to develop methods to increase their attention span by becoming effective listeners.

Most of the time people listen inefficiently. It is estimated that three fourths of each workday is spent talking and listening, and three fourths of what people do hear is heard imprecisely. The regret is that three fourths of what is heard accurately is forgotten within 3 weeks. Although listening is the most often used communicative skill, it is the one in which people have been given the least training. This presents a serious problem because the end product of listening is knowledge.

Listening involves sensing, and it goes beyond hearing or assessing only the spoken words. Good listeners think more broadly because they hear and understand more facts and points of view. Because good listeners look at problems with fresh eyes, they combine what they learn in more unlikely ways and are apt to develop new and valuable ideas. If given a choice, effective listeners focus on ideas rather than facts, because facts can be resurrected later.

Two important mental functions in effective listening are recall and comprehension. Recall is a have-or-have-not function involving memory. It is that portion of what is heard that can be restated later. In contrast, comprehension is a have-to-have function involving mastery or the portion of what is heard that is thoroughly understood and intelligently applied. A special kind of listening occurs when people are silent, attentive, and receptive. This third ear mulls over, interprets, speculates, posits, and reviews incoming information.

To be an effective listener, one must be motivated. In other words, one must have an interest in or reason for listening to what is being said. Effective listeners listen without prejudice to avoid ignoring or filtering out details or tuning out any speakers who do not match their own ideas or values.

The sonographer-student who wants to get the most out of classroom lectures must come to class prepared to listen. If all lesson assignments have been completed, he or she can simply concentrate on the subject being discussed. The sonographer-student should also view classroom lectures as give-and-take sessions between the instructor and students and use class discussion as a means of getting the facts straight or asking for explanations of any puzzling concepts.

Effective note taking

Because it is impossible to remember everything that is said in a lecture, it is critical to jot down only the important facts. Because writing is time consuming, note taking should be limited to key words or phrases to serve as reminders. After the lecture, notes can be reviewed and missing parts filled in.

By organizing in outline form the material covered in the lecture, the sonographer-student can develop his or her own personal study aid. He or she should make notes of the topics and the major points under each one. The importance of any phrases that an instructor repeats or writes on the chalkboard or overhead projector should be recognized and underlined in notes. The sonographer-student should summarize the sense of what an instructor says rather than try to include every word. Question marks should be written near anything that is unclear, and the instructor should be asked about it later. If necessary, notes should be rewritten to help establish the information more firmly. Notes should help the sonographer-student review a subject and provide correct and complete information. Flash cards, based on notes and arranged logically, provide another highly effective method to test understanding of a subject.

Skillful reading

Reading to comprehend is a complex and intellectual activity that can be achieved only through anticipation and evaluation of the material. Although speed-reading techniques may enable one to "read" large volumes of material, such techniques are worthless if comprehension is sacrificed.

A simple way to remember the main steps in effectively studying a reading assignment is based on the work of E. L. Thomas and H. A. Robinson. Their suggestion for students to maximize their studies is described as follows.

The PQRST method

Studying is a skill that can be learned. One of the most useful study strategies is the "PQRST" method.

P: PREVIEW

The student should scan the material first by looking at the images and reading the captions and charts. All of the material in the titles and subtitles of the chapter and all of the words in italics should be read, as well as any available summaries or objectives. Scanning enables the student to identify the main thought or general idea. If there is an accompanying workbook, the student should read the questions before the chapter text.

Q: QUESTION

The student should consider what the chapter is about and what major points the chapter makes. The objectives of reading the chapter should be understood so that one knows what is expected from him or her afterward. Questions in any workbook or manual that might accompany the text should be answered.

R: REREAD/REVIEW

The student should read the chapter carefully as many times as necessary to understand the material. It may be helpful to read only one page at a time and then recall as much of the material as possible. Performing the recall aloud uses two senses instead of one and enhances memory. Important points should be reviewed. What the student has read should be evaluated by relating it to existing knowledge. Notes should be taken, if necessary.

S: STATE

The student should state verbally, or in writing, the major points covered in the chapter. This process clarifies understanding of the material by using the student's own words to explain it—preferably to another student.

T: TEST

The student should test him or herself by reading the chapter objectives and seeing if he or she can perform all the skills without consulting the chapter. Any questions should be answered, and the activities listed in any course workbook should be completed. Once each of these steps has been completed, the student is ready for a mastery test of the material.

Reading technical materials

Different methods are required for reading technical material than for recreational reading. Looking up and learning new terms requires more time, as does taking notes of important points. By following the PQRST system, the sonographer-student can enhance his or her learning ability. If these steps are repeated until the subject is understood and the steps are spaced over several days, the material will be retained in both short- and long-term memory.

To firmly fix information in the student's mind, notes should be taken while reading, and the student should take advantage of using several senses to reinforce memory. The most logical way is to create an outline with main headings and notations under each heading. The student should put the main ideas (except for definitions) in his or her own words.

Instructors often assign outside reading of other books, pamphlets, and journal articles to add to their students' knowledge. The importance of becoming familiar with the institution's medical library cannot be overemphasized. Even after completion of a sonography program, a sonographer should set aside time each month for routinely reviewing periodicals and new books on sonography or related subjects.

Presenting material

If a sonographer-student is asked to give a journal review, the following suggestions will make the task easier and enable maximum learning:

- The topic heading should be listed, and under it the main points (subheadings of the article). Enough information should be provided to explain each point adequately.
- The title and page should be recorded for future reference (Index cards are useful for filing, easy retrieval, or rearrangement).
- Additional information that may have been found in other references should be included.
- A note should be made of any information that is puzzling as a reminder to discuss it in class or to look it up in another reference source before the presentation.
- A dictionary should be used to define unfamiliar words. A list or set of flashcards of such words and their definitions can be used to self-quiz.
- If the topic is a lengthy subject, the sonographer-student can work with a friend. In this way the material can be covered from a different perspective—keeping the audience interested—and rehearsed by testing each other's presentations.

If asked to make a case presentation, it is important that the sonographer-student review all available clinical information and add to it any relevant information derived from current resources such as journal articles. Box 3-2 lists the components of a case study or review and suggestions on its presentation.

Learning aids

Many tools are available to aid sonography students in learning the complexities of diagnostic medical sonography. The importance of the Internet cannot be emphasized too strongly.

BOX **3-2** Case Review

COMPONENTS

Case history	Official report
Requisition	Follow-up
Sonography data	Pathology review

Case history: The student-sonographer should include the patient's age, sex, symptoms, referral-route, and physical and laboratory findings.

Requisition: The student-sonographer should note any clinical question or questions, type of sonography study requested, and the referring physician's clinical comments.

Sonography data: The student-sonographer should arrange images in the order in which they were obtained during the examination. He or she should demonstrate normal structures first, then discuss abnormal structures or disease. The sonographer's impressions regarding size, location, consistency, technical difficulties, etc. should be noted.

Official report: The student-sonographer should include the final report, and compare or contrast it with the sonographer's impressions.

Follow-up: The student-sonographer should note sequelae of any sort; surgical or pathology reports, or both; and any additional diagnostic test results.

Pathology review: The student-sonographer should discuss the prevalence of abnormal pathologic findings and report them on any supporting journal articles. Describe those clinical symptoms of the patient that were most representative and whether or not the scans obtained sufficiently demonstrated the area of interest.

A whole world of knowledge is available with only a few keystrokes. Films and videotapes, CD-ROMs, and DVDs often are more valuable than written materials because they demonstrate action. Along with slides, they also may demonstrate rare diseases unlikely to be encountered in the normal course of a training program. To obtain maximum benefits, however, it is essential to know what to look for in any film or tape before viewing it.

Field trips

Sonographer-students can often get clearer impressions by observing rather than just reading about a subject or activity. To make the most of any field trip, they should learn in advance about the place they are visiting and what to look for once there. Afterward, they should be prepared to discuss as a group what they have seen.

Teaching machines

Sonographer-students who have been out of school for a few years often feel overwhelmed by the large amount and variety of educational hardware available in sonography programs. Calculators, computer terminals, software, and measuring devices are all learning aids that should be fairly easy to operate and use if the student takes the time to become familiar with the concepts, as well as the equipment.

Role-playing

For students inexperienced in actually working with patients and interacting with medical personnel, role-playing is one of the best available methods for gaining confidence. Sonographers are expected to maintain a comfortable flow of conversation with patients before, throughout, and after completion of all examinations. They also are required to communicate skillfully with physicians and other health professionals. When students act the roles of patient, sonographer, and physician, they often discover different approaches and solutions to common sonography problems. Role-playing also can prepare sonographer-students to better understand their patients by tuning in to nonverbal gestures, subtle meanings, inner feelings, and unstated messages.

Effective studying

Studying is much easier and more effective if it is planned. If a sonographer-student has been out of school for some time and is no longer in the habit of studying, establishing good study habits may be difficult at first. Study periods should be scheduled when the student is most alert and attentive, and the study environment should be arranged so that it is quiet enough to avoid distractions or interruptions. Finding a quiet place to study at home that is away from other residents should be a priority.

Ideally, a suitable study area should be well lighted, with sufficient space for writing and spreading books out conveniently. Propping books at a 30-degree angle when reading long passages can prevent eyestrain.

Everything should be assembled before studying begins. The student should keep the work area neat and provide simple comforts such as a straight-backed chair and a cool room to ease concentration and alertness.

Composing a study plan avoids wasting time. Also, a project should be finished before starting another. It is difficult to concentrate if the student skips from subject to subject while studying. Difficult tasks can be done first, but if the student is a procrastinator, an easy, interesting aspect of the study topic can be done first. If the student gets tired or bored, he or she should switch the subject or environment. A student who is no longer being productive should stop studying.

Longer study periods are best for organizing relationships and concepts, outlining, or writing papers. Shorter time intervals are more suitable for rote memorization, review, and self-testing. Even odd moments such as standing in a checkout line can be used to recall and review notes or flashcards. It is also advisable to do rote memory tasks and review details just before falling asleep.

Studying with a friend by quizzing each other, comparing notes, and predicting test questions can be beneficial. Some study-buddies even divide chapters, reporting what they each read and emphasizing the most important aspects of the material.

Cramming for a test is counterproductive as it can result in mental exhaustion. The student should start studying early and keep studying as he or she goes along. It is important for students to take care of themselves before an examination, too, by eating well and getting enough sleep and exercise the day before an examination.

Most important of all, a student should take a 10-minute break every 50 minutes.

TESTS AND EVALUATIONS

The sonographer-student must become accustomed to taking examinations or tests because they provide a method to evaluate progress and to prepare him or her for registry or certifying examinations after graduation. Much of the educational system has taught students to look for "the one right answer." This approach is fine for some situations, but too many people tend to stop looking after the first answer has been found. The following material describes the various types of tests used in sonography programs.

Objective tests

The most commonly used **objective tests** are written tests, which are answered by selecting a correct response from a group of alternatives or by filling in spaces. Objective tests can be presented in the following formats.

MULTIPLE-CHOICE
Questions are situational in nature, and usually only one answer is correct. Some multiple-choice tests, however, are constructed so that several answers may be correct. The sonographer-student is then expected to choose the best answer from a list of several options. He or she should look over the test to determine which approach is expected.

TRUE OR FALSE
A statement must be evaluated to see whether it is right or wrong.

COMPLETION
Missing words or phrases are included in a sentence. The sentence must be completed to make it true.

MATCHING
Two columns of words or phrases are provided, and the sonographer-student is asked to match each item in the first column with the related item in the second column. He or she should check to see if the number of answers equals the number of questions or if there are

more answers than questions. Then it must be determined whether answers may be used more than once.

Subjective tests

The most common form of **subjective test** is the essay test. The sonographer-student may be asked to (1) define or explain a term/concept or (2) describe how he or she would handle a given situation or solve a specific problem. Before writing, answers should be planned. Ideas should be expressed clearly and briefly. An outline format may be particularly effective in writing an answer.

Test-taking skills

Improving test performance requires many tips and tricks, but undoubtedly the most important of all is reading the instructions! Once this is finished, the following routine is recommended:

- The examination should be gone through once, and all the items about which the student is certain should be answered. This exercise may possibly provide answers to earlier questions that seemed difficult.
- The student should go through the examination again and answer any questions that are now obvious.
- For any remaining unanswered multiple-choice questions, the student should try to eliminate the obviously incorrect responses. Then he or she should choose the answer that first seemed right. When totally stumped, the answer "B" or "2" should be chosen, as they have been statistically shown to be the right answers. Teachers are reluctant to place the correct answer in either first or last position; instead they place it in the middle of seductive alternatives.

Once all test questions have been answered, it is a good idea to go through the whole test again. The student should check the choices to make sure they are still regarded as correct and that no clerical error has been made, especially if answers were recorded on separate answer sheets.

Testing equipment

Machine scoring requires the use of a preprinted answer sheet. Each question usually has three to six answer slots. One should read and follow the test instructions carefully and check that the answer selected correctly matches the appropriate question. Students should be aware that machine malfunctions can occur, causing an answer sheet to be incorrectly marked.

Computerized testing

Sonographer-students may be asked to use a computer terminal to take a test. In such tests, they usually receive immediate feedback on whether an answer was right or wrong. If wrong, the correct answer will probably be told. Because all certifying tests are now computerized, the sonographer-student should take as many computerized practice examinations possible to become comfortable and facile at using this testing medium.

TRANSITION FROM CLASSROOM TO CLINICAL SETTING

Clinical training and experience are among the most variable aspects of sonography programs in the United States. The clinical rotation is meant to help integrate, through actual experience, what was learned in the classroom. The design and implementation of clinical activities will be heavily governed by institutional regulations developed in response to legal, ethical, governmental, and financial pressures.

Scanning arts

Ideally, the sonographer-student should be provided with firsthand experience not only in the observation of, but also in the manipulation of, sonography equipment on a living patient. If regulations prohibit the use of live models or patients for scanning instruction, the use of scanning objects and "phantoms" may be substituted. The sonographer-student must practice until he or she has developed the requisite complex scanning skills on the basis of eye-hand coordination and has become familiar and proficient in using the equipment to make anatomic measurements.

Individual instruction is the exception rather than the rule in most sonography programs. However, a reasonable instructor-to-student ratio, as well as a reasonable student-to-machine ratio, should be in place. Learning to operate ultrasound equipment and to scan patients is no different from other eye-hand-coordinated activities such as playing the piano, tennis, or golf. Some group instruction is acceptable, but until the sonographer-student can relate "one-on-one," there is little hope of mastering the art and science of medical sonography. Although films and demonstrations are important, they are secondary to sensorimotor activities.

Scanning laboratories

The sonographer-student's first rotation from the classroom may be to the sheltered environment of a scanning-arts laboratory. This provides an opportunity to integrate classroom knowledge of the physical principles of ultrasound by using various types of ultrasound instrumentation. Scanning test objects or "volunteers," or both, provide hands-on experience in setting up an ultrasound unit, manipulating the transducer, positioning patients, making measurements of specified anatomic structures, and using various recording devices. As the sonographer-student actually performs the scanning protocols that have been studied, he or she will begin to appreciate how sonographers are required to tailor every examination to meet the needs of patients' individual body types. Through trial and error, but with the helpful direction of a clinical instructor, the sonographer-student should develop familiarity and confidence in scanning techniques before moving on to working with actual patients.

HOW TO GET THE MOST OUT OF CLINICAL ROTATIONS

Clinical instructors often use the time in the practice laboratory for role-playing sessions to develop the ability to converse with future patients, to answer their questions, to explain their own procedures, and to learn how to listen effectively. Having the chance to practice in a stress-free environment will provide a solid base for launching clinical skills.

Clinical observation and assistance

The next step may be a familiarization visit to a clinical site to observe day-to-day operations. While there, the sonographer-student may be asked to assist staff members by carrying out ancillary tasks such as helping the patients onto the scanning table or recording measurements and images as the sonographer directs. Once the sonographer-student can perform these tasks correctly, he or she can progress to the more independent phases of performing all aspects of the ultrasound examination under the direct supervision of either a clinical instructor or another registered sonographer.

Getting more "scan time"

Whether he or she is the sole sonographer-student or one of several such students on a clinical rotation, the main objective is to get a chance to scan patients. However, instructors realize that sonographer-students are there to learn all of the components of working in an imaging laboratory and not just the art of scanning. The sooner the student understands how the laboratory functions, the better the chances will be to be granted scanning experience.

Robert DeJong, radiology technical manager for ultrasound at the Johns Hopkins Medical Center, shared the following methods he teaches to gain increased scan time:

- "Arrive early and check the schedule to determine how many patients are scheduled and what types of examinations have been ordered.
- Meet with your clinical instructor and staff members to explain your goals.
- Explain to them what pathologies you are currently studying in class, and ask for the opportunity to scan any patients of that type.
- Be persistent, but also be present! Remember that staff will not go looking for you.
- Offer to help in any nonscanning tasks that might need to be done in order to create more time for scanning instruction.
- Ask permission to perform target scanning. Target scanning is scanning for a specific goal. One day it might be the kidney, another day the placenta or gallbladder.
- Ask permission to start the study by setting up the room, explaining the procedure, and positioning the patient.
- Ask permission to carry out target scanning while the staff sonographer is getting films checked, or to keep the patient in the room for an extra 5 minutes when the staff is going to lunch.
- Be alert, and recognize "nonscanning time." Nonscanning time is typically when the sonographer is doing paperwork, inputting into various computer programs, looking up the patient's history, or checking the study."

As the sonographer-student makes the classroom-to-clinical transition, his or her competence in meeting the educational objectives of the program will be evaluated. Remember that competency levels vary from student to student, so comparing oneself or competing with other students is unrealistic. Instead, the student should set his or her sights on performing better tomorrow than today.

Performance evaluations

Preliminary recommendations have been drawn up both by the Society of Diagnostic Medical Sonographers and by the American Institute of Ultrasound in Medicine regarding clinical performance, and the student's own sonography program may have adopted one of them (Box 3-3). Sonographer-students should understand what will be evaluated, how often evaluations will occur, and what type of evaluation instrument will be used. The sonographer-student should understand that clinical instructors will be rating their work habits, willingness to learn, speed of learning, and scanning prowess.

Most evaluations are divided into two categories: product and process competencies. Product competencies relate to the skills necessary to perform specialty sonographic examinations and cover a wide range of activities—from obtaining patient history to reviewing the sonographic images with the sonologist. Process competencies are universal skills (e.g., motivation, appearance, patient interaction) that transcend the various ultrasound specialties.

BOX **3-3**   Scope of Practice for the Diagnostic Ultrasound Professional

PREAMBLE

The purpose of this document is to define the scope of practice for diagnostic ultrasound professionals and to specify their roles as members of the health care team, acting in the best interest of the patient. This scope of practice is a "living" document that will evolve as the technology expands.

DEFINITION OF THE PROFESSION

The diagnostic ultrasound profession is a multispecialty field composed of diagnostic medical sonography (with subspecialties in abdominal, neurologic, obstetrical/gynecologic, and ophthalmic ultrasound); diagnostic cardiac sonography (with subspecialties in adult and pediatric echocardiography); vascular technology; and other emerging fields. These diverse specialties are distinguished by their use of diagnostic medical ultrasound as a primary technology in their daily work. Certification* is considered the standard of practice in ultrasound. Individuals who are not yet certified should reference the scope as a professional model and strive to become certified.

SCOPE OF PRACTICE OF THE PROFESSION

The diagnostic ultrasound professional is an individual qualified by professional credentialing† and academic and clinical experience to provide diagnostic patient care services using ultrasound and related diagnostic procedures. The scope of practice of the diagnostic ultrasound professional includes those procedures, acts, and processes permitted by law, for which the individual has received education and clinical experience, and in which he or she has demonstrated competency.

Diagnostic ultrasound professionals do the following:
- Perform patient assessments
- Acquire and analyze data obtained using ultrasound and related diagnostic technologies
- Provide a summary of findings to the physician to aid in patient diagnosis and management
- Use independent judgment and systematic problem-solving methods to produce high-quality diagnostic information and optimize patient care

Endorsed by:
- Society of Diagnostic Medical Sonography
- American Institute of Ultrasound Medicine
- American Society of Echocardiography‡
- Canadian Society of Diagnostic Medical Sonographers
- Society for Vascular Sonography

From Society of Diagnostic Medical Sonography: *Scope of practice for the diagnostic ultrasound professional*, Plano, Texas, 1999-2005, SDMS.

*Examples of credentials: registered diagnostic medical sonographer (RDMS), registered diagnostic cardiac sonographer (RDCS), registered vascular technologist (RVT); awarded by the American Registry of Diagnostic Medical Sonographers, a certifying body with National Commission for Certifying Agencies (NCCA) Category "A" membership.

†Credentials should be awarded by an agency certified by the NCCA.

‡Qualified endorsement.

BOX **3-4** Legitimate Topics for Student Evaluation of Programs and Courses

Classroom and clinical experience: can be discussed with academic and clinical instructors
Academic and clinical instruction: can be discussed with the program director
Clinical rotation: can be discussed with the medical director
Courses (most/least useful): can be discussed with the manager of the sonography program

Sonographer-students must become familiar with what is clinically expected of them if they are to successfully complete the practical portions of their training. Box 3-3 provides an example of the current scope of practice for sonographers. To avoid anxiety and fear, sonographers should be informed as to when evaluations will occur and whether the evaluation will be used for instruction or grading purposes. In either case, the instructor should review the evaluation with the sonographer-student, point by point, as soon as possible (while memory of the activity is still fresh) to obtain feedback and provide reinforcement. If the sonographer-student fails any of the program's goals and objectives, he or she should be given additional instruction and assignments and the opportunity to perform for reevaluation.

Often students are unaware that they have the right to evaluate their sonography programs and make suggestions and recommendations for improvement (Box 3-4).

Clinical competency

A competent sonographer must possess many diverse skills. The following list describes the minimum requirements of general proficiency:

- Extensive knowledge of the physical principles of diagnostic ultrasound to ensure the ability to recognize and overcome any scanning difficulties that may arise during an examination.
- A working knowledge of the mechanics and operational features of many types of ultrasound systems because of the broad-based nature of medical sonography.
- In-depth appreciation of pathology and pathophysiology, as well as the anatomy and physiology of pertinent body systems. Only with this type of educational foundation can sonographers develop the ability to tailor or redirect an ultrasound study to each patient's body habitus and disease process.
- The ability to survey and scan clinically relevant areas, correlating clinical information with sonographic findings.
- Recognition and recording of representative images and measurements of both normal and abnormal findings. Recognition of any indications that a more detailed examination is necessary.
- Evaluation of patients' clinical and laboratory histories in order to scan the proper anatomic areas and to know which images to record (those that demonstrate or rule out the clinical problem) for the sonologist's review.
- Familiarity with the differential diagnoses of common diseases in the patient population.
- The ability to function as part of the diagnostic team by becoming an assistant to or a resource for the physician.
- The ability to discuss procedures with the sonologist, referring physicians, and patients, as directed.

- The capability to assume the role of teacher to students, staff members, and patients.
- Willingness to engage in continuing education activities to ensure that proficiency is maintained.

EDUCATIONAL CURRICULA

Because of the multidisciplinary and dynamic nature of diagnostic medical sonography, it is crucial that students acquire not only the theory of the physical and applied principles, but also clinical knowledge and the skills that will permit them to achieve specialty performance objectives and perform at the level of responsibility expected of sonographers.

Programs of study

Several educational pathways are available to become a registered diagnostic medical sonographer (RDMS). Various types of sonography programs exist in this country. Some are formal educational programs and may be accredited; others are short-term, informal programs that provide limited education and focus on basic skills training. The latter type of program assumes that students will return to the workplace and continue their studies and training independently, but under the direction of their supervising physician. The availability of such options makes it important to distinguish the difference between education and training.

Most employers prefer to hire registered sonographers. Consequently, the educational program of choice is one that is accredited and will qualify the sonographer-student to take the national certifying/registry examinations and become credentialed in a chosen sonography specialty.

Education involves the process of systematically developing and cultivating knowledge, the mind, character, and skills through formal schooling, teaching, and instruction. In contrast, training is the systematic, practical instruction and drill in a subject that guides, conditions, or controls certain actions to bring about a desired condition. Before selecting a course of study, it is important to evaluate whether the sonographer-student will receive only education, only training, or both education and training. It is also important to learn in advance if a particular program meets the prerequisites of the American Registry for Diagnostic Medical Sonography (ARDMS) because students who complete nonaccredited long- or short-term training or on-the-job-training are ineligible to take the ARDMS examinations.

Three types of formal educational programs currently exist in the United States: hospital-based programs (1 year), community college programs (1 to 2 years), and baccalaureate degree programs (4 years).

Long-term training programs

Hospital-based programs were among the first formal programs offered to train sonographers. A diploma or certificate is usually granted on satisfactory course completion. Classroom activities often are limited to the appropriate sciences and usually are conducted on site, along with clinical rotations. The emphasis of the hospital-based program is on clinical performance.

In community college associate-degree programs and university-based baccalaureate programs, greater emphasis is placed on theory. Classes usually consist of nonscientific, as well as basic science, courses. The **didactic** or classroom sessions generally are held on campus, with clinical rotations occurring in area hospitals or clinics. The educational focus of these institutions is to provide a well-rounded educational experience that may serve as a springboard to advanced studies and employment in managerial or instructional positions.

Short-term training programs

These programs usually vary in length from 1 week to 3 months. They generally are proprietary programs that offer limited courses intended to familiarize the attendees with the operation and potential clinical usefulness of diagnostic ultrasound systems. This type of course requires its students to continue their training through self-study and supervised scanning in the workplace. This type of program, however, will not satisfy the requirements for ARDMS registration.

On-the-job training

In some remote settings, on-the-job training is the only available training option to providing a diagnostic ultrasound service for the community. Supplementary instructional videotapes, correspondence courses, and occasional visits by the manufacturers' application specialists are valuable resources. As with short-term training programs, the on-the-job–trained sonographer will be ineligible to apply for the ARDMS registry.

Summary

Humans are capable of three types of memory: immediate, short-term, and long-term. None of these memory systems operates totally independent of the other; that is, long-term memory depends on short-term memory, and short-term memory depends on immediate memory. Memory is improved when people learn and organize new facts and systematically relate them to their previously acquired knowledge.

Proper storage of information is the key to its retrieval. Experience has shown that the following steps must be followed to remember useful information:
Consciously decide to remember it
Repeat it to help fix its meaning
Refresh or review it at intervals
Understand it by searching for meaning
Artificial memory aids have been used for years and are widely accepted in learning certain types of material. However, the range of items that can be committed to memory in this fashion is quite limited. For the majority of learning situations, it is best to (1) deliberately intend to remember, (2) actively use as many senses as possible, and (3) refresh one's memory often.

In the education and training of sonographers, it is necessary to test not only students' comprehension of the material that has been presented but also their skills in manipulating the transducer on an endless variety of anatomically variable patients.

The final form of testing employs clinical evaluations that are based on such factors as performance, attitude, interpersonal relations, reactions to criticism, efforts to improve, appearance, health habits, punctuality, dependability, ethics, and day-to-day responses in the classroom.

Several types of educational and training opportunities are available to sonographers in the United States. Formal training can be acquired in hospitals, community colleges, and universities, and graduates are encouraged to take their registry examinations as soon as possible after completion of their training. Informal training is available through short-term programs (proprietary or nonproprietary), commercially sponsored customer courses, and on-the-job training. However, short-term training does not meet the requirements for registry examinations.

Supply and demand currently play pivotal roles in the education and employment of sonographers. It is assumed that informal, short-term education eventually will be phased out of existence if and when formal programs adequately meet the personnel needs of diagnostic medical sonography.

BIBLIOGRAPHY

Ellis DB: *Becoming a master student,* Rapid City, SD, 1993, College Survival.

General Ultrasound Online Educational Resource. Available at: *http://www.sonoword.com.*

Independent Learning Center: *Study guides and strategies: thinking critically.* Available at: *http://www.studygs.net/crtthk.htm.*

Joint Review Committee on Education in Diagnostic Medical Sonography (JRCDMS): *Standards and guidelines for an accredited educational program for the diagnostic medical sonographer, cardiac sonographer and/or vascular technologist.* Available at: *http://www.jrcdms.org.*

Lea JH: Developing competency-based clinical education in sonography, *Med Ultrasound* 5(1):1-4, 1981.

Lea JH: The value of role playing in sonography education, *Med Ultrasound* 7(2):81-82, 1983.

OB/GYN Ultrasound Online Educational Resource: Available at: *http://www.obgyn-net.*

Obstetrical Online Educational Resource: Available at: *http://www.thefetus.net.*

Society of Diagnostic Medical Sonography: *Scope of practice—diagnostic medical sonographer,* Plano, Texas, 2000, SDMS.

Society of Diagnostic Medical Sonographers Educational Foundation: *The scan,* Plano, Texas, 2004, SDMSEF.

University of North Carolina: *Improve your studying skills.* Available at: *http://caps.unc.edu/TenTraps.html.*

4

Sonographer Safety Issues

Learning Objectives

Students who successfully complete this chapter will be able to do the following:

- Discuss the prevalence, causes, and risks of musculoskeletal injuries (MSIs) in the field of sonography.
- Discuss ergonomic methods of prevention of MSIs.
- List the major components of a safe scanning environment.
- Name three strategies for combating unhealthy stress in the workplace.

Key Terms

burnout

compassion fatigue

ergonomics

musculoskeletal
  injuries (MSIs)

nonsteroidal
  antiinflammatory drugs (NSAIDs)

repetitive strain
  injuries (RSIs)

S ince its inception, the thrust of diagnostic ultrasound has focused on delivering high-quality diagnostic information as a way to improve patient care. Finding new clinical applications, scanning techniques, and improving image resolution have always taken center stage in the sonography community. Only recently has active attention been paid to the possibility that long-term scanning could be harmful to sonographers' health. This chapter identifies major health risks associated with performing ultrasound studies and recommends solutions to ensure a long and injury-free career for the diagnostic medical sonographer.

PREVALENCE OF MUSCULOSKELETAL INJURIES AMONG SONOGRAPHERS

For more than 40 years, sonographers have played a critical and often indispensable role in the research, development, and application of diagnostic medical sonography (DMS) to clinical medicine. One of the primary goals of sonography has been that of improved patient care. Unfortunately, equal concern and attention was not given to creating a safe working environment for sonographers. It would be 20 years before the question was first asked, *"Are there potential health hazards associated with long-term activity as a sonographer?"* It would take another 20 years before that question was studied, and the magnitude of the problem understood.

By the beginning of the twenty-first century more than three fourths of the sonography workforce reported experiencing pain while scanning, and one in four sonographers sustained career-ending injuries. Although their injuries were varied, a major contributing cause was the poor conditions in which they worked. The sonography community is now aware of the importance of **ergonomics**, the creation of a safe working environment, and is devoted to finding solutions to the work-related injuries and job-related problems encountered by sonographers.

CAUSATION AND MECHANISMS OF INJURY

Sonographers are often subjected to high-performance job pressures at workstations that were not specifically designed for them. Recent studies have shown that unless sonographers can work in a safe, efficient, relaxed manner, not only will their productivity suffer, they will also be at increased risk of developing what could have been avoidable work-related injuries.

Although it is true that specific workloads can be adapted to or tolerated by most individuals, if the individuals are not conditioned to the task and are constantly work-overloaded without sufficient rest or recovery, they risk pain and injury. Sonographers now appreciate that **musculoskeletal injuries (MSIs)** result from minuscule, cumulative trauma to human tissue and that it takes a combination of biologic and biomechanical factors to cause tissue breakdown. Studies have shown that a frequent source of muscle fatigue and potential injury exists whenever low levels of muscle contraction must be maintained for a long duration. These are the types of body demands that are often required when performing ultrasound studies. Besides the ergonomic and environmental stresses that may be present in the sonography workplace, additional risk factors that have been identified are stress, age, and gender.

BOX **4-1**   Common Work-Related Sonographer Injuries

Low back pain	Carpal tunnel syndrome
Tension neck syndrome	de Quervain syndrome
Shoulder bursitis	Trigger finger
Rotator cuff syndrome	Plantar fasciitis
Epicondylitis	Tarsal tunnel syndrome
Tendinitis	Sciatica

ERGONOMICS AND WORK-RELATED SONOGRAPHER INJURY

The most common work-related injuries among sonographers are tendonitis and tenosynovitis of the shoulder, neck, wrist, and back. These injuries are directly related to prolonged periods of arm abduction and muscle loading coupled with constant transducer pressure during scanning. Contributing to these **repetitive strain injuries (RSIs)** are (1) the use of poorly designed ultrasound equipment and stretchers; (2) improper body mechanics while scanning; (3) procedure duration; (4) inappropriate force; (5) insufficient rest/breaks; and (6) repetition of the same type of study for long periods during the workday. Clearly, changes and modifications in equipment and the duration and frequency of sonographic examinations are essential to prevent or significantly reduce such injuries. Sonographers must learn to protect themselves by avoiding situations that lead to MSIs, and sonography training should include instruction in safe scanning techniques, as well as information about injury and prevention.

The most common sites of sonographer pain or injury are the neck, back, shoulder, wrist, hands, fingers, and feet (Box 4-1). The primary causes of all of these injuries are associated with one or more of the following activities: repetition, force, and awkward postures. Awkward posture refers to the deviation of the skeletal bones and joints from a neutral or natural position (Box 4-2). The more often and the longer the duration that a joint deviates from the natural position, the greater the risk of injury. Specific activities leading to pain and injury areas follows:

• The use of prolonged pressure during transducer manipulation
• Shoulder abduction while scanning

BOX **4-2**   Specific Postures Associated with Injury

Neck (cervical spine)
  Flexion/extension (tilting head up to see monitor)
  Side bending (while reaching across the patient)
Shoulder
  Abduction/flexion (upper arm positioned out to the side > 30 degrees)
Wrist
  Flexion/extension (bending up and down while manipulating the transducer)
  Ulnar/radial deviation (bending the wrist to the side)
Low back
  Twisting at the waist (awkward posture) and static postures

BOX **4-3**   Signs and Symptoms of Developing Musculoskeletal Injury

> Pain
> Stiffness
> Numbness
> Decreased range of motion
> Tingling/burning
> Decreased grip strength
> Cramping
> Loss of muscle function

- Sustained twisting of the neck/back to reach over the patient or to reach equipment controls
- Static or awkward postures sustained for the duration of lengthy ultrasound procedures

PHYSIOLOGY AND SYMPTOMS OF WORK-RELATED INJURY

Sonographer work-related injuries typically include muscle strains and tears, ligament sprains, joint and tendon inflammation, pinched nerves, and spinal disc degeneration. MSIs can be difficult to diagnose, and although doctors can perform clinical tests for carpal tunnel syndrome (CTS), with many other MSIs, all there is to go on is whether or not someone is in pain, and pain is subjective. Box 4-3 lists the signs that a sonographer may be developing an MSI.

Pain is a messenger that indicates something is wrong. Pain can be both acute and cumulative, and for sonographers, cumulative workplace strain is the primary cause of injury. The first warning sign to take pain seriously is in *not knowing immediately* what brought on the current discomfort. To endure or ignore pain only perpetuates injuries, leading to work loss and, eventually, life-altering or career-ending disabilities.

SITES OF INJURY

Lower back pain

A high incidence of low back pain (LBP) is found in persons who sit or stand for long periods. Prevention requires maintaining correct posture alignment, reducing the duration of static postures, relaxing the musculoskeletal structures, and taking short breaks. Physical conditioning can make the difference between safety and injury; however, once injury occurs, it will take rest, massage, heat/ice, and flexibility and strengthening exercises to relieve any pain that is aggravated by work activities.

Upper back and neck pain

Nearly all back and neck pains are the result of repetitive strain on muscles and ligaments due to poor, awkward, or static posture. Pain symptoms typically range from brief, mild aches following a day of overexertion to crippling years-long misery. Back and neck pain is often resistant to painkillers, physical therapy, or even surgery. Prevention by sonographers involves adjusting the monitor for visual ease and properly positioning patients to maintain a safe, comfortable resting position for the scanning arm and shoulder. Psychosocial factors are often associated with upper back and neck symptoms, and the prevalence of sonographer injury is significantly influenced by the tendency to feel overworked. Lack of variation on the job, low control over time, and working in a highly competitive setting are frequently related to upper back and neck pain.

Thoracic outlet syndrome

Compression of nerves and blood vessels in the thoracic outlet region can cause pain in the neck and shoulder area and numbness and weakness in the arm/hand. Epidemiologic studies have shown thoracic outlet syndrome (TOS) to be associated with occupations that involve working in a static position for prolonged periods, as well as those that require maintaining awkward postures. TOS treatment includes relieving compression of the nerves and blood vessels in the thoracic outlet region and controlling and minimizing pain and other symptoms as much as possible to improve the overall quality of life. Conservative treatment is usually the first-line approach and includes physical therapy, postural training, muscle-strengthening exercises, and heat treatments with therapeutic ultrasound. Drugs may be used to control pain and muscle spasms. However, most patients with TOS improve with conservative treatment, and only a small number of patients require surgery.

Shoulder pain

The basic role of the shoulder, upper arm, elbow, forearm, and wrist is to place the hand in the appropriate position so that it can fulfill its function. Injury to the shoulder arises from joint instability and is caused by abduction of the arm greater than 30 degrees and by repetitive, excessive, or static force. To avoid shoulder pain, sonographers should position patients close to the edge of the scanning table/bed to narrow the reaching area and reduce arm abduction. Both the patient examination table and the ultrasound keyboard should be adjusted so that the sonographer's elbow can be positioned at a 90-degree angle.

Bursitis

Bursitis occurs with inflammation of the small sac of fluid (bursa) that cushions and lubricates an area between tendon and bone or around a joint. The condition is caused by overuse, repetitive motions, sudden injury, gradual degeneration, or aging. Continuous pressure or stress on a joint structure greatly increases the risk of developing bursitis. Symptomatology includes pain, tenderness, and stiffness near the affected bursa.

Sonographers most often experience bursitis in the shoulder of the scanning arm and should be cautioned that attempting to change the way one uses a joint to avoid bursa pain may result in muscle weakness in that area. The treatment of bursitis includes resting the painful area, applying ice, taking pain relievers if necessary, and doing gentle exercises and stretching to prevent stiffness. Aspiration of any excess fluid or application of a pressure bandage to the area is sometimes used to treat persistent bursitis. Antibiotic treatment may be necessary if the aspirate shows signs of bacteria. Severe and persistent bursitis may also be treated with an injection of corticosteroids to reduce inflammation.

Extremities

The upper extremities, especially the wrists and the hands, are an anatomically complex collection of bones, muscles, tendons, and nerves. All of these structures are essential to work activities and are increasingly subject to acute and chronic mechanical injuries (Box 4-4). Among sonographers, upper extremity injury is most often associated with the use of poorly

BOX **4-4**   Most Common Areas of Tendon Inflammation in Extremities

Upper extremities:	Lower extremities:
Shoulder	Leg
Rotator cuff	Knee
Biceps	Ankle
Elbow	Foot
Wrist	
Fingers	

designed transducers or improperly holding or excessively gripping the transducer. The resulting injuries are tendonitis, tenosynovitis, or tunnel syndromes. Additionally, damage to the elbow, epicondylitis (tennis elbow), or posterior impingement syndrome of the elbow can be sustained.

TENDONITIS

Lack of tendon elasticity and constant pulling on the tendon attachments to the bone make tendon attachments susceptible to microscopic low-level tearing. Such tearing produces the inflammation and irritation known as tendonitis. Tendonitis is variable, striking the most often used areas. Symptomatically, *tendonitis* ranges from aching pain and stiffness in the local area of the tendon to a burning sensation surrounding the entire joint around an inflamed tendon. Pain usually worsens during and after activity, and the tendon/joint area typically becomes stiffer the next day. With proper care, tendon pain should lessen over 3 weeks' time. However, the healing process continues beyond that period, and due to scar tissue formation, may not peak until approximately 6 to 8 weeks following the initial injury. Scar tissue initially acts as glue to bond the tissue back together, and in severe cases scar formation has been reported to prolong healing as long as a year. After 6 months, the condition is considered chronic, and it is much more difficult to treat. The initial approach to treating tendonitis is to support and protect the tendons by bracing any tendon areas that are being pulled on during use (Fig. 4-1). To lessen pain and minimize inflammation, it is important to loosen up the tendon before use.

DIGITAL TENDONITIS AND TENOSYNOVITIS

In the hand, inflammation of tendon sheaths can impede the tendon from gliding smoothly within its sheath. This is due to thickening or nodular development that prevents smooth extension or flexion of the finger. The finger suddenly may lock or *trigger*, extending with a snap. Trigger finger (flexor digital tenosynovitis) often coexists with carpal tunnel syndrome and occasionally with fibrotic changes of the palmar fascia. The major symptoms are aching or pain at the wrist and thumb, aggravated by motion. Tenderness can be elicited just distal to the radial styloid process over the site of the involved tendon sheaths. Rest, warm soaks, and **nonsteroidal antiinflammatory drugs (NSAIDs)** are only helpful in mild cases. For more severe conditions, local corticosteroid injections may be required. A rare hazard is tendon rupture.

CARPAL TUNNEL SYNDROME

The most commonly reported nerve entrapment syndrome is CTS, a repetitive motion injury. Females 30 to 60 years of age have the highest rates of CTS, which is caused by compression

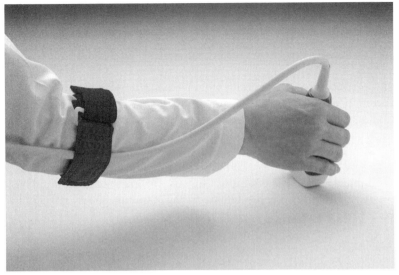

A

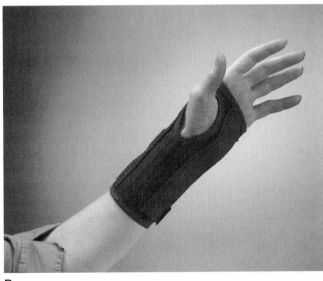

B

FIGURE **4-1 A,** Using a cable brace reduces the torque that the weight of the transducer causes to the hand during scanning. **B,** The use of a wrist brace alleviates the stress of extreme wrist flexion during scanning.

of the median nerve at the wrist, causing numbness. Importantly, highly repetitive motions are a greater risk factor than high-force motions. Individuals who repeatedly bend the wrist inward, toward the forearm, can be predisposed to CTS.

Symptomatology includes numbness, burning, tingling, and a prickling sensation over the palmar surface of the hand, thumb, forefinger, midfingers, and half of the ring finger. Some individuals experience a *shooting* pain extending from the wrist up the arm or down into the hand and fingers. With continued median nerve compression, many experience muscle weaknesses, making it difficult to hold objects with the affected hand. Eventually, the muscles atrophy, especially the fleshy part of the thumb. Untreated, this condition can result in permanent weakness, loss of sensation, or paralysis of the thumb and fingers of the affected hand.

Diagnosing CTS requires determining whether symptoms can be elicited by holding the hand in a position with the wrist bent for approximately 1 minute can elicit symptoms. Imaging studies may be indicated to rule out a tumor as the cause of compression. Electromyographic or nerve conduction velocity testing also has value in determining the severity of nerve damage. Treatment requires the use of splints, NSAIDs, injections of steroids, or surgery (in severe cases). Left untreated, the prognosis is poor and may result in permanent disability. Prevention requires the use of ergonomic equipment and room arrangements, use of proper body mechanics during scanning, and frequent breaks between patients.

DE QUERVAIN DISEASE

De Quervain disease is painful tenosynovitis caused by the relative narrowness of the common tendon sheath of the abductor pollicis longus and the extensor pollicis brevis. Symptoms include localized tenderness and swelling in the region of the styloid process of the radius and wrist pain radiating into the forearm and distally, into the thumb. Other findings may include decreased range of motion of the lower joint of the thumb and crackling noises over the tendon when moving it. With de Quervain disease, potential exists for symptoms in the arm other than those involving the tendon. These symptoms can result from the close proximity of the nerves, tendons, tendon sheaths, and fascia of the forearm to the site of inflammation. The major symptom of aching pain at the wrist and thumb is aggravated by motion. This condition occurs with repetitive use of the wrist, though it is occasionally associated with rheumatoid arthritis.

Diagnosis of de Quervain disease is based on the location of pain and the presence of swelling in the hand and decreased hand function. Rest or immobilization (splinting) of the injured part provides symptomatic relief. Heat or cold application (whichever is most beneficial) and NSAIDs may be indicated. Controlled exercise several times daily (progressively increasing with tolerance) is advised to prevent "frozen shoulder." Injection of corticosteroids within the tendon sheath may be helpful. Surgery is rarely necessary; however, a disabling complication of surgery performed for de Quervain disease is the development of a painful neuroma of the radial nerve. The most serious hazard associated with de Quervain disease is that of tendon rupture, which fortunately is rare.

PLANTAR FASCIITIS

The plantar fascia is a broad, flat ligament on the bottom of the foot extending from the front of the heel to the base of the toes. The purpose of this structure is to help maintain the arch of the foot (Fig. 4-2). Plantar fasciitis results from overuse and the repeated stress of using the foot. It can be caused by (1) any activities that increase weight and stress on the foot when working on hard floors or ground, (2) normal aging, and (3) being overweight. Wearing shoes with good arch supports is important, as are adequate cushioning and enough flexibility to easily bend under the ball of the foot.

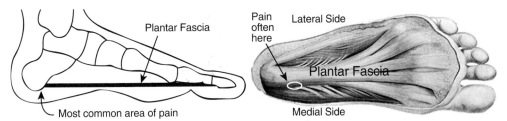

FIGURE **4-2** This anatomic drawing represents the appearance of the plantar fascia. An inflammation of the plantar fascia is called *plantar fasciitis* and often results in the development of a heel spur (a soft, flexible calcium deposit on the front and bottom of the heel.)

Plantar fasciitis, which is often confused with or considered the same as a heel spur, typically produces heel pain with the first few steps in the morning. This pain can be mild or debilitating and is usually located in the front and bottom of the heel. The condition can last a few months, be intermittent, or become permanent. If the plantar fascia becomes inflamed, it can produce arch pain. Treatment includes rest, ice, taping, strengthening and flexibility exercises, and orthotic devices. If unresponsive to treatment, extracorporeal shock wave therapy or surgery may be indicated.

TARSAL TUNNEL SYNDROME

The tarsal tunnel is a structure in the foot formed between the bones of the foot and overlying fibrous tissue. Within this tunnel lies the posterior tibial nerve. Tarsal tunnel syndrome results from pressure on, or compression of, the posterior tibial nerve. Symptoms include a painful burning, numbness, or tingling sensation in and around the ankles, which sometimes extends from the base of the foot and heel to the toes. Similar to CTS in the wrist, tarsal tunnel syndrome is related to standing for long periods. Treatment begins with antiinflammatory medications and possibly cortisone injections into the area around the nerve. Orthotics and changes in footwear may also help to relieve the symptoms. If none of these measures help, a surgical procedure called a tarsal tunnel release may be necessary. When a tarsal tunnel release is performed, an incision is made to open the tarsal tunnel and decrease pressure on the posterior tibial nerve. This surgery is similar to a carpal tunnel release in the wrist.

PREVENTING WORK-RELATED PAIN

The work-related MSIs that have plagued the sonography sector could actually be eliminated by staying in good physical condition, by following the ergonomic principles of designing a workplace and equipment that place body parts in the optimum position for working, and by observing safe scanning body mechanics.

Frequent rest and exercise are the primary steps in preventing MSIs. Sonographers should train just as serious athletes do to reduce or prevent the risk of injury. Sonographer exercise and stretching programs have been developed to help strengthen and support the torso and the upper extremities—the two areas most severely affected. A wealth of information regarding these and other appropriate exercises is posted on the Society of Diagnostic Medical Sonography website *(http://www.sdms.org)* in the "Work Zone" section.

In forward-thinking ultrasound settings, sonographers are provided with wellness programs that deliver useful and informative instruction. Monthly or bimonthly meetings focus on musculoskeletal safety and prevention, exercise, and the importance of stretching. Such programs can be developed in-house or contracted out, but both are more successful when there is positive support and reinforcement by the institution's administration.

The second step is to correct unsound work habits, especially the external stresses of exertional force, posture, and contact or static stress.

The third step is to correct any of the existing ergonomically unsound aspects in the sonography workplace.

ELIMINATING THE RISK OF INJURY

It will take time to convince and educate not only the majority of sonographers but instructors, hospital administrators, and equipment manufacturers that sonography is a high-risk occupation, the safety needs of which must be actively addressed (Box 4-5). Until then, sonographers must assume the task of protecting themselves and their career potential (Table 4-1).

To prevent injury, it is advisable for sonographers to do the following:
- Rest their arms on something during scanning. Specially designed scanning bolsters are available (Fig. 4-3); however, a rolled-up towel, glove box, or even the patient's body can also serve the purpose.
- Do not grip or push the transducer too hard.
- Never reach out to their side or in front of their body more than 30 degrees (Fig. 4-4).
- Alternate standing and sitting to prevent or avoid escalation of symptoms.
- Keep patients as close as possible to the edge of the examination table to allow the sonographer's scanning arm to be kept low and close to the body.
- While scanning in a seated position, use only adjustable chairs that allow the proper straight alignment of the spine (Fig. 4-5).
- Position the feet wide enough apart, when standing, to maintain whole body alignment.
- Avoid leaning toward the patient while scanning. If it is necessary to lean toward the patient to perform the examination, the patient is *too far away*.
- Take short breaks during an examination to relax the neck and shoulders and refresh the blood flowing to the muscles. This is important because decreased blood and oxygen flow to muscles can cause fatigue and set the stage for injury.
- Stop periodically during scanning to rest tense and contracted muscles.
- Vary the types of examinations so that easy examinations are scheduled before and after lengthy, complicated ones.
- Perform shoulder, wrist, and arm stretching exercises periodically throughout the day.

BOX **4-5**   Sonographer Self-Help Checklist

Step 1. Awareness
Step 2. Behavior modification
Step 3. Mandatory frequent breaks during the workday
Step 4. Modification of scan techniques (changing hands, posture, sitting/standing)
Step 5. Evaluation by a physical therapist

TABLE **4-1**   Injury/Risk Checklist

ACTION	INJURY RISK	SOLUTION
Reaching	Shoulder/neck	• Position equipment as close possible. • Position patient as close to operator as possible. Area to be scanned should be aligned with operator's shoulder. • Reduce reach to 30 cm or less. • Avoid extending arm over control panel/keyboard. • Never scan with arm extended away from body.
Twisting	Back/neck	• Distribute weight evenly on both feet when standing. • Use abdominal muscles to support torso when sitting. • Position display screen and control panel directly in front of operator.
Portable studies	Back/arm/wrist	• Lock leading wheels to steer more easily. • Avoid twisting motions of the trunk while steering equipment. • Hold wrists straight when pushing equipment.
Flexion/extension	Wrist/upper arm	• Maintain wrist in a neutral position. • Provide support for the wrist of the scanning arm.
Transducer grip	Hand/wrist	• Grip transducer only tight enough to maintain control. • Select transducers with flexible, lightweight cables. • Use a cable brace to support transducer cables. • Do not drape cables over shoulder or around neck; let them hang freely. • Avoid a pinching grip. Change/vary grip during scanning to distribute stress evenly over multiple muscle groups.
Posture	Back/foot	• Avoid static positions, alternate standing and sitting. • Stand with weight evenly distributed. • Sit with both feet on the floor, using abdominal muscles to support torso; do not slouch or slump.

• Take breaks during the day as a safety factor.
• Engage in regular programs of stretching and strengthening to reduce MSI symptoms.

IDENTIFYING AND ASSESSING WORKPLACE STRESS

Ergonomic stress

Numerous studies have shown that physical working conditions can be a source of stress. They also have revealed that it is much easier to fix the workplace than the worker, and this factor should be a major consideration in the design of all sonography settings.

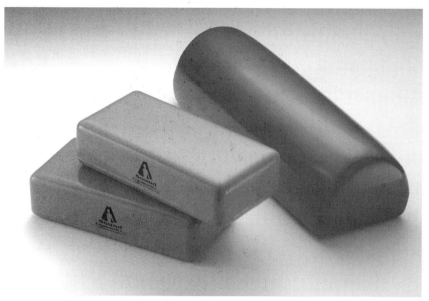

FIGURE **4-3** These ergonomically designed cushions are used to support and improve the natural alignment of the upper arm, reducing shoulder/neck strain and fatigue.

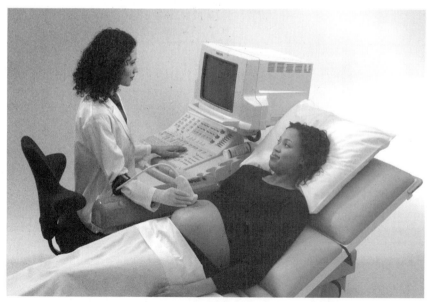

FIGURE **4-4** Demonstration of proper arm positioning during scanning activities. Cushions of various sizes, used alone or in combination, prevent the scanning arm from being "suspended" in the air, eliminating arm and shoulder muscle stress.

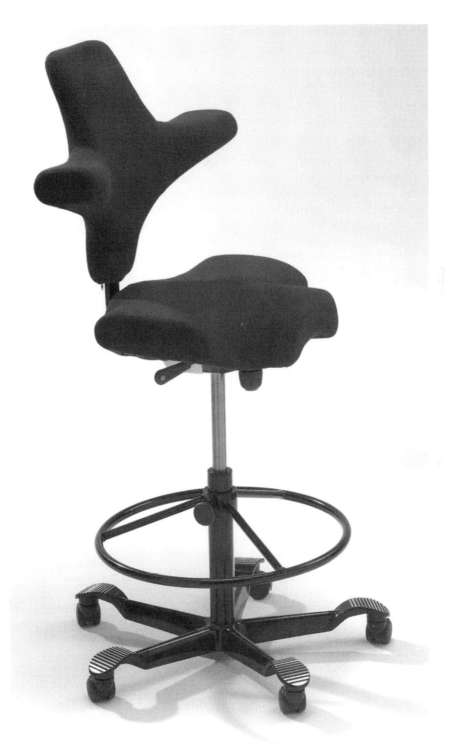

FIGURE **4-5** The HAG Capisco ergonomic chair is designed to encourage neutral positioning of the spine and shoulder, as well as the ability to move more freely while seated. It offers the support necessary to reduce the stress of awkward postures during scanning. Other important features are an adjustable seat; a broad, stable, and mobile base; and a unique backrest that provides support whether sitting forward, sideways, or backwards.

Imaging equipment, patient examination tables, and sonographer chairs should be designed with maximum flexibility, height adjustability, and proper support. Existing workplaces that are not designed with ergonomics in mind should be evaluated for their risk and injury potential, as well as focusing on ergonomic stress.

Environmental stress

Lighting, air quality, and overcrowding are three important environmental stress factors. Improper room luminance can be a major headache for imagers, causing eyestrain and increased fatigue. High ambient lighting can produce glare and reflect off the screen, degrading image contrast and possibly leading to misinterpretation. Standard office lighting, especially fluorescent lighting, is too bright for safe eye-friendly scanning. The use of full-spectrum bulbs on a rheostat (dimmer switch) is highly advised. In windowed scanning environments it is important to have adequate light-blocking blinds, shades, or curtains and to position the imaging equipment parallel to windows to prevent display screen glare. Walls painted in dark matte earth tones and dark flooring also are desirable, as they are efficient light absorbers.

A frequent source of sonographer complaint is eyestrain. Although eyestrain is prevalent among sonographers, it is preventable. The strategies for reducing eyestrain are simple and involve basic eye care, workplace lighting design, and eye-conscious work habits. Basic eye care begins with a thorough eye examination. If corrective lenses are indicated, sonographers should mention the type of work they do.

Older sonographers may find it difficult to focus on the display screen because they may be developing presbyopia, a focusing deficit afflicting many people in their late 30s or early 40s and virtually everyone older than age 45. Bifocal or progressive lenses are often prescribed to correct this condition. However, the lenses prescribed for normal reading distances (14 to 16 inches) are not effective for the viewing distance to an ultrasound display screen. To compensate and achieve better focus, bifocal wearers often tilt their heads back to see the screen. After a 6- to 8-hour day, such abnormal posture can lead to back and neck problems. Wearing single-vision lenses that are designed for middle distance only will allow maintenance of a more natural head and neck position during scanning activities. For added insurance, the top of the monitor should be positioned at eye level so that the eyes are looking *downward* to see the screen.

Eyestrain and fatigue can also be the products of long workdays and a lack of breaks. A simple strategy for reducing eyestrain involves taking frequent breaks and observing the 20-20-20 rule, described in Box 4-6. The Occupational Safety and Health Administration (OSHA) further recommends 10-minute rest breaks for every 2 hours of scanning, along with proper positioning of an adjustable display screen so that individuals can select their own best viewing angle.

Air quality

Research conducted into the possible links between poor air quality and worker ailments has been ongoing for the past 30 years. Studies have revealed that a range of 2000 to

BOX **4-6**   The 20-20-20 Rule

For every *20* minutes of scanning,
Look *20* feet away, for *20* seconds.

4000 negative ions per cubic centimeter is the ideal ion concentration of indoor environments. Achieving and maintaining such a balance are beneficial in creating a healthy ecosystem where humans thrive. Unfortunately, the construction and furnishings of modern working environments often act as a vacuum for negative ions.

Sonography workplaces, particularly those housed in modern buildings, suffer from poor air quality, largely due to their steel and concrete construction; sealed windows; and reliance on air-conditioning and heating. In air quality studies, many buildings of this type yield an average of only 25 to 50 negative ions per cubic centimeter, a number far less than recommended (>1000 ions/cc). It is the use of certain construction materials, lack of fresh air, and use of synthetic fibers in clothing and furniture that absorb the charge of negative ions within the environment. Additional negative ion depletion can be attributed to the presence of fluorescent lighting, electrical and electronic equipment, display monitors, and overcrowding.

When considering air quality, negatives are positive! Negative ions released into the air quickly attach themselves to airborne particles such as dust, dander, smoke, allergens, smog, and pollution. Consequently, these floating particles become too heavy to remain airborne, quickly falling to the ground. When negative ions are created, ozone is produced. Ozone (which is electrically bonded to oxygen) oxidizes and neutralizes the harmful aspects of the chemicals that make up pollution. Additionally, ozone acts as a powerful germicide, quickly destroying bacterial molds and small fungi.

One solution for counteracting the poor air quality found in modern buildings is the introduction of negative air ionizers. Used beneficially for many years in the closed and artificial atmospheres of submarines and spacecraft, where negative air ionizers were employed, the inhabitants experienced fewer colds, less absenteeism, and more alertness. Further studies confirmed that the use of negative air ionizers stimulated the reticulo-endothelial system, improved resistance to disease, acted on the human capacity to absorb and use oxygen, and sped up the oxidation of serotonin in the blood.

Overcrowding

The problem of overcrowding in the ultrasound workplace is most severe when studies must be carried out in intensive care units or emergency departments. Space in these areas is at a premium and is often a tangle of electrical cords and monitoring/respiratory equipment. Finding space and available electrical outlets is only the first obstacle; the second is to be able to conduct the study without having to awkwardly bend, reach, or stretch while scanning the patients in their hospital beds. Therefore it is important to evaluate all scanning areas—not just those within the department. All daily laboratory operations should be evaluated with an eye toward risk prevention, and the safe-scanning techniques covered earlier must be mandated.

Common workplace stressors

Following are the most common stressful workplace situations:
- Conflict: develops when a sonographer's fundamental values conflict with those of the employer (e.g., performing incomplete or extended patient examinations).
- Role ambiguity: triggered when sonographers are unclear of the employer's expectations.
- Role overload: results from too much to do in too little time.
- Nonparticipation: develops when sonographers have no say in important decisions that affect the quality or quantity of their work.

- Underutilization: occurs when sonographers find themselves in jobs that do not begin to tap their potential. When they question why they are working in such a setting or complain repeatedly of being bored, they are actually expressing their stress.
- Resource inadequacy: exists when there is a lack of sufficient resources to perform a task to the level of expectation (e.g., being confronted with new or unfamiliar equipment but being denied access to training, orientation, or even an instruction manual).

Solutions to workplace stressors

Sonographer stress can be obvious or subtle. It can be triggered by such things as a lack of professional identification and respect or anxiety about performing complete and accurate examinations. Work-related communication problems, struggles to follow hospital policies, and scheduling problems are typical stressors, as well as the ethical and legal conflicts with which sonographers and other health care professionals are confronted. Some sonographers mistakenly pursue the unrealistic goal of achieving perfection as a way to alleviate these problems. They begin working late and ignore meal times, breaks, and even vacations, believing that this will make them better sonographers and, in fact, indispensable. Instead, they should examine the unpleasant aspects of their situation and search for *realistic* solutions to bring back a healthy balance to their professional lives.

Whether it is long- or short-term stress, there is a potential for wearing out the body, increasing susceptibility to illness and delaying healing. A short list of some of the physical challenges that come from being "stressed out" consists of: fatigue, chronic headaches, irritability, changes in appetite, memory loss, low self-esteem, withdrawal, tooth-grinding, cold hands, high blood pressure, shallow breathing, nervous twitches, lowered sexual drive, and insomnia or other sleep pattern changes.

INTERNALLY GENERATED STRESS

Internally generated stress is stress *that we cause ourselves* and is a major factor in the development of sonographer burnout and compassion fatigue. Though it can have great relevance to sonographer injuries, it is infrequently addressed. To fully appreciate these concepts, it is important to define and understand the positive, as well as the negative, aspects of stress.

Stress has been defined as anything that stimulates and increases a person's level of alertness. In order to enjoy healthy, productive, and enjoyable stimulation, individuals should determine their *optimum* level of stress. Obviously, too little stress would result in a boring life, while too much stress could be unpleasant, tiring, and even a health risk.

For sonographers, it is important to identify the short- and long-term stresses present in their workplace and understand how to handle or counter them. Here is an example of short-term stress: During job stimulation lulls, boredom, lack of concentration, and loss of motivation can occur. Once the job pace picks up, these feelings disappear.

Long-term stress is potentially far more serious. Initially, challenges and stresses in the workplace can be faced with energy and positive and effective responses. Over time, however, victims of long-term stress begin to feel frustrated, irritable, and fatigued. They develop health problems and watch helplessly as the quality of their work begins to suffer. Continued high stress often carries with it feelings of failure and leads to frequent absences due to various ailments. As this stage is reached, stress victims start to distance themselves from their coworkers and employer and may begin looking for a new job. Without relief, high levels of long-term stress eventually can lead to depression, burnout, and compassion fatigue.

Burnout

The relatively new concept of stress as a mental and physical illness was not introduced until the mid 1970s, by endocrinologist Hans Selye. Nevertheless, a substantial volume of research and publications have now shown that individuals who work in abusive environments and are unsuccessful at changing them become prime candidates for the particular stress effect called **burnout**.

Burnout is a state of chronic work-related stress that is easier to prevent than it is to treat. Especially prevalent in the health care and helping professions, victims of burnout become poorly motivated, let their job performance slide, and frequently call in "sick" because of dissatisfaction with their job. Though devoted to their patients and their profession, sonographers who are asked to do too much in too little time and without adequate equipment and backup eventually develop feelings of anger, hopelessness, and fatigue. If these symptoms are recognized and caught in time, something as simple as a change of hours, duties, or locations often solves the problem.

Having a positive attitude is an effective, short-term way of dealing with job stress. Rationalizing that the stressful conditions may be temporary and that speaking to the employer may bring about a desired change can actually lower stress levels. Other stress strategies include getting extra sleep; engaging in regular exercise (workouts are excellent *stress eaters*); talking to coworkers or friends about what is troubling; or indulging in a special treat such as a massage, movie, or favorite food. Avoidance is another effective coping strategy, as are the words *"no"* or *"later."*

Compassion fatigue

The newest term in the lexicon of serious potential stresses is **compassion fatigue**, which results in a lessening or loss of sympathy for the misfortune of others. This is caused by overwork and excessive emotional demands. Compassion fatigue is unique to those in the health care and caregiving professions. For years, the focus of compassion fatigue was reserved for policemen, firemen, and emergency medical technicians. However, studies have now shown that those who provide health and home care and overextend themselves by assuming too much responsibility for their charges are also at risk. Whenever sonographers feel trapped between their patients' needs and the demands of their department, the more intensely they feel about this conflict, the more vulnerable they are to developing compassion fatigue (Box 4-7). If the condition inexorably sets in, a self-protective, dangerous emotional detachment can develop.

Unlike burnout, rest or change of scene cannot alleviate compassion fatigue (Box 4-8). Overcoming compassion fatigue requires changing one's perspective on the needs one tries to meet and honestly inspecting the true motivation behind the wish or need to help and support others. As caregiving professionals, sonographers must learn to empathize without absorbing their patients' pain. Discussing their feelings with a trusted and objective colleague or professional is an important step toward destressing.

Awareness is the key to coping with any kind of stress. It allows identification of the stress and the chance to develop a change in attitude. It allows analysis of responses to stress and

BOX **4-7**   Symptoms of Compassion Fatigue

Conflicted feelings about loyalty to patients vs. departmental policies
Constantly thinking of work problems when away from the job
Emotional detachment
Unusual reactions to daily problems
Grief over loss of ideals
Physical or mental exhaustion, or both
Sleep problems
Cynicism
Anger
Frustration
Feelings of isolation and hopelessness

can sometimes lead to solutions that can change the stressful situation itself. Only when the situations cannot be changed should sonographers begin to weigh the pros and cons of staying at a job or moving on.

Victims of compassion fatigue can only recover when they realize that their primary need is to care for themselves, and they cannot be "cured" until they are willing to make serious life changes. The hard truth is that compassion fatigue is a one-way street from which the only hope for a "cure" is to back up.

BOX **4-8**   Strategies for Combating Compassion Fatigue

Establish and maintain good professional boundaries
Empathize, but be detached enough to be objective
Maintain healthy habits: rest, exercise, breaks, and diet
Give oneself permission to *do nothing* and to *relax*
Discuss compassion fatigue and air grievances at staff meetings
Learn to recognize the triggers of compassion fatigue
Know one's limits and do not overstep bounds

Summary

The concerted effort to raise awareness of sonographer injuries was launched in the year 2000 by pioneering sonographer Joan Baker. At that time, it was estimated that one of every five sonographers would suffer career-ending, work-related injuries.

Now, 5 years later, there are still sonographers unaware of the risks they take every workday by trying to adapt to ergonomically unsound environments and equipment. They are ignoring early warning symptoms of muscle and joint tenderness or pain, and they are adopting exaggerated scanning postures without realizing that they will only exacerbate the problem. Within a few years, they will be destined to join the ranks of sonography's walking wounded unless they can be made aware of the dangers.

As with any potential danger, the best cure is prevention. So while we, the sonography community, try to educate ourselves, our employers, and equipment manufacturers, we must not forget how imperative it is that the students of today and the future be taught not only how to scan, but how to scan safely. This topic, and the growing volume of information about it, must be added to every DMS educational curriculum.

The same amount of attention and concern must be focused on the dangers of stress in the sonography workplace. No studies have been done on this subject yet, but everyone knows someone who is afflicted or who has had to leave the field because of stress-related emotional injuries. Clearly, stress is just as important in terms of preserving a sonographer's future in the field. However, it is a problem whose subtle symptoms are seldom recognized.

As sonography professionals, we have an obligation not only to keep ourselves physically and emotionally healthy but also to be alert and recognize workplace problems of all kinds. We must become actively involved in improving our chances for a long, rewarding, and safe career.

BIBLIOGRAPHY

Craig M: Occupational hazards of sonographers, *J Diagn Med Sonogr* 3:47-50, 1990.

Craig M: Sonography: an occupational health hazard? *J Diagn Med Sonogr* 1:121-126, 1985.

Gentry E, Baranowsly AB, Dunning K: *Accelerated recovery program (ARP) for compassion fatigue. Traumatology Institute (Canada). A division of Psych Ink Resources website.* Available at: *http://psychink.com/inpbcfat.htm.*

Occupational Safety and Health Administration regulatory text: *What you need to know about musculoskeletal disorders (MSDs).* Available at: *http:// www.osha-sic.gov/SLIC/ergonomics/index.html.*

Society of Diagnostic Medical Sonography: *Industry standards for the prevention of work-related musculoskeletal disorders in sonography.* Consensus Conference on Work-Related Musculoskeletal Disorders in Sonography. Plano, Texas, 2003, SDMS.

Society of Diagnostic Medical Sonography: *SDMS work zone: musculoskeletal injury (MSI).* Available at: *http://www.sdms.org/msi.*

Sound Ergonomics LLC website. Available at: *http://www.soundergonomics.com.*

Chapter 5

Patient-Sonographer Interaction: Basic Medical Techniques and Patient Care

Learning Objectives

Students who successfully complete this chapter will be able to do the following:

- Understand the obligations of the sonographer to patients, institution, and self.
- Discuss the patient care partnership.
- Describe patient reactions to illness.
- Understand how to measure vital signs.
- Discuss the care of patients with tubes or tubing.
- Discuss the safety considerations associated with patient care.
- List the components of good body mechanics.
- Describe the correct patient-transfer methods.
- Identify good health and hygiene practices.
- Discuss the sonographer's role in infection control.
- Identify the signs of cardiac arrest and airway obstruction.
- Define the ABCs of basic life support techniques.
- Discuss the impact of cultural beliefs on diagnosis and treatment.

Key Terms

automated external defibrillators (AEDs)

barrier devices

cardiac arrest

cardiopulmonary resuscitation

continuous chest compression CPR (CCC-CPR)

diastolic reading

Health Insurance Portability and Accountability Act (HIPAA)

(Continued)

Key Terms—cont'd

Heimlich maneuver

methicillin-resistant *Staphylococcus aureus* (MRSA)

nasogastric tube

National Patient Safety Goals (NPSGs)

purified protein derivative (PPD)

respiratory arrest

systolic readings

vancomycin-resistant *Enterococcus* (VRE)

Sonographers work under the direction of a physician-sonologist to obtain diagnostic images of the patients entrusted to their care. Sonography training teaches one how to operate ultrasound instruments and to decipher echo information returning from the patient's body. A sonographer should know how to provide basic care to patients. The current standard of care recommends using Standard/Universal Precautions in all direct patient contact activities (e.g., wearing gloves whenever in direct patient contact). However, for sonographers who find themselves in settings in which strict standard precautions are not practiced, it is important to wash hands before and after direct patient contact, whenever gloves are not worn or are unavailable.

SONOGRAPHER OBLIGATIONS

To fulfill the role of sonographer, one must be responsible to him or herself, to a department or institution, and to patients. From a physical standpoint the sonographer should be adequately rested and relaxed, practice good nutrition, and engage in exercise to promote his or her physical health. Maintaining good mental health also is important and requires recognizing his or her own needs, strengths, and limitations. A sonographer must recognize any anxiety or distress felt about any work-related situations that might interfere with job performance. Leaving personal or family problems at home is just as important as leaving work problems at work. A sonographer who is unable to resolve problems in either area should seek proper counseling. Because caring for patients can be emotionally draining, a sonographer should have a means of rejuvenating through physical exercise and enjoyable hobbies.

Developing a good self-image and viewing problems as challenges or opportunities, rather than stumbling blocks, makes it easier to accept criticism as a learning opportunity and not as a defeat. The sonographer will then have a sense of pride in his or her work and an eagerness to start each day.

PATIENT RIGHTS

In addition to having the necessary knowledge and skills to perform competent sonographic examinations, a sonographer is responsible for the type of care given to patients.

In 1973 the American Hospital Association (AHA) first adopted a Patient's Bill of Rights. Patient rights were developed with the expectation that hospitals and health care institutions would support these rights in the interest of delivering effective patient care. The AHA encouraged institutions to translate or simplify the bill of rights to meet the needs of their specific patient populations and to make patient rights and responsibilities understandable to patients and their families.

In 2004 the AHA replaced the Patient's Bill of Rights with a plain language brochure, *The Patient Care Partnership: Understanding Expectations, Rights and Responsibilities*. This brochure informs patients about what to expect during their hospital stay with regard to their rights and responsibilities.

The basic message is that patients have a right to expect the following:
- High-quality hospital care
- A clean and safe environment
- Involvement in their care
- Protection of their privacy
- Help when leaving the hospital
- Help with their billing claims

Health care providers know that all patients deserve to be treated with respect, dignity, and kindness. Sonographers must remember that patients' needs come first and learn to control any anger or frustration that might develop when working with patients. Sonographers are expected to discuss matters pertinent to patients only with authorized hospital personnel.

Sonographers should understand that patients have the right to information concerning their health care and to decision-making regarding their diagnosis and treatment. In some instances, patients may refuse care or tests, which makes it important that sonographers try tactfully to reason with them by explaining the nature of the examination as it relates to their problem or illness. If a patient continues to refuse an examination, he or she should be encouraged to contact the physician for a fuller explanation. Sonographers should provide reassurance that they will gladly reschedule the examination at a mutually convenient time if the patient decides to undergo the procedure.

In April 2001 the Department of Health and Human Services enacted the **Health Insurance Portability and Accountability Act (HIPAA)**. The HIPAA Privacy Rule became effective April 14, 2003. This ruling marked the first comprehensive federal protection for the privacy of health information. Pursuant to this act, all segments of the health care industry (including sonography) are charged with promoting enhanced patient privacy in the health care system. The HIPAA Security Rule, which required full compliance by April 21, 2005, is a federal law, and anyone not in compliance can face up to $250,000 in fines and jail time of up to 10 years.

The Privacy Rule was created as a national standard to protect individuals' medical records and other personal health information by doing the following:
- Giving patients more control over their health information
- Setting boundaries on the use and release of their health records
- Establishing appropriate safeguards that health care providers must achieve to protect the privacy of health information
- Holding violators accountable, with civil and criminal penalties that can be imposed for violation of patients' privacy rights
- Striking a balance when public responsibility requires disclosure of some forms of data (e.g., to protect public health)
- Enabling patients to find out how their information may be used and what disclosure of their information was made

- Limiting the release of information to the minimum reasonably needed for the purpose of the disclosure
- Giving patients the right to examine and obtain a copy of their own health records and to request corrections

A sonographer must understand the privacy procedures of his or her practice or hospital and provide patients information and answers to questions about how their information can be used. A sonographer is also tasked with securing patient records containing individually identifiable health information so that they are not readily available to those who do not need them. Any communications necessary for quick, effective, high-quality health care are considered *allowable communications.* These include communicating verbally with pertinent physicians and family members and using patient names to locate them in waiting areas.

In compliance with the HIPAA, sonographers must be careful to do the following:
- Put patient information away after hours
- Take files out of sight of any lingering staff and custodians
- Set screensavers on computers for the shortest time possible
- Take care that any conversations (including phone conversations) are not overheard by other patients
- Remove patient identification from any scans that will be used for publication or presentation
- Keep any patient charts filed with the names facing the wall to ensure that passersby or visitors to the ultrasound laboratory cannot see the names or any information on the charts.

Patients may request that students, other observers, medical personnel, and families leave the room during the sonography examination. If any patients elect to have friends or family members present during their examination, the sonographer should inform them of the hospital rules and any policies that govern such requests. Some sonographers say they feel uncomfortable having "outsiders" looking on while they are scanning, even though there may be no regulations prohibiting their presence. If this situation arises, a sonographer must give a truthful explanation to the patient if there is inadequate space for viewing or if the presence of observers hinders the sonographer's concentration and abilities. Often such situations can be eased if sonographers explain that they need time alone with the patient to prepare for the examination and to take a series of scans for evaluation purposes. In return for such cooperation, a sonographer could offer to call the observers into the examination room for their own "viewing." By following these suggestions, the discovery of unexpected pathologic findings can be controlled without causing anxiety to patients or their support group.

Another patient right involves the expectation of pleasant physical and emotional surroundings where the person's comfort, safety, and respect as an individual are ensured.

PATIENT ENVIRONMENT

One of the most important considerations in the design of an ultrasound facility should be the patient and the sonographer's physical surroundings. For safety and comfort the following features should be considered:
- Proper ventilation and comfortable temperature
- Adequate lighting

- Comfortable and safe furnishings
- Equipment in good working order
- Reasonable access to bathroom facilities
- A safe and private area for disrobing and storing personal articles

Usually it is the sonographer's duty to keep the examining room and equipment neat and clean. Any nondisposable medical equipment used by the patient should be properly cleansed immediately after an examination and returned to its proper place. The sonographer should contact housekeeping personnel for immediate services in case of accidental spills.

Emotional surroundings

An ultrasound facility should offer a climate in which the patient is treated as an individual. Staff members should introduce themselves to patients and explain what they will be doing for them. Patients should be oriented to any procedures such as filling out admission or consent forms. Patient privacy should be respected at all times, particularly during dressing and undressing, during performance of ultrasound scans, and during use of bathroom facilities. If patients require assistance at any of these times, the sonographer should provide it in a mature and completely professional manner.

A sonographer should allow patients to freely express their thoughts, opinions, or beliefs. He or she should be a good listener and not impose beliefs on the patient. In the event that the examination performed reveals serious illness or the threat of imminent death, patients may want to engage in spiritual practices or rituals. They should be shown respect for their wishes and provided assistance or privacy as indicated.

PATIENT CARE

Patient reactions to illness

Becoming a sonographer places one in a position to see the changes that disease and disability cause in people. A sonographer should understand that change is a series of gains and losses and that disease and disability interrupt the natural balance of the body and thus produce stress. Such stress can cause emotional reactions in patients. The following are among the important emotional reactions a sonographer may encounter.

ANGER
Anger toward others may be expressed verbally or physically.

ANXIETY
Feelings of apprehension may cause patients to be unwilling to adjust to their new situation and cry; fear being alone; or act suspicious, hostile, or withdrawn. Anxiety also can produce physical changes such as rapid pulse, increased blood pressure and respiration, headaches, nervousness, excessive perspiration, or rapid speech.

FRUSTRATION AND HELPLESSNESS
The longer it takes to diagnose and treat the illness, the more frustrated the patient can become. In American society, men are especially vulnerable to feelings of loss of control and independence because strength may be seen as a major asset in their self-image.

GRIEF

Grieving is the process of adjusting to the reality of a loss. Whether it is a loss of health or the loss of a pregnancy, patients are flooded with emotions. Shock, denial, anger, bargaining, guilt, and depression are common feelings that grieving patients must work through before they are able to accept their losses.

GUILT

Patients who feel that they are unable to perform their accustomed roles in life (such as mother or breadwinner) usually respond with anger (why me?) or view their loss as a punishment. Particularly in the area of loss resulting from pregnancy interruption, a woman tends to critically examine every aspect of her life to discover where she was at fault. The response to guilt can take many forms: withdrawal, blame, fault finding, or physical complaints.

DEPRESSION

Feelings of helplessness, sadness, or lack of vitality are characteristic of the depressed person. Severely depressed patients often complain of insomnia, early morning fatigue, loss of appetite, and numerous physical complaints.

DEPENDENCY

Some patients are highly demanding, whereas others show their dependency by an inability to follow directions or by attempting tasks beyond their capabilities.

SUSPICION

Feelings of mistrust may overcome some patients, making them fearful and feeling that everyone and everything is against them. Often, the one-on-one environment of the sonography laboratory encourages patients to talk about their feelings. Although a sonographer is not responsible for evaluating and treating patients' emotional reactions, he or she should share observations and concerns with the referring physician or charge nurse. By all means, a sonographer should try to be a good listener.

If a patient responds negatively to being scanned and becomes upset, sonographers should not get upset as well. Instead, they should try to be patient, understanding, and secure enough to let patients know they care.

Vital signs

The term *vital signs* refers to temperature, pulse, respiration, and blood pressure as indicators of the functioning of the body. During the course of a sonographic examination, sonographers may be required to assess the pulse, respiration, and blood pressure as part of the scanning protocol. Careful, accurate measurement of each of these parameters is essential.

As a part of the assessment of vital signs, the sonographer should observe the patient's total condition: color, skin temperature, and any comments about how the patient feels and reacts. If a sonographer has never worked with patients before, the following review will establish guidelines for taking vital signs.

Pulse

The pulse is the beat of the heart that can be felt as a vibration within the walls of the arteries. With each heartbeat, blood forced into the arteries causes them to swell or expand, producing arterial pulses that can be felt with the fingers.

BOX **5-1**   Average Heart Rates for Different Age Groups

AGE GROUP	BEATS PER MINUTE
Adult	60-100
Child	100-120
Newborn	140
Fetus	120-160

The most convenient site for taking the pulse is the radial artery, located on the thumb side of the wrist. However, other arteries close to the skin also provide pulse sites (e.g., temporal, carotid, mandibular, femoral, popliteal).

Pulse rate refers to the number of beats per minute, whereas rhythm refers to the time interval between beats. The sonographer should evaluate whether there is a smooth and regular rhythm as opposed to irregular rhythms with skipped beats. The strength of a pulse refers to its force and usually is described as bounding or weak and thready.

Substances such as coffee, tea, tobacco, or certain drugs can cause rhythm irregularities. Shock and hemorrhage can cause a weak, thready pulse, whereas fever can produce a bounding pulse.

The normal adult pulse rate is 60 to 65 beats per minute (bpm). Newborn infants have a pulse rate of 120 to 140 bpm, and women, children, and elderly patients usually have a slightly faster than normal pulse rate (Box 5-1). Athletes in good condition generally have a slower pulse—below 60 bpm.

Any variation of the normal rhythm of the heart is termed *arrhythmia* and includes premature beats or palpitations. Such irregularities may simply be a normal physical response or a sign of disease. Abnormally rapid pulse rates (>100 bpm) are termed *tachycardia.* Abnormally slow pulse rates (<60 bpm) are termed *bradycardia.* Exercise, strong emotions, fever, pain, and shock can all elevate the pulse. In contrast, resting, depression, and certain drugs (such as digitalis) can lower the pulse.

The pulse is felt by gently compressing the artery over a bony prominence in the area. One should never feel the pulse with his or her own thumb because it has a pulse of its own that interferes with obtaining an accurate reading of the patient's pulse.

An arterial pulse should be obtained as follows:
• The person taking the pulse should explain to the patient what he or she plans to do.
• The patient's arm should be in a comfortable, resting position.
• One should identify the location of the artery by placing his or her fingertips over the artery and pressing firmly enough to feel the pulsation (Fig. 5-1).
• The beats of the pulse (starting the count with zero) should be counted for at least 30 seconds. This number should be multiplied by 2 to obtain the beats per minute.
• If irregularities are noted (too fast/too slow), one should count the beats for a full minute and report the findings.

Respiration

The oxygen and carbon dioxide exchange that occurs in the lungs is referred to as *respiration.* The respiratory process begins with the delivery of oxygen to body cells via blood that has passed through the lungs. The cells give off accumulated carbon dioxide to the blood, which

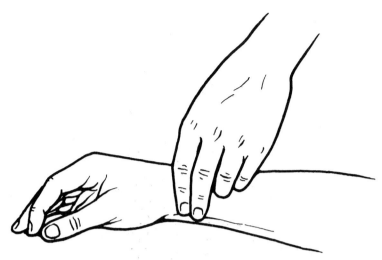

FIGURE **5-1** Taking a radial pulse. One should support the patient's arm in a comfortable position and never use the thumb to feel the patient's pulse.

returns it to the lungs. There, the potentially dangerous carbon dioxide wastes are exhaled out of the body in the act of breathing.

Breathing can be defined as the expansion (inspiration) and contraction (expiration) of the lungs. Normal breathing is quiet, effortless, and regular in rhythm; it occurs at a rate of 16 to 20 breaths per minute in the normal adult.

Rate, rhythm, and the depth and character of the respiration should be noted. The rate refers to the number of respirations per minute. Rhythm refers to the regular rate of breathing and a symmetric movement of the chest. Depth refers to the amount of air taken in with each respiration (normal, shallow, deep). Character refers to the quality of respiration (e.g., quiet, labored, wheezing, coughing).

Any injuries to the lungs, chest muscles, or diaphragm affect breathing. Noting any positions the patient may need to assume to breathe easily (e.g., sitting up or standing as opposed to lying down) is important. Any difficulty in breathing (dyspnea) or changes in the patient's color (cyanosis or pallor) should also be noted.

Respiration should be counted without the patient being aware of this task. The sonographer should watch the patient's breathing and count a breathing sequence (in and out) as one respiration. The count should be started at zero, and counting respirations should continue for at least 30 seconds. One should multiply the number by 2 to arrive at the respirations per minute. If irregularities are observed (rate, rhythm, patient appearance, or behavior), the respirations should be counted for 1 full minute and the findings should be reported.

Blood pressure

Blood pressure is the pressure that circulating blood exerts against arterial walls. It is produced by the pumping action of the heart. The pressure of blood within the arteries is highest whenever the heart contracts (called *systolic pressure*). Between beats, when the heart rests, arterial pressure is at its lowest (called *diastolic pressure*).

Heart activity can be heard as "thumping" sounds in the large arteries of the limbs. These sounds can be translated into numbers representing millimeters of mercury (mm Hg) on a manometer. When taking a blood pressure reading, the sonographer listens with a stethoscope and watches the numbers on a manometer.

The optimal adult blood pressure is less than 120/80 (120 indicating systolic pressure, 80 indicating diastolic pressure). Blood pressure changes occur because of the effects of aging on the heart and arteries.

- Normal ranges extend from 20 to 120 in young adults to systolic pressures of 130 to 140 in aging patients.
- Prehypertension is associated with pressures between 120 and 139 systolic and higher than 80 to 89 diastolic.
- Abnormally high blood pressure is termed *hypertension* (>140 systolic, and >90 diastolic). Even if only one reading, systolic or diastolic, is in the high range, it signifies high blood pressure. Abnormally low blood pressure is called *hypotension* (80/50).

Strong emotions, pain, exercise, and some disease conditions are factors that can increase blood pressure. Resting, depression, hemorrhage, and shock are factors that can lower blood pressure. Blood pressure readings also can vary from minute to minute and day to day because of changes in a patient's physical, mental, or emotional activity.

The volume of blood in the body and any resistance to the flow of blood through blood vessels also affect blood pressure. For example, hemorrhaging decreases blood volume, causing the blood pressure to fall. In contrast, fatty deposits develop within the blood vessels of patients with arteriosclerosis, causing resistance to blood flow and producing higher blood pressure readings.

The site for taking blood pressure is usually over a large artery in the arm or leg. The brachial artery of the upper arm is often selected, but arteries of the lower arm, thigh, and calf may also be used, depending on the accessibility of the limb and the patient's condition.

When the arm is used, the patient should either sit or lie down on his or her back, with the arm and blood pressure cuff at the level of the heart.

Wide varieties of blood pressure monitors are available: mercury/aneroid, digital, and multipurpose vital sign monitors. The most familiar of these is the sphygmomanometer (either mercury or aneroid), a cuff, and a stethoscope (Fig. 5-2).

Mercury manometers, which provide the most accurate measurements, show increments of 10 points, from 0 to 300. Aneroid manometers show units of 20, ranging from 20 to 300. Raising the silver column of mercury or the aneroid needle to 200 begins the procedure. A properly calibrated manometer will show the needle and mercury column at the zero mark on the mercury manometer (20 on the aneroid manometer) when not in use.

The cuff contains an inflatable rubber bladder that should be centered over the brachial artery, 1 inch above the elbow (Fig. 5-3). Cuffs should be wrapped snugly but not tightly. If the cuff is too loose, both systolic and diastolic readings will be heard higher than their actual values.

A stethoscope with a flat diaphragm is best for taking blood pressure. After using one's fingers to locate the brachial artery in the shallow depression where the elbow bends, one should place the diaphragm of the stethoscope over the artery without touching the cuff or the patient's clothing. Gentle application should be used because too much pressure can cause abnormally low diastolic sounds.

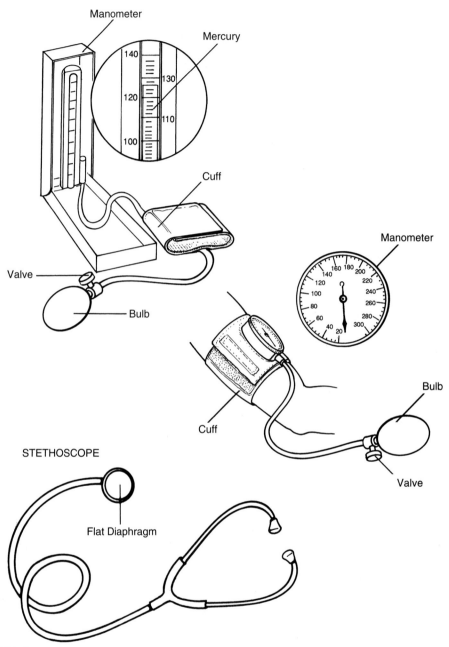

FIGURE **5-2** Instruments used for measuring blood pressure. Illustrated are the mercury and aneroid types of manometer and accessory equipment (stethoscope and cuff) required to accurately measure blood pressure.

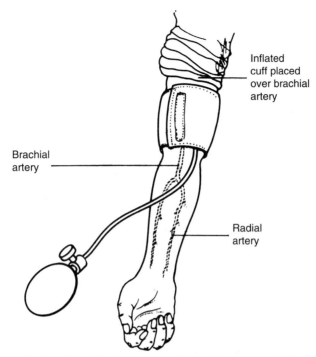

Inflated
cuff placed
over brachial
artery

Brachial
artery

Radial
artery

FIGURE **5-3** Correct positioning of the blood pressure cuff. Blood pressure cuff should be snugly wrapped approximately 1 inch above the bend of the arm. Stethoscope should be placed over brachial artery at bend of arm.

MEASURING BLOOD PRESSURE

The procedure for measuring blood pressure follows:

- The sonographer should explain the procedure to the patient in a private and noise-free environment.
- The patient should be resting for 5 minutes before the blood pressure is taken. If the patient has been actively exercising, the reading should be taken after 15 to 30 minutes.
- The sonographer should select and use the same site consistently because of variations in blood pressures if taken in different locations. Blood pressures also should be taken with the patient in the same position each time. A lying, sitting, or standing blood pressure can vary within the same individual.
- The patient's clothing should be removed, as necessary, to expose the site. The patient's arm should be positioned on a supporting structure (table or bed) at heart level while the blood pressure is being taken.
- The sonographer should ensure there are no leaks in the tubes, cuff, or valve and remember that using too small a cuff can result in pressure readings higher than normal.
- The sonographer should sit to take the blood pressure so that he or she can read the manometer at eye level. The manometer should read 0 before beginning.
- Air should be let out of the cuff, and the cuff should be applied just far enough above the patient's elbow to leave the space over the brachial artery free. The cuff should be wrapped firmly around the patient's arm and fastened securely on the last turn.
- The sonographer should locate the pulse in the artery and place the stethoscope directly over the point of strongest pulsation.

- Holding the rubber bulb in the palm of one hand, the sonographer should close the valve on the rubber bulb with a thumb and finger and rapidly inflate the cuff by pumping the bulb.
- The cuff should be inflated to about 20 to 30 mm Hg above the expected systolic reading. As the cuff pressure increases, it will shut off the flow of blood within the artery. Inflation of the cuff should take 7 seconds or less.
- The valve should be carefully loosened and the cuff should be deflated slowly and steadily. The sonographer should listen carefully for sounds of the first heartbeat (systolic pressure) and watch the mercury column or aneroid needle gauge for the points at which the sounds are first heard.
- About 2 to 3 mm Hg per heartbeat should be deflated until all sounds stop or there is a distinct change in the sound (diastolic pressure).

> *NOTE:* If the cuff is deflated too slowly, false elevated readings will result. If the cuff is deflated too quickly (5 to 10 mm Hg/heartbeat), false low readings will be obtained.

- When all sounds stop, the cuff should be deflated rapidly and completely to 0.
- The sonographer should not reinflate the cuff during the reading. If a reading must be repeated, all the air must be let out of the cuff and 15 seconds should lapse before inflating the cuff again.

INTERPRETING ARTERIAL SOUNDS

Arterial sounds are interpreted as follows:

- **Systolic readings** are the first sounds heard, as the cuff is deflated (blood resuming flow as the heart pumps).
- The last sound heard as the air is let out is the **diastolic reading** (blood flowing freely through the artery when the heart is resting).
- If one has difficulty hearing the diastolic sounds, the cuff should be completely deflated. After 15 seconds, the patient should raise his or her arm to drain the blood from the blood vessels of the lower arm. When the patient lowers the arm, the blood pressure can be retaken.

> *NOTE:* There may be distinct changes in the sounds heard between the systolic and diastolic sounds. Sounds may become muffled before stopping or may remain muffled down to 0. In this case, the diastolic should be recorded at the point when the change from clear to muffled is heard, as well as when the sound ends completely (e.g., 120/76/62). The reading should be written down promptly.

- The procedure should be repeated if one has any doubt about the reading. If the reading is elevated, it should be rechecked after 5 minutes. Briefly, the sonographer should explain the reason for a second reading to avoid alarming the patient and affecting the blood pressure.

Digital manometers were developed for professional use in hospitals, clinics, and doctors' offices. They provide automatic cuff inflation and take up to three pressure readings before averaging the total for the most accurate measurement. Wrist cuff monitors also are available. Their small size makes them ideal for portable work and for home monitoring practices.

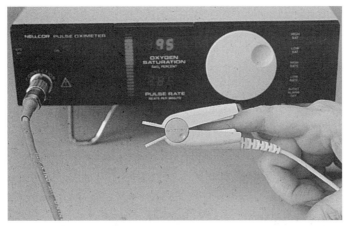

FIGURE **5-4** Pulse oximeters are used to detect oxygen problems before clinically noticeable in various settings (especially in surgery and intensive care). The pulse oximeter sensor is attached to the patient's skin (to the finger, nose, or earlobe) to measure the oxygen saturation level in the blood. Oxygen saturation should always be greater than 90%.

Continuous vital signs monitors also are widely used in hospital settings. They are designed to spot check or continuously monitor several critical parameters such as heart (pulse) rate, pulse oximetry, blood pressure, and temperature.

Pulse oximeters are used in various situations, especially in surgery and the intensive care unit (ICU). Pulse oximetry measures the oxygen concentration in arterial blood (Fig. 5-4). The normal range is 95% to 100%. Measurements are used to prevent hypoxia and to evaluate the effectiveness of treatment. A sensor is attached to the patient's finger, toe, earlobe, nose, or forehead. The sensor light beams pass through the tissues, and a detector on the other side measures the amount passing through the tissues. The oximeter then measures the oxygen concentration from this information. That value, and the patient's pulse rate, are displayed on the monitor. Oximeter alarms will sound if the oxygen concentration is low or if the pulse rate is too fast or too slow. Easily attached to IV poles or on rolling stands, these monitors may accompany in-patients who must be transported to the ultrasound laboratory.

Patients with tubes or tubing

IV infusion tubing, nasogastric suction, urinary catheters, and nasal catheters and cannulas for oxygen administration are the most common types of tubing a sonographer will encounter when working with hospital patients. Although he or she may not be responsible for starting any of the procedures associated with such equipment, knowing how to handle and care for patients who have such tubes in place is important.

Intravenous equipment

IV tubing connected to a plastic bag or bottle is used to infuse fluids into the patient's body. A needle or plastic catheter attached to the container is inserted into a vein. The flow of fluid is measured by a drip meter, and a clamp on the tubing is used to regulate the flow of the prescribed fluid (Fig. 5-5).

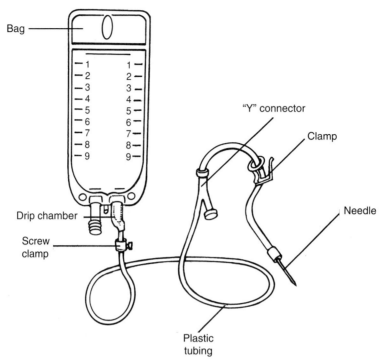

FIGURE **5-5** IV equipment. Plastic tubing leads from a solution-filled bag at one end and connects to a needle at the other end. Clamping the tubing controls the rate of flow.

Some institutions may use computerized infusion pumps to regulate drip rate. This device delivers a measured amount of fluid over a period of time. If problems occur, such as drops falling at an improper rate, bag emptying, infiltration within the patient's tissues occurs, or patient's arm position obstructs flow, an alarm sounds.

Unless specifically authorized, a sonographer should not change or regulate the amount of flow of a solution, although he or she may have to move some patients to and from the scanning table or bed or remove their clothing. The following guidelines should help in working with such patients.

- If the needle has been inserted in the patient's hand or arm, the sonographer should help the patient keep the involved arm straight.
- The bottle or bag should never be lowered below the level of the needle insertion when transferring or positioning the patient.
- The sonographer should watch for and immediately report any of the following:
  - The occurrence of nausea, vomiting, rapid breathing, or an increase in pulse rate—signs of circulatory overload that must be dealt with immediately
  - If no solution is passing from the bottle into the tubing even though solution is still in the bottle
  - When the plastic drip chamber is completely filled with solution
  - When blood appears in the tubing at the needle end
  - When all of the solution has run out of the bottle or bag or when it is almost empty

- Whenever the needle has deliberately or accidentally been removed
- Whenever the patient complains of pain or tenderness at the needle insertion site
- Any time a raised or inflamed area on the patient's skin or near the needle insertion is noticed, which may mean that the solution has infiltrated and is running into the adjacent tissues (the sonographer may be asked to close the clamp to shut off the flow of solution)
- Whenever the tubing becomes disconnected and the patient is bleeding freely from the connection site

Nasogastric tubes

Hospital patients commonly have a tube inserted into one nostril. Depending on the length of the tube, it may terminate in the patient's stomach or intestine. Such tubes can be used for feeding, to obtain specimens, to treat intestinal obstructions, to prevent or treat distention after surgery, or to drain fluids from the patient's stomach by suction (Fig. 5-6).

When a **nasogastric tube (NG tube)** is being used to drain substances out of the stomach or to collect a specimen, the patient is given nothing by mouth (NPO) because food would only be drawn back out through the tube. In caring for patients with NG tubes, it is important to never pull on the tube when moving these patients or changing their positions. If the patient begins to gag or vomit while the tube is in place, the sonographer should report it immediately.

Fluids can be removed from the patient's body through the tubes by gravity or suction. The outer end of the tube may have a clamp attached, or a plastic connection may link it to longer tubing attached to an electrical suction machine. Suction (by use of either a syringe

FIGURE **5-6** A nasogastric (NG) tube is inserted through one nostril and down through the esophagus until it reaches the stomach. A syringe or mechanical pump can be used to suction the stomach contents.

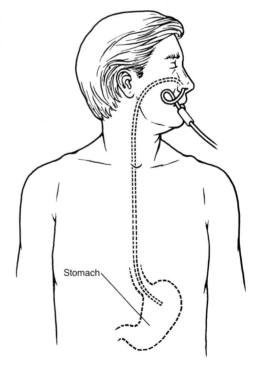

Stomach

or a machine) is often used to remove thick secretions that cannot be drawn out easily by gravity.

Rules for working with patients connected to mechanical suction machines follow:
- Any leakage in the tube or suction system should be reported.
- The drainage bottle should never be raised or opened.
- The tubing should never be disconnected.
- Any rapid increase in the amount of material being suctioned should be reported immediately.

Oxygen therapy

Oxygen may be administered to any patient experiencing respiratory difficulty (oxygen deficiency). The goal of such therapy is to lessen a low-oxygen concentration in the blood and to decrease the workload of the respiratory system.

The use of oxygen is associated with some hazards; oxygen should be considered a drug, and its dosage or concentration should be evaluated and ordered by a physician.

Although oxygen by itself cannot burn, contact with any combustible material (even a spark) causes it to ignite and burn or, in high concentrations, explode.

Delivery systems for oxygen therapy include in-room piping systems and oxygen tanks, or cylinders. If a laboratory is equipped with an in-room piping system, oxygen and suction usually are provided through wall outlets. Outlet connectors, which vary in shape, color, and connection methods used, are keyed to a specific gas or function (Fig. 5-7).

Oxygen may also be contained in large tanks or small cylinders. Large cylinders are usually used for patients requiring high flow rates or oxygen use over extended periods.

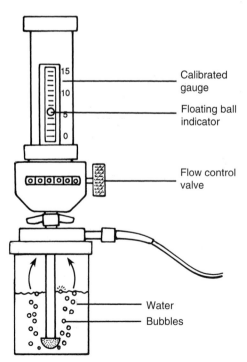

FIGURE **5-7** Wall-mounted oxygen flowmeters. Schematic drawing of a typical wall-mounted oxygen flowmeter. Water levels must be kept high enough to bubble as oxygen flows through the flowmeter.

Calibrated gauge

Floating ball indicator

Flow control valve

Water

Bubbles

These can be identified by size and the presence of a metal cap screwed onto the top of the cylinder to protect the valve from damage. Their size and a rectangular valve (without a handle), which has three holes on one side, can identify small cylinders.

These small cylinders are used during patient transportation or for short duration needs. Some ambulatory patients need continuous oxygen and may use over-the-shoulder slings or rolling stands to hold the tank when ambulating.

Because the gas contained within a cylinder is under extremely high pressure, the sonographer should *never* do the following when gas cylinders are in use:
- Transport a high-pressure cylinder unless it is secure in a cylinder cart
- Allow a cylinder to stand free; it must be secured to avoid falling and causing an accident
- Transport patients on a stretcher with a cylinder lying next to them
- Place a cylinder near a source of heat such as a radiator because it may cause an explosion

The delivery of oxygen to the patient may involve the use of either high- or low-flow devices. Among the low-flow devices are the nasal cannula or nasal prongs, nasal catheter, or simple oxygen masks.

The nasal cannula is used when a patient needs extra oxygen rather than a total supply of oxygen (Fig. 5-8, *A*). The prongs are inserted into the patient's nostrils and held in place by an elastic band around the patient's head. They are connected to the oxygen source by a length of plastic tubing.

A nasal catheter is a piece of tubing that is longer than a cannula. It is inserted through the nostril into the back of the patient's mouth. This method provides more effective oxygen delivery and is used when the patient must have additional oxygen at all times. The nasal catheter is fastened to the patient's forehead or cheek by a piece of adhesive tape to hold it steady.

Several different types of oxygen masks may be used. Among the most common types of masks are the following:
- *Simple mask.* A transparent mask with a simple nipple adapter that is fitted over the nose, mouth, and chin (Fig. 5-8, *B*).
- *Partial rebreathing or reservoir mask.* A low-flow device identified by the presence of a bag, which must remain constantly inflated by one third (Fig. 5-8, *C*).
- *Venturi mask.* A high-flow mask that provides the most reliable and consistent oxygen enrichment. The Venturi mask is identified by the presence of a hard plastic adapter with large "windows" on either side.

All oxygen masks, except the Venturi mask, require humidification, which is generally achieved by means of a humidifier (usually disposable) filled with water. The humidifier is connected to a threaded outlet at the bottom of the flowmeter or regulator. A small universal connector extends from the front or top of the humidifier for connection to the oxygen device.

The following precautions should be observed in working with patients receiving oxygen therapy.
- All fire regulations in effect at the institution should be observed.
- The flowmeter should be checked to ensure oxygen is being delivered to the patient. The water level in the humidifying chamber should be high enough so that it bubbles as the oxygen goes through it.
- The tubing connected to the oxygen source should be taped to the patient to help keep it from accidentally being pulled when moving the patient.
- The patient should not lie on the tubing and the tubing should not be kinked, which can slow or stop the oxygen flow.

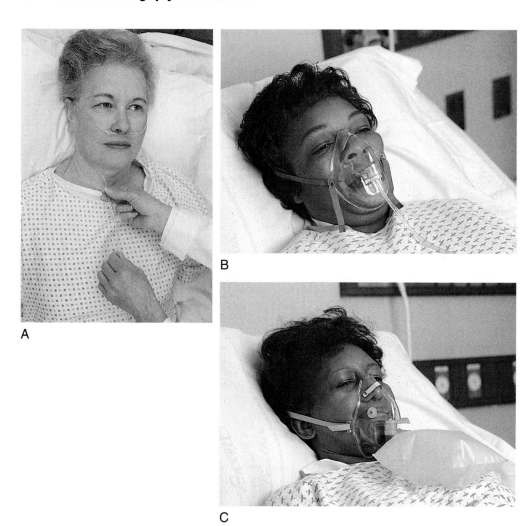

FIGURE **5-8** **A,** Nasal cannula. The two prongs of the cannula should be inserted a short distance into the patient's nostrils. An elastic headband behind the ears is used to keep the cannula in place. **B,** A simple oxygen face mask should cover the nose and mouth of the patient. Small holes in the sides of the mask allow oxygen to escape during exhalation and room air to enter during inhalation. **C,** Reservoir or partial rebreathing mask. This low-flow device is equipped with an inflatable bag.

- Inhalation therapy or respiratory therapy departments are responsible in most hospitals for the patient's treatment. They should be called to make any needed adjustments after checking with the patient's physician or nurse.

Catheters

The most common kind of catheter used for removing fluids from the body is the urinary catheter. The catheter (made of plastic tubing) is inserted through the patient's urethra and into the bladder (Fig. 5-9). Catheters may be used to obtain sterile specimens when patients are unable to urinate naturally or to determine how much residual urine remains in a patient's bladder after urination.

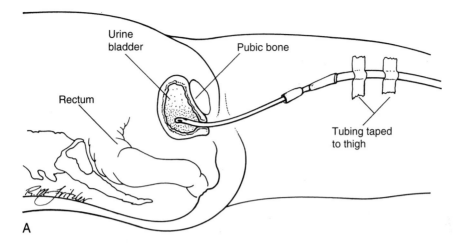

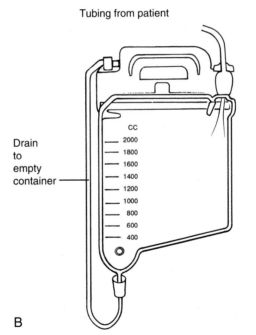

FIGURE **5-9** Catheterization equipment. **A,** A plastic/rubber urinary catheter is inserted through the urethra and into the bladder. **B,** Urine drains into a container.

A retention or indwelling catheter is a system used to provide temporary or permanent drainage of urine. A Foley catheter is commonly used. Foley catheters are specially designed as two tubes, one inside the other. The inner of the two tubes is connected at one end to a small balloon. After the catheter has been inserted, the balloon is filled with water or air so that the catheter will not pass out through the patient's urethra. Urine drains from the bladder through the outer tube and collects in a container attached to the patient's bed or table. Clamping or unclamping the tubing can control the flow of urine. Importantly, the catheter bag must always be positioned at a level lower than the patient's urinary bladder. Catheterization is a sterile technique, and the catheter drainage system should consist of a closed sterile system.

As with other patient tubing, the catheter should be taped to the patient (inner thigh in this case) at all times and should be checked periodically for kinking or to ensure that the patient is not lying on the tubing and obstructing the flow of urine out of the body.

Another use of the urinary catheter involves patients scheduled for obstetric or gynecologic sonography. Some of these patients are unable to fill the bladder naturally or maintain a full bladder for the duration of the examination. As a result, they must be catheterized to instill fluid into the bladder, with the tubing clamped off until the end of the sonography study. Bladder filling is not required for transvaginal examinations.

Because of the short length of the female urethra, the risk of urinary tract infection is increased with catheterization. For this reason, it is unwise to use catheterization as a routine method of filling the bladder of patients scheduled for pelvic sonography, unless there is a clinical indication to do so. Only trained and authorized personnel should perform any catheterization procedure.

Wound drains

After surgery, a patient may have a drain or wick placed within a wound to allow for drainage. Sonographers must anticipate and avoid the possibility of pulling or dislodging such drains during patient positioning or transfer.

Colostomies and ileostomies

Surgical treatment of patients with disorders of the intestinal tract may result in the construction of a colostomy (an opening into the colon) or an ileostomy (an opening into the ileum). In such patients, a loop of intestine is brought out of the body through a surgical incision on the abdominal wall; the opening allows drainage of feces. The colostomy or ileostomy opening (stoma) is covered by plastic disposable bags or pouches that are held in place by a double-faced adhesive or special glue. These appliances may require frequent changing because of the constant flow of liquid feces that is especially prevalent during the immediate postoperative period.

When performing abdominal sonography on such patients, it is wise to have a small supply of appliances on hand because it may be necessary to remove and later replace the devices to gain unobstructed access to the surface of the abdominal wall. These procedures should be followed:

- Clean rather than sterile technique is used whenever removing or changing these dressings or bags. However, wearing gloves is preferred.
- The old appliance should be gently removed and the area cleansed around the stoma. A folded gauze pad should be taped around the stoma to absorb any discharge and to protect the scanning surface during the examination.
- Contents of the old appliance should be flushed into a toilet. Then one should dispose of the old appliance in a plastic bag to prevent cross-contamination.
- Before applying a new bag, one should cleanse and dry the skin around the stoma so that the appliance can be securely fastened to prevent the escape of discharge or odors.
- If gloves are not worn, one should wash his or her hands and clean the patient area.
  Sterile technique is indicated if it is necessary to scan in the area of open wounds.

The use of gloves and sterile gel is then required. If it is necessary to scan over the open wound itself, this can be accomplished by applying sterile gel to the area and covering it with a protective thin plastic film. An additional layer of sterile gel is then applied to the top of the film to ensure an airless contact with the transducer and the scanning surface.

Dressings

Dressings are applied as covers to wounds to protect them from further injury or infection and to absorb drainage. During the course of a sonographic examination, the sonographer is required to remove and replace dressings. Because sterile dressing changes are usually the responsibility of the nursing staff, the sonographer should always check, before removing or replacing a dressing, to determine whether wound isolation precautions are in effect. If wound isolation precautions are not required, the following steps should be carried out:

- The sonographer should wear gloves or wash hands before working in the wound area or use sterile scanning media to prevent wound infection.
- Care should be exercised when removing a dressing to avoid dislodging a scab or causing the patient pain.
- Any adhesive tape used to secure new dressings should not be irritating to the patient's skin.
- Any unusual circumstances regarding the wound (e.g., bleeding, drainage, odor, or patient complaints of pain, burning, or itching) should be reported.
- Soiled dressings (and gloves) should be discarded properly, and the sonographer should wash his or her hands thoroughly after caring for the patient.

ASSISTING PATIENTS ON STRICT BED REST

Occasionally, patients on strict bed rest are brought to the ultrasound department for diagnostic testing. During their examination, it may be necessary to provide them with bedpans, urinals, or emesis basins.

Bedpans

Female patients use bedpans for voiding and bowel movements. Males use them only for bowel movements. Bedpans are usually made of plastic or stainless steel and should be part of the laboratory's or department's available equipment. Metal bedpans are often cold and should be warmed with water and dried before given to the patient. In many instances, the use of a fracture pan is a better option, as it is smaller, easier to position under the patient, and more comfortable for the patient.

When handling bedpans and their contents, medical aseptic, Standard/Universal Precautions, and Bloodborne Pathogen Standards should be followed. If the patient is of childbearing age and experiencing heavy vaginal bleeding, the contents should be inspected for the presence of any products of conception and reported. Any unusual color, amount, or condition of the wastes should also be reported to the charge nurse. The sonographer may be required to save the specimen for laboratory testing. If not, the contents should be disposed of properly, and the bedpan should be properly cleansed and disinfected before storing.

Urinals

Male patients use urinals for voiding. Usually constructed of plastic, urinals have a cap on the top and a hooklike handle. The patient should stand, if possible, to urinate. Otherwise, he can sit on the side of the scanning table/bed or lie down on the bed.

The same safety precautions used for handling bedpans also apply to handling urinals. After use, any unusual odor, color, or other observations of the urine should be reported to the charge nurse and the contents of the urinal disposed of properly. The urinal should be cleansed, disinfected, and returned to storage.

Emesis basins

Vomiting often accompanies illness or injury. If the patient feels nauseated, turn his or her head well to one side to prevent aspiration of vomit. Place an emesis (kidney-shaped) basin under the patient's chin. Provide the patient with water to cleanse his or her mouth. Observe the emesis for color, odor, and any undigested food. If the appearance resembles dark "coffee grounds," it is evidence of undigested blood and should be reported to the charge nurse. It may be necessary to save a specimen for laboratory study, so the sonographer should not discard the emesis until cleared to do so. The emesis should be removed by following the same safety principles described earlier.

SAFETY PROVISIONS

Patient safety

The Joint Commission on Accreditation of Healthcare Organizations (JCAHO) has developed a program to promote specific improvements in patient safety. **The National Patient Safety Goals (NPSGs)** highlight problem areas in health care and describe solutions to those problems. Accredited organizations are evaluated for continuous compliance with the requirements of the NPSGs. The goals address the safety-related areas of the following:
- Medication
- Infection control
- Surgery and anesthesia
- Transfusions
- Restraints and seclusion
- Staffing and staff competence
- Fire safety
- Medical equipment
- Emergency management
- Security

   Of particular interest to sonographers is the July 2004 requirement of compliance with practicing Universal Protocols by all accredited hospitals and office-based surgery facilities. Applicable to all operative and invasive procedures, the principal components of the Universal Protocols include the following:
- Preoperative verification process
- Marking of the operative site
- Taking a "*time out*" immediately *before* performing the procedure to reverify that it is the *right* site, *right* procedure, and *right* patient

   Complete information on this vital initiative is available at *http//www.JCAHO.org,* under the topics of NPSG, Universal Protocol, Infection Control, Sentinel Events, and Standards.

   Sonographers should anticipate the safety needs of their patients, themselves, their coworkers, and their laboratory environment. A quick response to an emergency can be ensured by posting fire and disaster plans, committing them to memory, and carrying out periodic reviews.

Special precautions are necessary for patients prone to medical emergencies or accidents. Knowing the location of the crash cart and other emergency equipment in the department is essential. Recognizing the fact that unconscious or sedated patients are not responsible for their own safety should prompt sonographers to use side rails, close supervision, and restraints if necessary. Double-checking patients' identity by matching their identification bracelets to their charts is another form of ensuring patient safety.

When performing sonography examinations on children, or when children accompany the patient to the sonography laboratory, the sonographer must consider their natural curiosity. Children's inclination to explore the environment by climbing, touching, and tasting without awareness of inherent dangers can threaten their safety.

Patients may be confused or disoriented because of medications, the effects of aging, or emotional disturbances. Such patients are not responsible for their own safety. To prepare them for any activity, they should be given any instructions clearly. Extra time should be allowed for them to adjust to any changes in position before being moved.

Elderly patients may suffer from poor vision or hearing and may be unable to recognize danger or warning signals. Because their reaction times are slower than those of younger patients, they may require additional assistance in almost every physical activity.

When working with patients in wheelchairs or on stretchers, the sonographer should make it a practice to lock the brakes or lift the foot rests, or both. Proper body mechanics should also be used when transferring patients to and from wheelchairs or stretchers.

Patient safety devices frequently are used to provide postural support or restraint when patients are weakened or disabled by illness, confused by the effects of medication, or prone to accidents and injuries. If a safety device must be removed during a sonography procedure, the sonographer should ask a coworker to help with the patient until the device is reapplied.

Treatment restraints require a doctor's order and are generally used to keep confused patients from disrupting or dislodging equipment such as intravenous or nasogastric tubes. Such restraints may take the form of mittens or soft ties around the limbs. Because the use of restraints may cause patients to feel agitated or confused by their limited ability to interact with their environment, sonographers or their delegates should stay with the patient until the person is ready to leave the sonography area.

In most institutions, restraints must be ordered by a physician or charge nurse and cannot be arbitrarily applied. Therefore it is important that both the sonographer and his or her patients understand that such devices are used for protection and never as a means of punishment.

SONOGRAPHER SAFETY IN THE PATIENT CARE ENVIRONMENT

Often sonographers become so focused on imaging and caring for their patients that they overlook the obvious need to provide safety for themselves. Some general considerations for sonographer safety follow:

- He or she should use good body mechanics and be sure to obtain adequate help for lifting or moving heavy objects or patients.
- The sonographer should be aware of the isolation policies of the institution to protect himself or herself from exposure to infection. The wearing of gloves and the use of other protective equipment are strongly urged whenever the sonographer is in direct patient contact.
- Electrical equipment must be properly grounded for its environment.
- The use of extension cords or ungrounded adapters with electrical equipment should be avoided.

- Periodic inspections of cords or wires should be carried out to check for fraying or defects.
- Electrical cords should not be allowed to contact wet or damp areas of the patient's anatomy (e.g., gel- or oil-coated abdomen).
- Only safety-inspected and approved devices should be used for warming scanning media such as oils or gels; extreme care is warranted if such items are "warmed" in a microwave oven.
- The sonographer should remove and properly dispose of any items likely to cause accidents (e.g., needles, razor blades).
- Oxygen or other gas containers should be secured to prevent them from falling; smoking in areas where oxygen is used should be prohibited.
- The sonographer should know where a fire alarm is located and how to report a fire to authorities.

Body mechanics

Body mechanics can be defined as the use of correct movements during the performance of any activity. Because back injuries are frequent complaints of sonographers, one must prevent self-injury while positioning, lifting, and transporting patients. Not only will good body mechanics protect the sonographer from injury, they also will reduce fatigue and allow the sonographer to use his or her body more efficiently and effectively. An added bonus is that the use of good body mechanics also protects patients from injury. Initially the sonographer may find that it requires a conscious effort to maintain proper body alignment, but as the concept is used on a daily basis, it should become second nature.

Suggestions on the use of good body mechanics when lifting heavy loads follow:
- The sonographer should maintain good posture, which is essential to developing good body mechanics.
- He or she should always evaluate a situation before acting/deciding what needs to be done and whether help is necessary.
- The sonographer should always explain to patients what he or she plans to do.
- Any objects or hazards should be removed before moving backward or during the transfer of patients.
- The sonographer should be sure his or her feet are a shoulder length apart to provide a strong base of support. Weight should be distributed evenly. The sonographer should stand with one foot slightly forward for balance and have the toes of the leading foot pointed in the direction of the activity (Fig. 5-10).
- The sonographer can prepare for the activity by keeping his or her back straight and being ready to bend at the hips and knees. The large muscles of the thigh should be used instead of the smaller muscles of the back for any lifting activities. Before the lift, the sonographer should tighten abdominal and pelvic muscles, tuck buttocks in, and keep the head and chest up.
- The sonographer should never bend sideways from the waist or hip for any activity. When turning, he or she should always pivot the feet and never twist.
- The sonographer should not attempt to lift a heavy load alone if he or she is unsure it can be done safely.
- The sonographer should always position him or herself as closely as possible to whatever is being lifted and never reach for a load.

FIGURE **5-10** Correct posture for lifting heavy loads. Feet should be placed one shoulder length apart, with weight evenly distributed, to provide a strong support base.

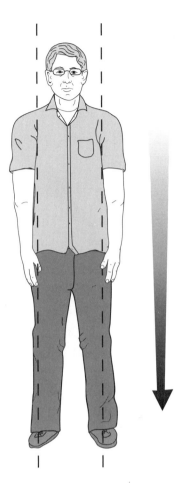

- He or she should lift smoothly and avoid jerky movements. If lifting with the help of another person, a signal such as lifting on the count of 3 should be prearranged.
- The sonographer should lower his or her body to the object being lifted by bending the knees, not the back (Fig. 5-11). Straighten the legs while lifting the object. If he or she must start a lift with a slightly curved back, the large muscles of the legs should take over. Whenever possible, the sonographer should push, pull, or roll an object instead of lifting it.

   Good body mechanics are equally important whenever moving, transferring, or ambulating patients. To prevent a patient fall when moving or transporting a weak patient, it is advisable to use a gait belt as a transfer aid. Gait belts are usually made of canvas, nylon, or leather. The belt is placed around the patient's waist, over clothing, with its buckle in front. The belt should be snug, with just enough room to get one's fingers under it. The sonographer's hand should be brought up from the bottom of the belt (palm away from the patient) to help grasp the belt firmly. Some belts provide a handle for the transport person to hold onto, which improves coupling during the lifting of the patient.

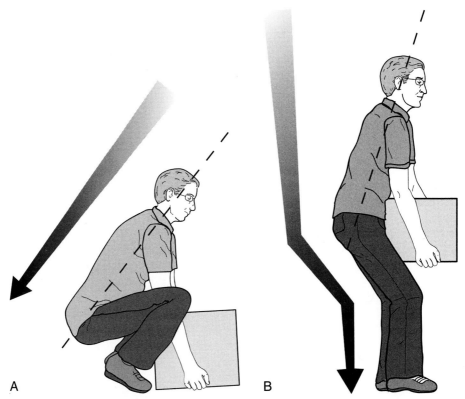

FIGURE **5-11** Proper body mechanics for lifting. **A,** The back should be kept straight, and the large muscles of the thigh should be used in lifting instead of the smaller muscles of the back. **B,** Before the lift, one should tighten abdominal and pelvic muscles, tuck buttocks in, and keep head and chest up.

The techniques that follow can prevent injury to the sonographer and patients whenever it is necessary to move them.

Moving the patient up in bed or on the scanning table

- The sonographer should be sure the table or bed is locked so that it will not slide. If possible, the bed should be adjusted to elbow height for the most comfortable position. Then the sonographer should relate what he or she plans to do and give instructions on how the patient can help.
- The sonographer should slide or pull, rather than lift, the patient whenever possible. If the patient is unable to cooperate or is heavy, a colleague should help. A lifting or turning sheet placed underneath a patient from shoulders to buttocks is helpful in such situations (Fig. 5-12).
- The sonographer should remove any pillows from the head of the table or bed and help the patient bend the knees, with instructions to press the feet firmly on the bed.
- The sonographer should stand with one foot slightly ahead of the other as he or she slides one arm under the patient's shoulders and the other under the thighs. The patient should be kept as close to the sonographer's body as possible.

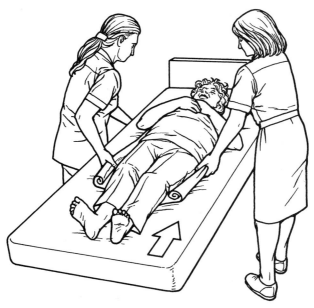

FIGURE **5-12** Using a lifting/turning sheet to move helpless patients. It is advisable to slide or pull, rather than to lift, helpless patients. With the help of a colleague, this technique affords the safest way to move patients who are heavy or unable to help themselves.

- On the count of 3, the sonographer should have the patient push with his or her feet as the sonographer shifts weight from the back leg to the forward leg. The sonographer should then slide the patient up on the table or bed.
- The sonographer should replace the pillows to make the patient comfortable and put up side rails if necessary.

Turning patients toward the sonographer

- The sonographer should have the table or bed at elbow height and stand as close to the bed as possible.
- Using a rocking motion of the legs, the sonographer should shift the weight from one foot to the other as he or she rolls the patient onto the side. Once again, a turning sheet will save time and energy.
- When the sonographer turns the patient toward him or her, the sonographer should check to see that the patient has ample space to turn. Then the patient should bend the knees slightly, placing the far leg over the one nearest the sonographer. The sonographer should ask the patient to fold his or her hands across the chest. The sonographer should place one of his or her hands on the patient's far shoulder and the other on the far hip, and pull the person toward him or her. For patients who are able to pull themselves up, the sonographer can raise the side rails for the patient to hold onto.
- The sonographer should maintain the patient's alignment by placing a pillow at the back to prevent the person from rolling over. Then the pillow should be placed under the patient's head for comfort.

Turning patients away from the sonographer

- The sonographer should raise the side rails on the side the patient will turn toward.
- He or she should stand at the side the patient is turning from (side rails down on this side). The patient should bend his or her knees slightly, placing one leg over the other so that the feet point away from the sonographer. The patient should fold his or her arms across the chest.
- The sonographer should slip one of his or her arms under the patient's back and far shoulder. The other arm should be placed as far as possible under the patient's hips. The sonographer should gently roll the patient onto his or her side as the sonographer draws an arm toward himself or herself, using a rocking motion of the body and shifting weight from the back leg to the forward leg, moving body weight in the same direction as the patient is moving. For patients who can turn themselves, the sonographer should raise the side rails, which patients can grab to pull themselves up.
- The sonographer should support the patient's alignment by placing a pillow at the back to prevent the person from rolling over. Then the pillow should be placed under the patient's head.

To transfer a semiambulatory or nonambulatory patient onto and off of scanning tables, beds, or stretchers, as well as in and out of wheelchairs, the following general safety considerations apply:

- The sonographer should explain the procedure and allow the patient to help as much as possible.
- The sonographer should ensure that the transfer vehicle is close to the patient and that its wheels are locked.
- The sonographer should use good body mechanics, with sufficient personnel to help perform the transfer safely.
- The sonographer should remember that ambulating a person who has been in bed for prolonged periods requires a gradual approach to upright activities.

Assisting patients to and from table or bed

- Once the patient is sitting upright, the sonographer should move the person to the edge of the bed, with instructions to "dangle" the legs over the side (Fig. 5-13).
- The sonographer should stand facing the patient, supporting weight evenly on both feet. The patient should be asked to slide to the edge of the bed with the feet flat on the floor or on a stool. The sonographer should give the patient a few minutes to adjust.
- The sonographer should have the patient hold onto his or her shoulders or, if the patient is weak, his or her arms. One should place his or her hands under the patient's arms, and on the count of 3 pull the patient forward, shifting weight from the forward foot to the backward foot (Fig. 5-14).

In assisting patients to and from a wheelchair, the sonographer should always keep his or her center of gravity at the patient's center of gravity. If patients are weak, the sonographer must control their hips and shoulders during the transfer and not attempt to transfer patients who are unable to bear any of their own body weight. Instead, he or she should get help.

Wheelchair transfers

- The sonographer should explain the procedure to the patient.
- He or she should position the wheelchair close to the bed, either parallel to it or at a slight angle (Fig. 5-15). The sonographer should lock the wheels and position the footrests up and out of the way.

FIGURE **5-13** Assisting the patient out of bed or off a scanning table. One should always allow a weak patient to dangle the legs over the edge to regain equilibrium before attempting to move him or her.

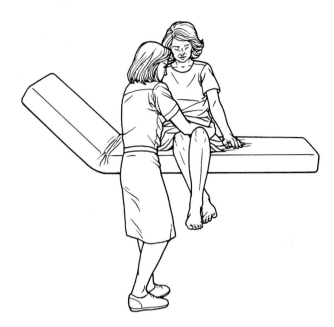

FIGURE **5-14** Assisting patients to and from a bed or scanning table. The sonographer should provide support under the arms of the patient and rotate or shift his or her weight as the person is brought closer to the sonographer.

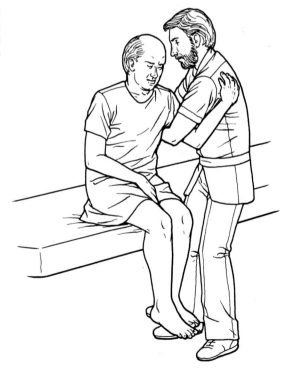

- The patient should be moved to the edge of the table or bed in an upright position, with the legs over the edge. With the patient's hands on the sonographer's shoulders, the sonographer should place the hands and arms under the patient's arms.
- The sonographer should assist the patient from the bed (with feet on the floor) as he or she rotates weight from the forward foot to the back foot.
- The sonographer should pivot or step sideways toward the chair and always pivot his or her entire body and the patient's entire body. One should not twist the back.
- Lower the patient into the chair by lowering the body, bending at the knees and hips as the patient sits down (Fig. 5-16). The sonographer should keep his or her shoulders level with the patient's shoulders. For patients able to help, have them grasp the arms of the wheelchair to support their own weight while sitting down and back into the chair. Once the patient is properly positioned in the chair, fold the footrests down and position the patient's feet on the footrests.
- When reversing the transfer (from chair to table or bed), the sonographer should bring the chair next to the table/bed and lock the wheels. They should lift the patient's feet and fold the footrests up and out of the way.
- The sonographer should have the patient place both hands on the arms of the chair and help the person stand as outlined in Figure 5-16.
- The standing patient should be turned so that his or her back is to the bed. The patient should move backward until he or she can step up or sit on the table or bed. Then the individual should be assisted to lie down and swing the legs up onto the bed.

Stretcher transfers

- The sonographer should wheel the stretcher next to the bed, aligning the head of the stretcher with the head of the bed. Pillows and bed linens should be moved out of the way.
- If possible, the sonographer should adjust the bed height to the height of the stretcher. The stretcher and bed wheels should be locked.
- The sonographer should stand on the far side of the stretcher and have the patient bend the legs and place the feet flat on the bed. He or she should instruct the patient to use the arms to help push himself or herself over and onto the stretcher.

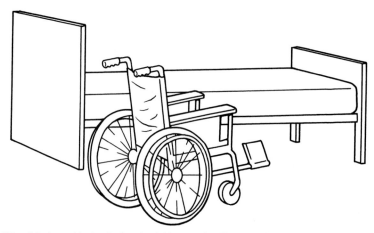

FIGURE **5-15** Wheelchair positioning before bedside transfer. The wheelchair should be parallel or at a slight angle to the bed, with wheels locked and footrests up and out of the way.

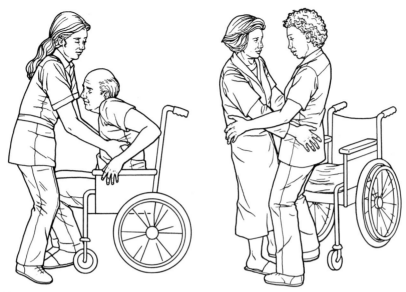

FIGURE **5-16** Moving patients to and from a wheelchair. One should bend at the knees and hips when lowering or raising a patient. The sonographer should keep his or her shoulders level with the patient's shoulders and enlist the person's help, if possible, by having him or her support his or her own weight when rising or sitting in the wheelchair.

- For a helpless patient, the sonographer should position a durable sheet under the person from knees to shoulders. With the help of at least one other individual, the sonographer should roll the sheet close to the patient's body. Grasping the roll, on the count of 3, they should lift slightly and pull the patient onto the stretcher. They should be careful not to drag the patient's head (Fig. 5-17).
- When proper positioning on the stretcher has been accomplished, the patient should be covered with a sheet; a pillow should be placed under the person's head and the side rails should be raised.

> *NOTE:* If the patient has tubings or drains, the sonographer should take special care to avoid pulling them out or disconnecting them.

INFECTION CONTROL

Preventing the spread of harmful microorganisms is a basic concern in all health care settings. Toward that end, the Centers for Disease Control and Prevention (CDC) and the Occupational Safety and Health Administration (OSHA) have established minimum standards for infection control. Formerly titled *Universal Precautions (Protocols),* the most recent recommendations are now called *Standard Precautions* (Box 5-2).

Standard Precautions should be used for contact with potentially infectious blood and certain body fluid. The use of barriers such as gloves, gowns, and masks is advised to provide

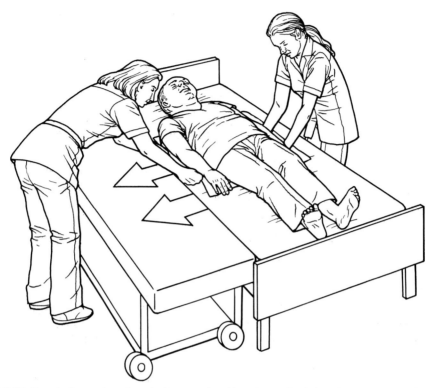

FIGURE **5-17** Transferring patients from bed to stretcher. Use of a "pulling" sheet is recommended whenever transferring patients who cannot help themselves.

protection for sonographers (or other health care workers). All health care institutions should provide personal protective equipment and instructions in their proper use to all employees.

Infection can be defined as the invasion and subsequent multiplication of microorganisms within the body, resulting in localized cellular injury. Infections can be restricted to a body part (local) or can involve the entire body (systemic). Normally, the human body is capable of protecting itself from infection, but age, nutritional states, stress, fatigue, medications, general health, and the presence of disease or injury can lower the body's natural resistance.

A cycle of infection is created when a pathogen (source) finds an environment in which it can grow (reservoir) (Fig. 5-18). Humans and animals are common reservoirs for both pathogenic and nonpathogenic microbes. Those who harbor disease organisms without signs or symptoms of infection are considered carriers and can pass the pathogen on to others.

Pathogens seek portals of exit, which might be through the respiratory, gastrointestinal, urinary, or reproductive tracts; breaks in the skin; or blood. Once pathogens find a portal of exit, they must be transmitted to another, susceptible host via a portal of entry in order to survive. The entry portals are the same as exit portals. When successfully transmitted, the only way to halt the infection is to break the chain of infection.

BOX **5-2** Standard Precautions (Tier One)* for Use with All Patients

- Standard precautions apply to blood, all body fluids, secretions, excretions, nonintact skin, and mucous membranes.
- Hands are washed if contaminated with blood or body fluid, immediately after gloves are removed, between patient contact, and when indicated to prevent transfer of microorganisms between patients or between patients and environment.
- Gloves are worn when touching blood, body fluid, secretions, excretions, nonintact skin, mucous membranes, or contaminated items. Gloves should be removed and hands washed between patient care.
- Masks, eye protection, or face shields are worn if patient care activities may generate splashes or sprays of blood or body fluid.
- Gowns are worn if soiling of clothing is likely from blood or body fluid. Perform hand hygiene after removing gown.
- Patient care equipment is properly cleaned and reprocessed, and single-use items are discarded.
- Contaminated linen is placed in leakproof bags to prevent skin and mucous membrane exposure.
- All sharp instruments and needles are discarded in a puncture-resistant container. CDC recommends that needles be disposed of uncapped or a mechanical device be used for recapping.

From Perry AG, Potter PA: *Clinical nursing skills and techniques,* ed 5, St Louis, 2002, Mosby. Originally modified from Centers for Disease Control and Prevention, Hospital Infection Control Practice Advisory Committee: Guidelines for isolation precautions in hospitals, *Am J Infect Control* 24:24, 1996.
*Formerly Universal Precautions and Body Substance Isolation.

FIGURE **5-18** The cycle of infection. Infection can develop if the cycle remains intact; that is: 1) The Agent (pathogen) finds a Host, a Reservoir, and 2) a Portal of Entry. 3) A Method of Transmission and Portal of Exit complete the chain. The chain of infection can be broken when aseptic techniques are employed.

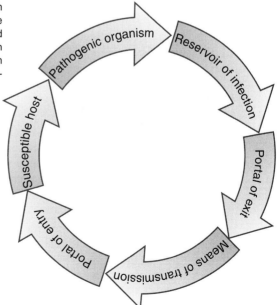

Nosocomial infections

Special emphasis should be placed on nosocomial infections, which are infections acquired during a stay in the hospital. Nosocomial infections are caused by normal flora or by pathogens transmitted to the patient from another source. Normal flora become pathogens when transmitted from their natural location to another site or host. (Example: *Escherichia coli*, normally found in feces and the intestines, could be spread to and infect the urinary tract by poor wiping after bowel movements.) If hand washing is poor, *E. coli* can spread to anything the hands touch and, in turn, be transmitted to other people.

Because microbes can enter the body through equipment used in treatments, therapies, and diagnostic tests, such equipment must be properly cleansed or sterilized. The most common sites for nosocomial infections are the urinary and respiratory systems, wounds, and the bloodstream. Many patients are already weakened from disease or injury. They may have surgical wounds or open skin areas. Both infants and the elderly are more susceptible to infections; also, their bodies are often unable to fight these infections effectively. Practicing medical and surgical asepsis, isolation precautions, and the CDC's Bloodborne Pathogen Precautions (BPPs) offers the best way to help prevent the spread of nosocomial infections (Box 5-3).

Blood and bodily fluids, secretions, and excretions are all potentially infectious materials if the health care worker is exposed to these substances by any penetration of the skin. OSHA formulated the BPP standards in 1991 (OSHA: 29CFR 1910.1030) to reduce the health risk to health care workers. The standards are based on a combination of engineering and work practice controls, personal protective equipment, training, medical surveillance, and other requirements to minimize the risk of disease transmission (Box 5-4).

The nosocomial transmission of tuberculosis (TB) is well documented, but such transmission in the United States has generally been low. That risk may be increased in health care facilities in communities with (1) high rates of HIV, (2) high numbers of persons from TB-endemic countries, and (3) a high prevalence of TB infection.

Sadly, the transmission of TB in health care facilities has been primarily caused by incomplete implementation of recommended TB infection control measures, which were established by the CDC. If a sonographer works in a setting described earlier, he or she should be given a baseline **purified protein derivative (PPD)** skin test as part of a comprehensive TB screening program in the facility. This test should be repeated annually for any sonographer with the potential for exposure to TB.

Two other emerging problems involve nosocomial infections. The first is caused by **methicillin-resistant *Staphylococcus aureus* (MRSA).** This antibiotic-resistant infection usually develops in hospitalized patients who are elderly or extremely sick or who have an open wound such as a bedsore or tubing such as urinary catheters or IV catheters. Patients at great risk are those experiencing a prolonged hospital stay; receiving broad-spectrum antibiotics; being hospitalized in an intensive care or burn unit; spending time close to other patients with MRSA; having recent surgery; or carrying MRSA in the nose without developing illness.

The second infection is **vancomycin-resistant *Enterococcus* (VRE).** Over the past decade, VRE has rapidly emerged as a health care–associated pathogen in U.S. hospitals, where many outbreaks have occurred and VRE has become endemic. Because the infection can rapidly spread from one health care facility to another, following the CDC guidelines and cooperating with other health care facilities and state and local health departments can be effective in controlling this important antimicrobial-resistant pathogen.

BOX **5-3** Bloodborne Pathogen Precautions

Standard Precautions: Use Standard Precautions for the care of all patients.

Airborne Precautions: In addition to Standard Precautions, use Airborne Precautions for patients known or suspected to have serious illnesses transmitted by airborne droplet nuclei. Examples of such illnesses include the following:
- Measles
- Varicella (including disseminated zoster)*
- Tuberculosis†

Droplet Precautions: In addition to Standard Precautions, use Droplet Precautions for patients known or suspected to have serious illnesses transmitted by large particle droplets. Examples of such illnesses include the following:
- Influenza
- Pneumonia
- Meningitis
- Other serious bacterial respiratory infections spread by droplet transmission including the following:
  - Diphtheria
  - Mycoplasma pneumonia
  - Pertussis
  - Pneumonic plague
  - Streptococcal pharyngitis or scarlet fever in infants and young children
- Serious viral infections spread by droplet transmission including:
  - Adenovirus*
  - Influenza
  - Mumps
  - Parvovirus B 19
  - Rubella

Contact Precautions: In addition to Standard Precautions, use Contact Precautions for patients known or suspected to have serious illnesses easily transmitted by direct patient contact or by contact with items in the patient's environment. Examples of such illnesses include the following:
- Gastrointestinal, respiratory, skin, or wound infections or colonization with multidrug-resistant bacteria judged by the infection control program, based on current state, regional, or national recommendations, to be of special clinical and epidemiologic significance.
- Enteric infections with a low infection dose or prolonged environmental survival including the following:
  - *Clostridium difficile*
  - For diapered or incontinent patients: enterohemorrhagic *E. coli 0157:h7*, *Shigella*, hepatitis A, or rotavirus
- Respiratory syncytial virus, parainfluenza virus, or enteroviral infections in infants and young children
- Skin infections that are highly contagious or that may occur on dry skin including the following:
  - Diphtheria (cutaneous)
  - Herpes simplex virus (neonatal or mucocutaneous)
  - Impetigo
  - Major (noncontained) abscesses, cellulitis, or decubiti
  - Pediculosis
  - Scabies
  - Staphylococcal furunculosis in infants and young children
  - Zoster (disseminated or in the immunocompromised host)*
- Viral/hemorrhagic conjunctivitis
- Viral hemorrhagic infections (Ebola, Lassa, or Marburg)

Modified from Perry AG, Potter PA: *Clinical nursing skills and techniques,* ed 5, St Louis, 2002, Mosby. Originally modified from Centers for Disease Control and Prevention, Hospital Infection Control Practice Advisory Committee: Guidelines for isolation precautions in hospitals, *Am J Infect Control* 24:24, 1996.
*Certain infections require more than one type of precaution.
†See *CDC Guidelines for Preventing the Transmission of Tuberculosis in Health-Care Facilities.*

BOX **5-4**   OSHA Standards for Reducing Occupational Exposure to
              Bloodborne Pathogens

1. Gloves must be worn when there is a reasonable expectation that the employee may contact blood, for example, during venipuncture.
2. Contaminated needles and other sharps must be placed in puncture-resistant containers properly labeled as a biohazard; when the containers are full, they are to be sealed and disposed of properly.
3. Contaminated needles should not be bent, sheared, recapped, or removed from the syringe after use.
4. Reports to OSHA of needle-stick injuries are required, and the health care agency must provide medical evaluation and follow-up.
5. Hepatitis B vaccination is to be made available to all employees who have occupational exposure.
6. Training and education must be offered to high-risk workers concerning precautions for prevention of exposure and use of personal protective equipment.
7. Each facility must have an infection control plan, including methods for the reduction of the health care worker's exposure to biohazardous wastes.
8. Facilities must have engineering and work practice controls to eliminate or minimize employee exposure. Controls may include sharps disposal containers and self-sheathing needles.

Modified from Perry AG, Potter PA: *Clinical nursing skills and techniques,* ed 5, St Louis, 2002, Mosby. Originally modified from Occupational Safety and Health Act: Bloodborne pathogens, *Federal Register* 56(235):64, 175, 1991.

Standard precautions

Microorganisms grow best wherever they find sufficient food, moisture, and warmth. They can enter the body through the nose, mouth, or breaks in the skin. Organisms also can be transported on soiled equipment and supplies, discarded tissues and linens, and the hands of health care professionals. For this reason, health care professionals must observe medical aseptic techniques when dealing with patients. Following the CDC's guidelines in Box 5-3 will ensure the safety of patients and staff members.

Medical asepsis can be practiced in two ways: (1) general medical asepsis, which concerns all the measures taken to keep health care workers, patients, and the environment clean to prevent the spread of germs and (2) isolation precautions that are carried out to confine disease-producing germs.

When working with patients, the following *general* precautions should be taken.

- The sonographer should wash hands before and after each direct patient contact, *even if wearing gloves.*
- Clean patient linens should be kept away from the sonographer's "dirty" uniform.
- Used linens should be disposed of in a hamper or bag, never on furniture or the floors.
- Wound dressings should be discarded in the proper place.
- The scanning environment should be kept clean, and only clean items should be allowed to touch the patient.

A part of general cleanliness also involves a sonographer's personal hygiene. The following checklist describes the personal practices that every sonographer should observe.

- He or she should stay healthy and get adequate rest and good nutrition.
- He or she should bathe daily and wash hair at least every week. A hairstyle that is appropriate for germ control should be worn.

- Fingernails should be kept short and clean underneath the nails. NOTE: Chipped nail polish, porcelain, or other types of artificial nails are not permitted because they can harbor/spread bacteria and are a threat to patients' health.
- Hands should be washed after every direct patient contact, *even if wearing gloves.*
- The sonographer should wear clean uniforms or laboratory coats daily and not wear costume jewelry because it can harbor germs.
- He or she should not come to work when ill, especially with a communicable disease.
- The sonographer should cover his or her mouth and nose when coughing or sneezing and discard tissues promptly in an appropriate container.

Isolation techniques

When patients develop infections, special steps are taken to prevent the spread of the organisms. Because sonographers may be requested to perform bedside examinations on such patients or care for patients with impaired immunity, they must understand and be prepared to carry out the following general isolation precautions. Institutional policies may vary, so the following suggestions are simply guidelines for working in an area where isolation precautions are being used:

- The sonographer should organize all necessary supplies before entering the patient/ isolation area to provide sonographic examinations. Working under isolation precautions can be time consuming and frustrating; thus it is particularly important to avoid leaving the area for forgotten supplies.
- Hands should be washed before and after each patient contact *even if wearing gloves.* This is the single most effective means of preventing the spread of infection. It is important that the sonographer wash his or her hands again after contact with any patient excretions or secretions before touching the patient again.
- The sonographer should use a paper towel to turn faucets on or off.
- If the sonographer must remove dressings to perform the sonographic examination, the dressings should be properly bagged for disposal, using supplies provided within the unit.
- All gloves used during an examination must be discarded in an appropriate container before leaving the isolation area.
- Gowns should be discarded in a designated hamper before leaving the isolation area.
- Masks should cover the nose and mouth and be put on before entering the isolation area, and they should be removed or discarded before leaving the isolation room. Whenever a mask becomes moist, it should be changed because it no longer provides an effective barrier to the spread of germs.
- Masks should be used only once. *A mask should never be lowered around one's neck and then reused.*
- Ultrasound equipment must be cleansed before entering the isolation unit. Sterile transducer covers and scanning agents should be used when performing studies on patients in isolation, and all equipment should be disinfected after use.

Taking protective measures

GLOVES

Gloves are worn as protection from the patient's pathology and to protect the patient from any microbes on one's hands. The gloves must not be damaged when one puts them on (Fig. 5-19). Long fingernails, rings, and just plain carelessness can cause pinpricks, cuts, or tears, allowing blood, fluids, secretions, or excretions to enter the glove and contaminate one's hand. Important considerations when gloves are required include the following:

- Hands should be dry before putting on gloves.
- Any gloves that are punctured, torn, or cut should be discarded and replaced.
- Gloves should cover the wrists. If wearing a gown, gloves must cover the cuffs.
- Gloves should be used only once and discarded after use.
- Whenever gloves are exposed to blood, bodily fluids, secretions, or excretions, the sonographer must put on a new pair of gloves.
- When removing gloves, ensure that the inside part is on the outside because the inside is considered clean. Wash hands immediately after removing gloves.

One more important fact about gloves must be addressed. Health care professionals with ongoing exposure to latex products, especially gloves, may develop an allergy to latex. Latex allergies should be suspected in anyone who develops the following symptoms after latex exposure:

- Nasal, eye, or sinus irritation
- Hives
- Shortness of breath
- Coughing/wheezing
- Unexplained shock

Anyone who experiences these symptoms, be it sonographer or patient, should be evaluated by a physician because further exposure could mean a serious allergic reaction.

An FDA-approved test is available to diagnose allergic contact dermatitis. A special patch containing latex additives is applied to the skin and checked over several days. Positive reactions are shown by itching, redness, swelling, or blistering where the patch covered the skin.

Once an allergy to latex develops, special precautions are necessary to avoid latex exposure. The alternatives to latex gloves are synthetic, low-protein, and powder-free gloves. OSHA's BPP Standards require hand washing after removal of gloves or other protective equipment. This helps minimize any powder or latex remaining in contact with the skin.

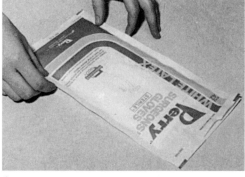
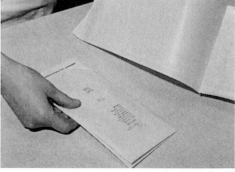

A   B

FIGURE **5-19** Open gloving. **A,** The sonographer should perform hand hygiene. When obtaining gloves, the correct size is important. **B,** The sonographer should open the outer wrap to expose the folded inner wrap.
(*continued*)

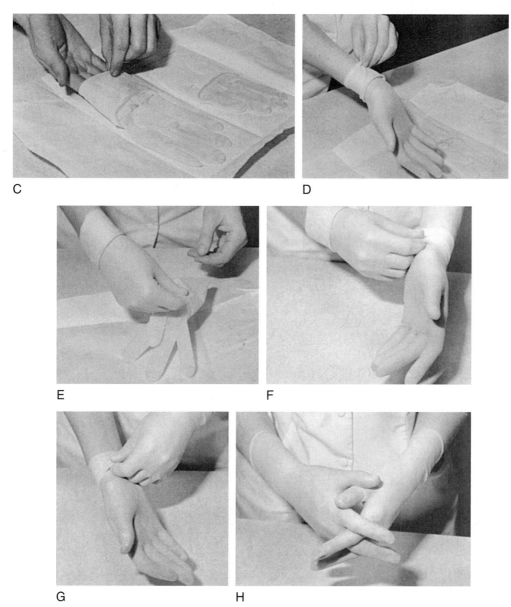

FIGURE **5-19, cont'd C,** He or she should expose gloves with open ends facing oneself. **D,** When putting on the first glove, only the inner surface of the folded cuff should be touched. **E,** Using the gloved hand, the sonographer should grasp the second glove under the cuff. **F,** The sonographer should put on the second glove and unfold the cuff. **G,** He or she should insert fingers under the cuff of the first glove and unfold the cuff. **H,** Gloving complete. One should keep hands in front of his or her body and at a safe distance from the uniform to avoid contamination.

GOWNS

The most common protective clothing is the gown. However, aprons and shoe and leg covers may also be required in some instances.

- Gowns must be long and large enough to completely cover the sonographer's clothing.
- If the gown becomes wet, it is contaminated and should be removed and replaced.
- The inside and neck of the gown are clean; the outside and waist ties are contaminated.
- If required to also wear a mask, the sonographer should wash his or her hands and put the mask on before donning the gown.
- Watches and jewelry should be removed before donning a gown. Long uniform sleeves should be rolled up.
- The gown should cover the sonographer's clothing/uniform and be snug around the neck. The gown should be overlapped at the back and snugly tied at both the neck and the back.
- Masks should be put on *before* the gown.
- Gloves should be put on only *after* the sonographer has gowned.
- When the sonographer is ready to ungown, he or she should remove the gloves first and then undo the gown ties.
- He or she should wash hands and untie the neck strings, being careful not to touch the outside of the gown.
- The gown should be pulled down from the shoulders, turning it inside out as it is removed.
- Holding the inside shoulder seams of the gown, the hands should be brought together and the gown rolled away from the sonographer, while keeping it inside out.
- The sonographer should wash hands and use a paper towel to open doors.

MASKS

Masks are used for airborne particle and droplet protection. Breathing can cause masks to become moist or wet. When this happens, the mask is contaminated. It should be discarded properly and replaced with a new mask.

- Before putting on the mask, the sonographer should wash his or her hands.
- The sonographer should not touch the part of the mask that will touch his or her face.
- The upper strings should be tied in back, over the ears and toward the top of the head.
- The top of the mask should fit snugly over the sonographer's nose. If glasses are worn, the mask should fit under the bottom edge of the glasses.
- The sonographer should wash his or her hands again before working with the patient.
- When finished, remove the gloves first, then untie the bottom strings, followed by the top strings.
- Holding the top strings, remove the mask and bring the strings together so that the inside of the mask folds together.
- The sonographer should discard the mask properly and wash hands.

EYE PROTECTORS AND FACE SHIELDS

To protect the mucous membranes of one's eyes from patient pathogens, the sonographer may be asked to wear goggles or a face shield along with a face mask. Once his or her work with the patient is finished, the sonographer should discard any disposable eyewear and clean any reusable eyewear with soap, water, and a disinfectant before using them again.

Preparing a sterile field

When invasive procedures are scheduled in the ultrasound laboratory, sonographers must obtain the proper sterile pack/tray for the procedure. A sterile field should not be prepared until just before the procedure (Fig. 5-20). The sonographer should follow these steps:
• Select a flat work surface that is clean, dry, and above waist level.
• Wash hands thoroughly.
• Place the sterile linen-wrapped pack (which contains a sterile drape) on the work surface.

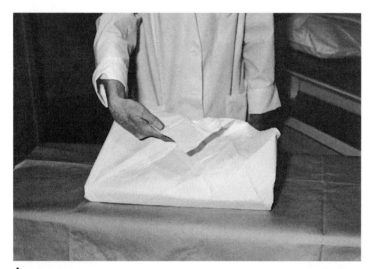
A

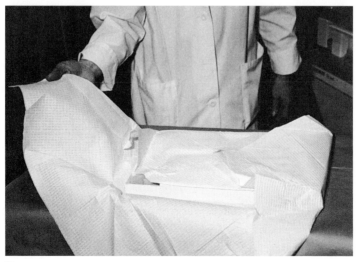
B

FIGURE **5-20** Preparing a sterile field. **A,** The sonographer should open the first corner away from himself or herself. **B,** He or she should open one side by grasping a corner tip. (*Continued*)

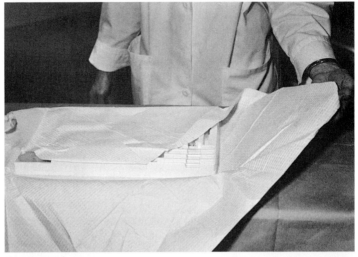

C

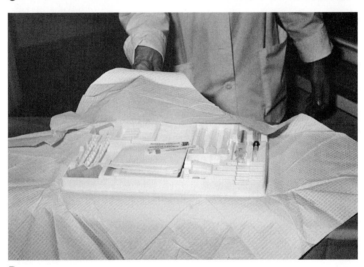

D

FIGURE **5-20, cont'd C,** Then he or she should open the second side in the same manner and **D,** pull the remaining corner toward himself or herself. If there is an inner wrap, it should be opened in the same manner. A sterile field is now established.

- Remove the tape seal and unwrap both layers. The opened package wrapper can be used as a sterile field.
- Starting with the outermost flap of the drape, open it while keeping the arm outstretched and away from the sterile field.
- With the other hand, grasp the adjacent corner of the drape and hold it straight up, over the work surface, and away from the body.

- Holding the drape, position the bottom half over the work surface.
- Place the top half of the drape over the work surface last.
- Add the sterile items by following the directions, and place them directly on the field or transfer them with sterile forceps.
- DO NOT place any objects within a 1-inch border of the drape, or they will have to be discarded.
- Wear sterile gloves while preparing items for the field. The sonographer can touch the drape, but sterile items must be handed over by an assistant. Gloves may not touch the wrappers of the sterile items.

Types of isolation

The five specific types of isolation are: strict, respiratory, enteric, wound-skin, and reverse isolation.

STRICT ISOLATION

This protects others from patients' germs and is used to prevent the spread—by contact or airborne transmission—of highly contagious diseases (e.g., streptococcal pneumonia, smallpox, diphtheria). Gowns, gloves, and masks must be worn, and all articles used must be disinfected or disposed of properly. In some cases, protective eyewear is also required.

RESPIRATORY ISOLATION

This is used to protect others from germs in the patient's nose, mouth, throat, and lungs. It is used for disease spread by droplets that are coughed, sneezed, or breathed into the air (e.g., chickenpox, mumps, tuberculosis, scarlet fever, meningococcal meningitis). Gowns and gloves are not necessary, but washing hands and wearing masks are required. Contaminated articles must be disposed of properly or disinfected.

ENTERIC PRECAUTIONS

These are used in diseases involving ingestion of disease-producing microorganisms (e.g., hepatitis, AIDS) to protect others from germs in the patient's bowels, bladder, and stomach. Hand washing and wearing gowns and gloves for direct contact are necessary. Wearing masks is not. All contaminated articles should be disposed of in specially provided bags or they should be properly disinfected.

WOUND-SKIN PRECAUTIONS

These are necessary to protect others from germs in patients' wounds or any other heavily contaminated areas (e.g., burns, staphylococcal or streptococcal infections). Their use is intended for infections that are spread by direct contact with wounds, linens, or dressings. Hand washing is required, and gowns and gloves must be worn. Masks are necessary only if dressings are removed to perform the sonography examination. Articles contaminated with urine, feces, or vomitus should be bagged or disinfected.

REVERSE (PROTECTIVE) ISOLATION

This protects patients from the germs of others. It is used with persons who have extremely impaired resistance (e.g., patients on chemotherapy, steroid therapy). Hand washing and the wearing of gowns, gloves, and masks are required.

Cleansing of the ultrasound equipment and the use of sterile transducer covers and scanning media are indicated.

EMERGENCY MEDICAL SITUATIONS

Heart attacks and choking because of obstructed airways are frequent causes of accidental death. Choking occurs especially in children, who are known to put "everything" into their mouths. Although most sonographers perform their examinations in a medically supervised setting, it is important that they be familiar with basic lifesaving measures as they await a response to their emergency alert. If classes in lifesaving techniques are not included in a sonographer's training, he or she is urged to investigate instructional sessions offered by the local chapter of the American Red Cross.

Choking but conscious patients

An obstructed airway is a critical emergency because it can cause anoxia, which can lead to brain damage and death within 4 to 6 minutes. The universal gesture of a choking person is a sudden, agitated placement of a hand to the neck. Other signs of choking are the inability to talk, cry, or breathe followed by the patient becoming cyanotic. Coughing often causes the object to pop out and relieve the symptoms. Importantly, when a person begins to suffer from lack of oxygen, the throat muscles relax, which may make it easier to dislodge foreign objects. If the patient is unable to remove the foreign object, the sonographer can assist by performing the Heimlich maneuver.

The **Heimlich maneuver** is a choking rescue technique used to clear an obstruction of the airway caused by a foreign object in adults and children older than 1 year of age (Table 5-1). Involving abdominal thrusting motions, the technique can be performed with the patient standing, sitting, or lying down (Fig. 5-21). Abdominal thrusts should only be used on conscious adults and are contraindicated on pregnant, markedly obese, or recent abdominal surgery patients. Such patients require chest thrusts to force the air out of the lungs and create an artificial cough. For infants younger than 1 year old, the procedure is limited to rescue back blows and chests thrusts (Fig. 5-22). When visible, obstructing foreign objects can be seen, a finger-sweeping maneuver is used to manually remove the foreign body from the mouth. The finger-sweeping technique may also be necessary when the patient with an obstructed airway is unconscious.

The Heimlich maneuver can also be self-administered. If one is choking, he or she should do the following:
- Make a fist with one hand.
- Place the thumb side of the fist above the navel and below the lower end of the sternum.
- Grasp the fist with the other hand.
- Press inward and upward, quickly.

If the thrust did not relieve the obstruction, one should press the upper abdomen against a hard surface (a chair back, table, or railing). Then he or she should use as many thrusts as needed.

All of these techniques are contraindicated for patients with incomplete or partial airway obstruction or when the patient can maintain adequate breathing and can dislodge the foreign body by coughing effectively. It is only when a patient cannot speak, cough, or breathe that immediate action must be taken to dislodge an obstruction.

(*Text continued on pg. 123*)

TABLE **5-1**   Choking or Airway Obstruction Emergency

TECHNIQUE	ADULT	CHILD 1-8 YR OLD	INFANT YOUNGER THAN 1 YR OLD
HEIMLICH OR CHOKING RESCUE PROCEDURE			
Conscious patient	Tell patient you will try to dislodge the foreign body.	Have the child stand. Perform abdominal thrusts using the adult technique, but WITH LESS FORCE.	Whether the infant is conscious or not, place him or her face down, straddling your arm, with the infant's head lower than his or her body.
	Stand behind the patient and wrap your arms around his or her waist. If the patient is standing, place one of your feet between the patient's legs so you can support the patient's body if he or she loses consciousness.		Resting your forearm on your thigh, deliver 4 back blows with the heel of your hand, between the infant's shoulder blades.
	Make a fist with one hand. Place the thumb side against the patient's abdomen, slightly above the umbilicus and well below the sternum.		If the obstruction is not dislodged, place your free hand on the infant's back. Support the infant's neck, jaw, and chest with your other hand and turn the infant over onto your thigh.
	Grasp fist with free hand and squeeze patient's abdomen 6-10 times, with quick **inward-upward** thrusts, forceful enough to create an artificial cough that might dislodge the obstruction.		Position the fingers of your free hand on the infant's sternum.
	Repeat thrusts until object is expelled or the patient loses consciousness.		Then, place your middle and ring fingers next to your index finger and lift the index finger off the infant's chest. Deliver 4 chest thrusts as you would for chest compressions, but more slowly. As with a child, never perform a blind finger-sweep.

(Continued)

TABLE **5-1** Choking or Airway Obstruction Emergency—cont'd

TECHNIQUE	ADULT	CHILD 1-8 YR OLD	INFANT YOUNGER THAN 1 YR OLD
Unconscious patient	Call for help and place the patient in the supine position.	Place the child in the supine position.	
	Begin CPR if necessary. If rescue breathing is unsuccessful, reposition the patient's head and try again.	If the child is large, kneel astride his or her thighs. If the child is lying on a scanning table, stand by the child's side.	
	If still unsuccessful, kneel astride the patient's thighs.	Deliver abdominal thrusts as you would for an adult patient, but with LESS FORCE.	
	Then, place the heel of one hand on the top of the back of the other hand, which should be placed outstretched with the palm down.	Never perform a blind finger-sweep on a child because it would risk pushing the foreign body farther back into the airway.	
	Rest your hands between the patient's umbilicus and the tip of the xiphoid process at the midline.		
	Push in and up with 6-10 quick abdominal thrusts.		
	After the thrusts, open the patient's airway by grasping the patient's tongue and lower jaw between your thumb and fingers.		
	Lift the jaw to draw the tongue away from any foreign body.		
	If the object can be seen, remove it by inserting your index finger deep into the throat at the base of the tongue. Using a hooking motion, remove the object.		
	DO NOT use blind finger-sweeps because your finger may act as a second obstruction.		
	After the object is removed, perform rescue breathing.		

TABLE **5-1** Choking or Airway Obstruction Emergency—cont'd

TECHNIQUE	ADULT	CHILD 1-8 YR OLD	INFANT YOUNGER THAN 1 YR OLD
	Check for spontaneous breathing and a pulse. Proceed with CPR if necessary. If the object is not removed, try rescue breathing anyway. If you cannot, repeat the abdominal thrusts until you clear the airway. *Conscious pregnant or obese patient* Stand behind the patient and place your arms under the patient's armpits and around her or his chest. Place the thumb side of your clenched fist against the middle of the sternum, avoiding the rib margins and the xiphoid process. Grasp your fist with your free hand and thrust with enough force to expel the foreign object. Continue until the patient expels the obstruction or loses consciousness. *Unconscious pregnant or obese patient* Place patient in supine position. Kneel near the patient's side and place the heel of one hand at the bottom of the patient's sternum. The long axis of your hand should be aligned with the long axis of the patient's sternum. Place the heel of your free hand on top of the other hand, making sure your fingers do not touch the patient's chest. Deliver thrusts forcefully enough to dislodge the object.		

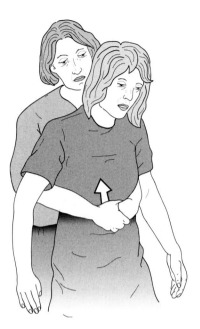

FIGURE **5-21** Applying the Heimlich maneuver. Abdominal thrusts may be applied to choking patients in either the standing or supine position.

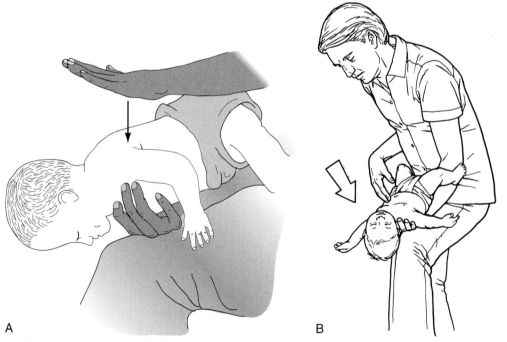

A   B

FIGURE **5-22** Performing the Heimlich maneuver on infants. **A,** Infant is held face down, on the forearm, and supported with one hand. Blows are delivered to the infant's back between the shoulder blades. **B,** Infant is held face up on one's thigh while chest thrusts are delivered, using two or three fingers.

Cardiopulmonary resuscitation

Throughout the ages, man has tried to revive unconscious or dying humans. The first recorded attempt at resuscitation (about 800 BC) can be found in the Bible, where "Elijah actions" are described:

> " . . . lay upon the child and put his mouth upon his mouth, and his eyes
> upon his eyes, and his hands upon his hands; and he stretched himself
> upon the child; and the flesh of the child waxed warm."

   In Medieval times the application of heat or flagellation was used to warm a cold body or elicit some response from an unconscious patient. In 1530, use of an ordinary fireplace bellows was recommended to blow hot air and smoke into a patient's mouth, and this became the accepted practice for the next 300 years. Not until the early nineteenth century, when medical authorities had a better understanding of respiratory system anatomy, did they realize that overdistention of the lungs by bellows could be fatal. That practice was discontinued and replaced by rolling patients from stomach to side—16 times a minute— and applying pressure to the patient's back while he or she was prone.

   The U. S. military advocated mouth-to-mouth resuscitation during World War II. By 1950 the American Red Cross began programs to educate the public in the new technique of **cardiopulmonary resuscitation (CPR).** CPR is an emergency technique used on patients whose hearts have stopped or who are not breathing, or both. The next major step would not occur until 1960, when closed chest massage was introduced. The crucial element of this technique was the delivery of oxygen to the brain by developing minimally increased blood circulation. The first guidelines to perform CPR were based on this technique.

   During the Vietnam War, the U.S. Army introduced CPR to the public for the first time, and the American Red Cross quickly began another campaign to teach the method to the American people.

   CPR was designed to counteract **cardiac arrest**, when heart and breathing stop suddenly without warning. Today, CPR is performed on all hospital patients whose heart or lungs have stopped working, unless a written "do not resuscitate" (DNR) order has been signed.

   Increasingly, CPR training teaches continuous chest compressions or the use of defibrillators and barrier devices when performing CPR. However, at the time of this writing, these practices are not universally practiced in *every* ultrasound setting. Therefore the following material explains the techniques of rescue breathing and CPR and ends with the introduction of the latest thinking on improving the practice of CPR.

CPR OVERVIEW

Basic CPR requires no special equipment other than a hard surface on which to place the patient. Complications can occur if CPR is performed incorrectly. Possible complications include gastric distention (too much air delivered during ventilation), fractured ribs, lacerated liver, and punctured lungs.

   Importantly, most patients who suffer sudden cardiac arrest develop ventricular fibrillation and require defibrillation. Because CPR alone does not improve their survival chances, one must assess the patient and call a code or contact EMS before starting CPR. Timing is critical, and the sonographer's role is to keep the patient alive until advanced cardiac life support can begin.

RESCUE BREATHING

A patient may experience difficulty breathing for many reasons. Heart attacks, strokes, seizures, and fainting are among the more common causes. In cases of **respiratory arrest**, breathing stops, but the heart still pumps blood for several minutes. Rescue breaths must be given before beginning chest compressions to help circulate blood in a patient whose heart has stopped beating (Fig. 5-23). As a rescuer, one must quickly determine what has happened to a patient and then follow the general lifesaving procedures summarized in Table 5-2.

CHEST COMPRESSIONS

When a person's heart stops beating, blood no longer circulates throughout the body and blood no longer has a supply of oxygen. In such situations, it is vital that CPR be initiated within the first 4 minutes of the event.

Mouth-to-mouth resuscitations and manual cardiac compressions do not restart a heart that has stopped. What CPR does do is keep the patient alive until more advanced and aggressive treatment can be administered.

To position oneself properly to perform chest compressions on an adult, elbows should be straight and shoulders directly over the patient's chest. Enough pressure should be exerted to depress the sternum about 1½ to 2 inches. Pressure should be released without removing one's hands from the chest.

If a patient appears unresponsive to rescue breathing, it is important to recheck for signs of circulation (e.g., breathing, coughing, movement). If there no signs of circulation, chest compressions should be initiated.

BASIC CARDIAC LIFE SUPPORT

Importantly, CPR done *improperly* on a person whose heart is still beating can cause serious injury. DO NOT perform CPR unless the following conditions exist:
- The patient has stopped breathing.
- The patient does not show signs of circulation (e.g., normal breathing, coughing, or movement in response to rescue breathing).
- No one with more training in CPR is present.
  For basic life support, it is helpful to think **ABC**:

Airway,
Breathing
Circulation

As part of its ongoing efforts in this area, the American Heart Association (AHA) has developed information to improve survival from sudden cardiac arrest. Called the *Chain of Survival,* the concept advocates the following:
- Early access
- Early CPR
- Early defibrillation
- Early advanced life support

More complete information is available to instructors and students at: *http://www.americanheart.org* under the topic Statement on the Chain of Survival.

The AHA and the American Red Cross are two organizations that have long been involved in establishing and teaching the basic life-saving procedures in practice today. Through the

(*Text continued on pg. 130*)

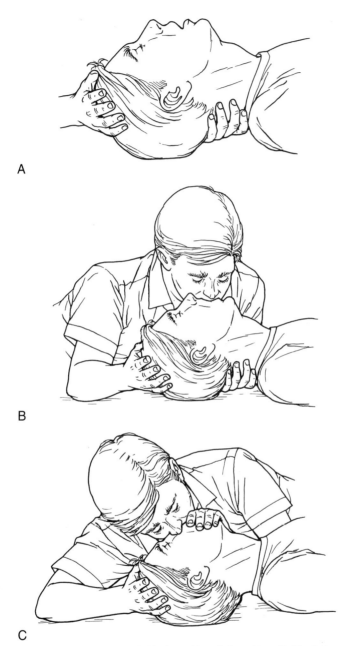

A

B

C

FIGURE **5-23** Methods of artificial ventilation. **A,** Backward head-tilt position. **B,** Mouth-to-mouth resuscitation technique. **C,** Mouth-to-nose resuscitation technique.

TABLE **5-2**   Cardiopulmonary Resuscitation

TECHNIQUE OR SYMPTOM	ADULT	CHILD 1-8 YR OLD	INFANT YOUNGER THAN 1 YR OLD
ABC	Open patient's **airway,** check for **breathing,** assess for circulation, and **call** for help before beginning compressions.	Same as adult CPR. CPR is appropriate only if the child is not breathing.	Generally the same as for adults and children, but with some variations. If the infant is not breathing, call for help and give rescue breaths for 1 min.
Injury assessment	Check for injuries, especially to the head or neck. If suspicious, move patient as little as possible to reduce risk of paralysis. Place the patient in a supine position on a hard, flat surface. When moving the patient, roll the head and torso as a unit. Avoid twisting/pulling the patient's neck, shoulders, and hips. Kneel near the patient's shoulders to have easy access to head and chest. Use the head-tilt, chin-lift maneuver to open the airway. Avoid placing your fingertips on the soft tissue under the patient's chin, as this may inadvertently obstruct the airway. *Check for breathing* while keeping the airway open. If the patient starts to breathe, keep the airway open and continue checking until help arrives.	Same as adult.	Same as child.
Rescue breathing	*Rescue breathing,* or ventilations, should be performed if the patient does not start breathing after you have opened his or her airway.	Open airway using head-chin lift. Follow adult procedure. Give rescue breaths for 1 full min.	Open airway using head-lift.

(Continued)

TABLE **5-2**   Cardiopulmonary Resuscitation—cont'd

TECHNIQUE OR SYMPTOM	ADULT	CHILD 1-8 YR OLD	INFANT YOUNGER THAN 1 YR OLD
	Pinch the patient's nostrils with the thumb and index finger of the hand on his or her forehead.		Take a deep breath, and tightly seal your mouth over the infant's nose and mouth. Deliver a gentle puff of air. If the infant's chest rises and falls, then the amount of air is sufficient.
			Continue rescue breathing with 1 breath every 3 sec.
	Use a barrier device if available. Take a deep breath and place your mouth over the device (or the patient's mouth), creating a tight seal.		
	Give 2 full ventilations, taking a deep breath after each to allow time for his or her chest to expand and relax to prevent gastric distention. Each ventilation should last for 1½ to 2 sec.		
	If unsuccessful, reposition the patient's head and try again. If still unsuccessful, a foreign body may be obstructing the airway.		
	Check for loose dentures or any other objects that might be causing an obstruction. Follow instructions for clearing an airway obstruction.		
	Assess circulation by keeping one hand on the patient's forehead so that the airway remains open. With your free hand, palpate the carotid artery nearest you, by placing your index and middle fingers in the groove between the trachea and sternocleidomastoid muscle of the neck. Palpate for 5-10 sec.		

(Continued)

TABLE **5-2** Cardiopulmonary Resuscitation—cont'd

TECHNIQUE OR SYMPTOM	ADULT	CHILD 1-8 YR OLD	INFANT YOUNGER THAN 1 YR OLD
	If there is a pulse, DO NOT begin chest compressions. Instead, perform rescue breathing at a rate of 12/min (or 1 every 5 sec). After 12 ventilations, recheck the patient's pulse. If there is no pulse, start chest compressions.		
Chest compressions	Be sure your knees are far enough apart to provide stable support. Locate the rib margin with your free hand and move your fingertips along the sternal notch. Place your middle finger on the notch and your index finger next to your middle finger. Your index finger should now be at the bottom of the sternum. Put the heel of your other hand on the sternum, next to the index finger. The long axis of the heel of your hand will be aligned with the long axis of the sternum.	Position the heel of one hand about 2 fingers' width above the tip of the sternum. Place the free hand on top of the other and lock fingers of both hands together. Raise fingers so that they do not touch the child's chest and recheck for circulation. Using less force than with adults, compress the sternum 1 to 1½ inches. Count "1&2&3&4&," giving a downward thrust with each number. Give 5 chest compressions. Then give 1 rescue breath. Repeat this cycle 12 times (1 min), then check again for signs of circulation such as coughing, moving, or	Place 2 fingers on the infant's sternum, about 1 finger-width below the nipple line. Press with gentle force, compressing the sternum about ½ to 1 inch. Give 5 chest compressions. Then give 1 rescue breath. Repeat the cycle (5:1) 12 times (about 1 min). Check for signs of circulation or movement in response to rescue breaths. If no signs of circulation, continue CPR until help arrives or signs of circulation are present or breathing is restored. Compression rate should be 100/min.

(continued)

TABLE **5-2**   Cardiopulmonary Resuscitation—cont'd

TECHNIQUE OR SYMPTOM	ADULT	CHILD 1-8 YR OLD	INFANT YOUNGER THAN 1 YR OLD
	Take the first hand off the notch and put it on top of the hand on the sternum, making sure you have one directly on top of the other, and that your fingers are not on his or her chest. Lock your elbows. Keep arms straight and shoulders directly over your hands. Using the weight of your upper body, compress the patient's sternum 1½ to 2 inches by delivering pressure through the heels of your hands. After each compression, release pressure and allow the chest to return to its normal position so that the heart can fill with blood. DO NOT change your hand positions during compression as you might injure the patient. Perform 4 complete cycles of 15 compressions and 2 breaths. Check the carotid pulse. If there is no pulse, perform CPR and a pulse check. Adult compression rates should be 100/min.	normal breathing in response to rescue breaths. If still unsuccessful, continue CPR until help arrives or signs of circulation are present and breathing is restored. Compression rate should be 100/min. Ratio of compressions to ventilations should be 5:1.	Ratio of compressions to ventilations should be 5:1.

years, these procedures have changed in response to medical advances and experience gained. Therefore health professionals must stay current, and one of the best ways to do so is to routinely check the websites of these organizations. Clearly, the best way to learn and master critical life-saving techniques is to take a formal CPR course.

Emerging techniques and trends

BARRIER DEVICES

Today, **barrier devices** (disposable airway equipment) are available to prevent direct contact with a patient's mouth and blood, secretions/excretions, and bodily fluids. Masklike barrier devices, as well as mouth-to-mouth barrier devices, have added an element of safety for the person performing rescue breathing. The barrier device is placed over the patient's mouth and nose to form a tight seal. Then the standard breathing protocol is begun.

CONTINUOUS CHEST COMPRESSION CPR

The University of Arizona's Sarver Heart Center has introduced a new breakthrough method of performing CPR. This method, called **continuous chest compression CPR (CCC-CPR)**, is easier to learn and perform than the standard CPR techniques that have been in use for more than 40 years.

CCC-CPR emphasizes chest compressions and eliminates the need for mouth-to-mouth breathing.

The Arizona studies found that stopping chest compressions to give mouth-to-mouth breaths may actually be more harmful than helpful. Standard CPR techniques call for performing 15 chest compressions followed by two mouth-to-mouth breaths. The compressions act to move oxygenated blood through the body and to the organs. When the compressions are stopped to begin rescue breathing, no blood is moved and the organs are essentially starved. Another drawback to standard CPR is that it takes longer to administer the breaths than previously thought. An additional consideration is the possible reluctance to perform CPR because of the perceived risks associated with mouth-to-mouth breathing.

The CCC-CPR technique involves positioning the patient on the floor, placing one hand on top of the other, and placing the heel of the bottom hand in the center of the patient's chest. With elbows locked, *forceful* chest compressions are then delivered at a rate of 100/min.

AUTOMATED EXTERNAL DEFIBRILLATOR

In patients with sudden cardiac arrest, the latest advance is that of the increased access to **automated external defibrillators (AEDs)**. These devices administer an electric shock through the chest wall to the heart of the patient. The devices have built-in computers to (1) assess the patient's heart rhythm, (2) judge whether defibrillation is necessary, and (3) administer the shock. Audio and visual prompts are provided to guide users through the process. Many public places (e.g., schools, airports, airplanes, malls, gyms, golf courses, large office buildings) now have AEDs on their premises.

NOTE: AEDs are used on adults and children between the ages of 1 and 8.

ASSISTING PATIENTS WITH SPECIAL NEEDS

Elderly patients

The emotional needs of the aging person are a primary concern. Patients in this age group are not really much different from those in any other, but because of the physical and social changes associated with aging, their ability to cope and maintain a positive outlook is decreased. The losses experienced by aged patients are numerous and wide ranging: loss of spouse, family, friends, job, familiar environment, pets, and health and vigor. An accumulation of such losses can create problems in coping with or adapting to change in ways that maintain independence and a sense of well-being.

The feelings of well being, of being needed, and of loving and receiving love are diminished for the aging patient. A positive self-image, feeling important, and enjoyment of meaningful personal and interpersonal relationships are all challenged by losses.

The sonographer should be consciously aware of the fact that age brings losses. Most elderly persons can cope and adapt if losses come gradually. When losses come too rapidly, however, they become overwhelming, bringing intense feelings of loneliness and frightening thoughts of loss of independence and privacy.

Sensory changes (e.g., diminished vision and hearing) that occur with age can lead to an inability to respond to the environment, preventing the perception of danger signals. Eventually such a lack of sensory stimulation leads to the confusion and withdrawal that is so common in elderly patients. By demonstrating concern and preparing elderly patients for their sonograms, the sonographer can increase their feelings of control over their situation and help to decrease their level of stress.

Some memory loss is common with aging, producing slower reactions to questions, directions, and decision making. The sonographer can overcome this problem by slowing the rate at which he or she gives instructions, communicating in a quiet environment with minimal activity, and providing extra time for response.

Despite the negative aspects of aging, there are many potential rewards in dealing with elderly patients. A lifetime of living has given them a wealth of knowledge and experience; therefore asking their opinions or advice can result in useful suggestions concerning what will work best for them. Elderly patients can provide sonographers a chance to practice the almost lost art of listening, if sonographers just encourage them to talk about their experiences. Talking about their experiences and accomplishments makes them feel that their lives had a purpose. By boosting their self-esteem and independence, one can make the elderly patient a more cooperative patient.

Touching and receiving affection are important. A smile, a pat on the arm, and a squeeze of the hand are just as essential as food and shelter. These gestures help to ease the loss of human contact that relocation or death may have brought into the lives of elderly patients.

Patience, caring, and sensitivity are the keys to working with all patients, but especially with the elderly. Respecting the elderly and treating them as adults, not children, is important. By planning an examination with the sonographer's own individual needs in mind, everyone will benefit from the experience.

Multicultural backgrounds

Only recently has the medical community begun to realize the full impact of a patient's culture on his or her recovery. In some cultures, illness is looked on as the will of God or as a punishment for sins. In others, illness is attributed to outside forces.

ETHNICITY

Beliefs about nutrition and dietary practices, illness (its causes and cures), as well as religious beliefs about illness and death, are just as important as special anatomic considerations or disorders specific to a particular cultural group.

In working with patients from other cultures and backgrounds, it is easy to develop cultural biases because of language barriers, physical appearances, or differing religious beliefs and mores. A cultural bias is a tendency to interpret words or actions according to some culturally derived meaning assigned to it. Identifying a cultural bias was once easy because patient populations were relatively homogeneous and people were comfortable doing things *the American way*. Today, however, with the arrival of increasing numbers of immigrants and refugees, America has become more multicultural, more a part of the global village that is our planet. Consequently, sonographers must develop an understanding of multicultural variables and their effects (Box 5-5).

Treatments and cures vary widely from one cultural group to another. Black and Latino cultures have long used roots, potions, and herbs for treating sickness. Some credit the use of charms, amulets, and faith healers with driving away evil spirits. Native American women may not seek early prenatal care because they believe that pregnancy is a natural, normal process. To many multicultural patients, a hospital or clinic is associated with illness and death. Once the sonographer recognizes the roles that cultural differences can play, he or she will begin to understand why former patients may have reacted in a way he or she perceives as inappropriate to his or her concept of "normal."

RELIGION

Religious beliefs about illness can play strong roles in the reactions of Jews, Roman Catholics, Mormons, Christian Scientists, Seventh-Day Adventists, and Jehovah's Witnesses. Such religions may dictate behaviors with wide-ranging impact on the patient's diet; consideration of abortion; or acceptance of medication, treatments, or surgery.

DISTANCE

One evident area of cultural bias concerns the distance people believe is appropriate when communicating and physically interacting with one another. Americans generally divide distance into four zones: intimate, personal, social, and public. Such biases are significant to sonographers because sonography procedures take place within such personal and intimate zones. A patient from another culture might resent being "embraced" by a sonographer who was merely trying to assist him or her onto the scanning table. In contrast, there are cultures in which patients refuse to even speak to a sonographer unless they are literally toe-to-toe and would be offended by a sonographer who unwittingly stepped back or withdrew from them. Patients who regard distances differently expect sonographers to respect their customs.

TIMING

The right time and the correct time are not always synonymous to all patients. Although most American sonographers are compulsively punctual and expect their patients to be the same, in some South American and South African cultures an appropriate amount of tardiness is considered normal. The result is that such patients feel no obligation to apologize for being late. In fact, they would be offended if a sonographer appeared rushed or hurried during their examination and would consider such behavior insulting.

BOX **5-5**   Multicultural Patient Variables

The patient population in the United States is becoming increasingly multicultural. Health care and all of its support systems must develop more cultural awareness and avoid imposing an alien value system on multicultural patients and their personal support system—their families.

VARIABLE	EXPLANATION
Cultural background	Differences and similarities between patient and sonographer
Definitions	Specific cultural definitions and concepts relating to health and the causes of illness and injury
Medical practices	"Folk medicine" or tribal practices
Attitude	Customs and practices regarding health care, relationships, and interactions (e.g., personal space, eye contact, and modesty)
Socioeconomic status	Economic level of patients or family
Environmental factors	Contributing factors such as substandard nutrition and housing that may affect the patient's chief complaint or related disorders
Terminology	Specific names, terms, or slang related to illness (e.g., "bad blood," "proud flesh," "mal ojo")
Language barriers	Differences in language of patient/family and sonography staff
Body concepts	Attitudes regarding nudity/modesty; male-female interactions
Physical/health concepts	Reactions to pain, aging, death, childbirth, abortion, mental retardation, or mental illness
Moral-ethical concepts	Attitudes regarding sexual expression, homosexuality, incest, or illegitimacy
Dietary customs	Religious or cultural concepts about food and how they relate to specific illnesses; dietary taboos
Physical appearance	Attitudes about obesity; adaptability to special therapeutic diets; cleanliness and grooming
Religion	Importance of religious beliefs and practices
Group identity	Importance and type of family structure; traditional male-female roles
Visible differences	Physical differences related to ethnic background (e.g., black, Native American, Oriental)
Inherited conditions	Disorders specific to cultural groups (e.g., sickle cell anemia, Tay-Sachs disease)
Demographics	Number of people belonging to a group in the same geographic area as the health care facility
Prejudices	Within the same cultural group or directed to "outsiders"; stereotyping of other cultural-ethnic groups
Racial-cultural differences	Mixed families: mixed races, religions, or cultural backgrounds

The American concept of "first come, first served" also is alien to cultures in which the oldest or the sickest patients are seen first, or in which the highest-ranking patients or female patients receive preferential treatment.

Cultural biases can be so deep-seated that individuals are not consciously aware that they have them; thus it will take an astute sonographer to recognize and consider such facts when attempting positive patient interactions.

Religious and ethnic mores may play an important role whenever sonographers are asked to perform highly intimate examinations involving the heart or reproductive organs. Male sonographers, in particular, face such biases more frequently than do their female counterparts. If the patient's reluctance to submit to such sonographic examinations cannot be overcome, it may be necessary for the sonographer to call in a chaperone or trade places with a physician or another sonographer of an acceptable gender.

PREJUDICE

Another form of culturally derived bias is prejudice. It may be based on race, ethnicity, sexual orientation, or appearance. A sonographer must be constantly aware of the injurious effects of such discrimination and make every effort to understand the personal biases of patients, as well as his or her own. In some cases, one may even be expected to defuse potentially hostile situations for those who cannot overcome such feelings.

Summary

Providing competent and excellent patient care in today's health care environment has never been more challenging because the majority of patients are either better educated and more demanding or are newcomers to the United States, with differing cultural and religious views on how they should be treated. Today's sonographers must connect with a diverse group of patients and meet their needs while competently and efficiently carrying out their diagnostic studies.

Patients expect their care to be reliable . . . to get what has been promised to them. They expect prompt responses to their requests. Patients want assurances that everything will be all right while they are under a sonographer's care, especially if they are subjected to unfamiliar or threatening procedures. They expect sonographers to not only be proficient but also empathetic and to focus on them as human beings. Finally, they expect to be cared for in clean, up-to-date, quiet, and efficiently run surroundings.

Most diagnostic medical ultrasound programs do an excellent job of helping students develop good technical skills. However, equal attention must be focused on helping students develop a humanistic approach to dealing with their patients. Additionally, patient care education must continue after graduation. For, regardless of whether the sonographer is a student or a veteran, he or she will never get a *second* chance to make a good *first* impression.

BIBLIOGRAPHY

American Heart Association: *CPR and emergency cardiovascular care*. Available at: *http://www.americanheart.org*.

American Hospital Association: *Patient's bill of rights. Catalog no. 157759, Chicago, 1992*. Available at: *http://www.aha.org*.

American Hospital Association: *The patient care partnership: understanding expectations, rights and responsibilities*. Available at: *http://www.hospitalconnect.com/aha/ptcommunication/partnership/index.html*.

American Red Cross Health and Safety Services. Available at: *http://www.redcross.org/services/hss/*.

Centers for Disease Control: *Standard/Universal Precautions*. Available at: *http://www.cdc.gov*.

Medline Plus Medical Encyclopedia: CPR for infants and children. Available at: *http://www.nlm.nih.gov/medlineplus/encyclopedia.html/ency*.

OSHA: *Bloodborne pathogen standards*. Available at: *http:/www.osha/gov*.

Perry AG, Potter PA: *Clinical nursing skills & techniques, ed 5*, St Louis, 2004, Mosby.

Purtilo R: *Health professional/patient interaction, ed 3*, Philadelphia: 1984, WB Saunders.

Sarver Heart Center CPR Research Group: *Be a lifesaver with continuous chest compression CPR*. Available at: *http://www.heart.arizona.edu/publiced/lifesaver.htm*.

Chapter 6

Communications and Critical Thinking Skills

Learning Objectives

Students who successfully complete this chapter will be able to do the following:

- Define communication and the components necessary for communication to occur.
- Compare and contrast verbal and nonverbal communication
- Identify communication barriers.
- Explain how culture and religion can influence health and illness.
- Discuss various approaches used in communicating with patients who require special assistance.
- List the advantages and disadvantages of sonographer reports including the creation of images (films and tapes) for patient use.

Key Terms

body language

communication barrier

communication triad

nonverbal communication

self-actualization

self-esteem

social conversation

supportive communication

verbal communication

Communication can be defined as exchanging information by sending and receiving messages. True communication, however, involves more, including the ability to receive, interpret, and respond appropriately and clearly to messages. To be effective communicators, sonographers must develop not only communication skills but also the ability to listen and convey interest, compassion, knowledge, and information.

BASIC SURVIVAL NEEDS

According to psychologist Abraham Maslow, the basic needs of humans for survival and functioning are as follows:

- Physical needs
- Safety and security
- Love and belonging
- Self-esteem
- Self-actualization

Maslow arranged these needs from the lowest to highest levels and postulated that lower-level needs must be met before higher-level needs could be achieved. Picturing these needs in the shape of a pyramid, with physical needs forming the base of the pyramid, is helpful (Fig. 6-1).

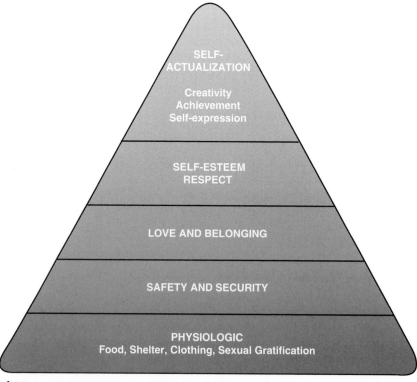

FIGURE **6-1** Maslow's basic needs pyramid concept is best demonstrated in the form of a pyramid constructed of basic needs ranging from the lowest (base) to the highest (apex) levels. Successful performance requires satisfying the lower needs before attempting to satisfy the higher needs.

Physical needs

If sonographers apply these needs to their patients, they identify physical needs as oxygen, water, food, elimination, rest, and shelter. Without sufficient quantities of any of these needs, a patient could die.

Safety and security

Safety and security needs are best defined as protection from danger, harm, and fear. Many patients fear using the health care system. The strange procedures and frightening equipment, having their body subjected to examinations, and the pain and discomfort associated with surrendering themselves to diagnoses and treatments are factors that patients consider. Explaining the following can ease compliance and gain a patient's trust:
- The reason for a procedure
- Who will be doing it
- How it will be performed
- What sensations or feelings to expect

Love and belonging

Humans thrive when they feel love, closeness, affection, belonging, and meaningful relationships with others. Many patients, especially children and the elderly, can be slow to recover or can even die if this need is not being met. Not only family and friends but also members of the health care profession can provide this important need.

Self-esteem

Self-esteem can be defined as belief in one's self. It is achieved only when people feel that others value them. When patients are ill or injured, they may feel that they are not productive or attractive, especially if disease or injury results in amputations or deformities. They lose self-esteem by feeling that they no longer have any value.

Self-actualization

Self-actualization is the ability to experience one's potential. It involves learning, understanding, and setting and reaching goals. As the highest level of need, it is rarely, if ever, met. Fortunately, this need can be postponed without becoming a threat to life. Many people constantly pursue learning and understanding throughout their adult lives. Sonographers have an opportunity to influence patients and to encourage them to learn all that they can about their illness, by providing personal observations and recommending appropriate resources.

COMMUNICATION CHARACTERISTICS

As mentioned earlier, communication can be defined as exchanging information by sending and receiving messages, as well as having the ability to receive, interpret, and respond appropriately and clearly to messages. To be effective communicators, sonographers must develop communication skills and the ability to listen and convey interest, compassion, knowledge, and information.

Several components are required for communication to occur:
- A sender (the originator of the message or idea)
- A message channel (verbal or nonverbal means of transmitting the message or idea)

BOX **6-1**   Effective Patient Communication

> The following suggestions are important in establishing and maintaining good patient communication.
> *Organize* one's thoughts in order to present them in a logical and specific manner.
> *Use common words*, and avoid those that may have more than one meaning.
> *Be concise*, and stay on the subject. Do not wander. Avoid unrelated or unnecessary information.

- A receiver (someone to receive and interpret the message)
- An interaction (feedback that results from the receiver's response)

Communication is successful only when both the sender and receiver understand the message the same way. In effective communication, senders and receivers often use both verbal and nonverbal communication. **Verbal communication** includes the transmission of words in either verbal or written form, whereas **nonverbal communication** consists of eye contact, facial expressions, body movements and posture, tone of voice, and touch. In some instances the message the patient wishes to impart is contradicted by the accompanying nonverbal "expressions." As a worker in the health care profession, the sonographer will find himself or herself involved in many types of communication and the need to properly assess and understand it (Box 6-1).

Social conversation is an automatic type of communication that people use out of habit. Usually consisting of polite or friendly exchanges of factual or social information (chitchat), such conversation is superficial and flows easily from one topic to another. Social conversation does not provide significant information, identify problems, or result in solutions. Nevertheless, social conversation is important in establishing a relationship with patients and creating a climate of **supportive communication**.

Supportive communication is more goal oriented and information bearing than social conversation. Important patient information is discussed—how patients feel—and any problems that concern them can be shared. The purpose of supportive communication is to help relieve patient anxiety, anger, or frustration and to learn about any unmet patient needs. By talking through such concerns, the sonographer can often to help patients resolve their problems. However, supportive communication can be successful only if the sonographer really understands the patient and assists that understanding by means of the following skills:

- *Listening:* Listening carefully to the *message,* as well as the words the patient is speaking, is important.
- *Observing:* The most important facet of any nonverbal communications is the awareness of the true message that the patient may be sending. Sometimes this type of communication is more accurate than the verbal message. For example, when patients are eager to communicate, they maintain eye contact. Lack of eye contact often represents uncomfortable emotions such as anxiety, depression, and embarrassment. **Body language** in the form of yawning, drumming the fingers, shrugging the shoulders, or rolling the eyes sends the message *"I am uncomfortable," "I would rather not be here,"* or *"Hurry up!"* Sonographers must be sensitive to the feelings that patients express by both words and actions.
- *Responding appropriately:* When a listener exhibits attentiveness and interest, patients feel more at ease in talking about their problems and concerns. Anything a sonographer says

to the patient should relate to what the patient has just told the sonographer, either verbally or nonverbally. Providing feedback encourages patients to keep talking about their concerns until they have talked them out or reached some decisions.

- *Maintaining silence:* Sonographers should allow patients and themselves to be silent in order to give patients the chance to decide what to say or not to say. The sonographer should evaluate the silence. Is it heavy, sad, tense, or comfortable? Silence can also mean that a patient does not want to talk anymore. Sonographers must impress on their patients that this is all right, too.
- *Clarifying:* Sonographers should check the statements they heard or the cues they observed to be sure they understand their patients. Patients' knowledge that their sonographer understands their communication is important. Sonographers should avoid ambiguity because it creates communication problems.
- *Repeating:* Repeating ideas or statements the patient has communicated serves to clarify the message and allows patients to change their minds or reinforce their viewpoints.
- *Gathering information:* The sonographer should attempt to obtain as much information about patients as possible by asking questions that are open ended and cannot be answered with a simple yes or no response.
- *Summarizing:* By verbally listing or reviewing the ideas that patients express, the sonographer allows them to take a more objective look at their comments. This can be especially helpful with patients who have difficulty making decisions.
- *Accepting:* Patients should be encouraged to express negative feelings or thoughts even if the sonographer disagrees. The sonographer must realize that he or she can appear judgmental.
- *Touching:* A pat on the shoulder or touches on the hand are nonverbal gestures of support. The sonographer should be sure that the patient does not have any objections to being touched.

COMMUNICATION FACTORS

Barriers

Anything that interferes with the communication process constitutes a barrier. Both verbal and nonverbal barriers exist, and they can be communicated by either senders or receivers. One common **communication barrier** is that of talking too fast. Using slang, medical vocabulary, or broad generalizations can also make it difficult for the receiver to know what the sender is trying to say.

Sonographers must avoid "talking down" to patients or speaking in hostile or insulting tones. Such behavior makes patients defensive and unable to understand messages. Strong feelings such as anger or prejudice toward the person who is speaking can also cause misunderstanding of what is being said. Listeners often miss parts, or all, of a message when they are distracted by their concern about their problems. Labeling patients as "complainers" or "disoriented" only encourages listeners to ignore or misunderstand what these patients are saying.

Language can be a communication barrier if the sender and receiver speak different languages. The sonographer should keep in mind that smiling is a universal language technique and use hand signals if possible. If the sonographer tries to speak a few words in the other person's language, it will be appreciated and will gain cooperation.

Cutting off communication

Whenever a listener prevents a conversation from starting or continuing, or moving from a social to a supportive level, the communication is cut off. Common reasons why listeners do this are embarrassment, feeling threatened, or distrust of the sender. Such tactics may be conscious or subconscious. The following examples are responses that will stop or cut off communication:

- *Judgmental responses.* Telling patients they should not feel angry or afraid or that there are people in worse situations only leave the patient feeling guilty or ashamed for complaining.
- *Arguing.* Debating with patients instead of learning what they are thinking is counter-productive.
- *Solving.* The sonographer should avoid offering advice or answers before patients have the chance to think of their own solutions.
- *Interrupting.* Cutting off patients before they have a chance to have their say puts the sonographer at risk of receiving only part of the message and giving an inappropriate response.
- *Changing the subject.* Patients feel that a sonographer does not want to listen to him or her when the sonographer deliberately changes the subject before a topic is completed.
- *Distractions.* Sonographers must guard against showing by body language or behavior that they are disinterested.
- *False assurances.* Kidding or falsely cheering patients out of a situation only makes the sonographer feel more comfortable. It deprives the patient of working through a problem and possibly finding solutions or making decisions.
- *Untruthfulness.* The sonographer should never fabricate or construct excuses to avoid confronting patients with unpleasant news.
- *Evasion.* The sonographer should not focus patients' attention on their signs or symptoms simply to reassure them or to avoid being questioned about whether they are going to die.
- *Avoidance.* The sonographer should not redirect patient questions to someone else, thereby indicating that he or she cannot or will not answer.
- *False reassurance.* The sonographer should avoid telling patients not to worry—that everything will be all right—just to prevent them from talking about their fears. The sonographer really does not know that everything will be fine. By saying these things, he or she may prevent patients from working through their fears or working out solutions to their problems. Instead, the sonographer should show respect for patients by a willingness to listen without judgment to their concerns and feelings. Correct information that is as true and as factual as possible should be given. If the sonographer does not know the facts or is not free to discuss them, he or she should find someone who is authorized to give that information. The sonographer's patients must trust their honesty.

Exploring attitudes and feelings

A patient's physical state (e.g., being tired, cold, rested) or emotional state (e.g., being sad, happy, confident) can greatly affect the ability to carry on with supportive communication. Both sonographers and patients can be affected. A sonographer who does not feel well may become irritated by the patient's behavior and not really listen to—or may even avoid— the patient. When patients do not feel well, they often become angry or stubborn. In such instances it is helpful to realize that this may not be the right time to work out a problem. If the sonographer becomes aware that this is happening, he or she should take a break, seek help, and try to be careful about what is said. Strong negative emotions such as anger and crying are particularly difficult to handle in such circumstances.

The sonographer should realize that these same situations can occur with co-workers, family, or friends. When problems cannot be resolved, when the sonographer senses hard feelings or anger among coworkers, when the sonographer cannot seem to communicate with a supervisor, he or she should step back and evaluate the situation. The sonographer should examine what happens when he or she talks to others and how the sonographer feels about him or herself and the other person. The sonographer can use the same techniques of developing supportive communication with patients to help communicate effectively with coworkers, family, and friends.

PATIENTS WITH SPECIAL COMMUNICATION PROBLEMS

The ability to communicate relies heavily on the five senses, especially hearing, seeing, and touching. Patients who cannot hear or see not only have difficulty communicating but also may become confused. When working with patients with any sensory losses, sonographers should plan to use the patient's remaining senses to their fullest.

In working with elderly or hospitalized patients, the sonographer may encounter confusion. The causes of the patient's confusion may range from too little stimulation of the patient's five senses to physical causes such as too little oxygen, poor nutrition or fluid intake, medications, or infections. The following material offers suggestions on working with patients who have experienced a loss of hearing or eyesight, who have speech disorders, or who are confused or disoriented.

Hearing-impaired patients

If the sonographer's department has a sign language interpreter, he or she can arrange for that person to be present to speak directly to the hearing-impaired patient. If no sign language interpreter is available, the sonographer can do the following:
- Determine if the patient is using any hearing aids. Then, face the patient directly and on the same level if possible. Use facial expression, body gestures, and touch to enhance communication.
- Speak in a normal fashion without shouting. Be sure that the light is not shining in the eyes of a patient who is trying to read lips.
- Reduce background noises when carrying on conversations with the hard-of-hearing patient. Do not eat or chew anything while talking.
- Be sure to get the patient's attention before speaking. Never talk from another room.
- If the patient has difficulty understanding something, find another way of saying the same thing rather than repeating the original words.
- Use a pad and pencil whenever necessary. Consider learning sign language as a personal goal if deaf and hard-of-hearing patients constitute a significant portion of one's patient population.

Visually impaired patients

The sonographer can follow these guidelines:
- Determine whether the patient wears any prescribed corrective lenses. Always treat the patient's glasses with care if they must be removed during the examination. To prevent scratches, never place the glass side directly on a hard surface.

- When ambulating or transferring patients, have them hold on to an arm while leading the way. Visually impaired patients will sense the sonographer's movements but must be warned of any steps or hazards.
- Use touch and tone of voice to help communicate with the patient.
- Ask blind patients how they are used to doing things for themselves and then allow them to continue unless their actions would interfere with their safety.

Speech-impaired patients

The sonographer can follow these guidelines:
- Encourage patients to express themselves through any means possible. To improve their speaking ability, patients must try to talk, write, and read as much as possible, even if they make mistakes.
- Keep patients a part of the social world by talking while performing their examination. Encourage coworkers to do so, also.
- If the patient has difficulty understanding communication, be sure to stand where visible and speak slowly and clearly in a normal tone of voice. Use common vocabulary and short, simple sentences. Give directions or requests in a simple manner, repeating or rephrasing the directions as necessary. Use simple gestures or pantomime for clarification.
- For patients who have difficulty speaking, provide ample time for them to organize what they want to say. Do not hurry or pressure them. Watch for clues or gestures if the patient's speech cannot be understood.
- Be patient. Becoming upset only adds to the patient's frustration. Assist patients with words they cannot say, but do not speak for them. Give them a chance to try to say the words.
- Do not treat patients as children. Respect them as the adults they are.
- Use supportive communication (verbal or nonverbal) to help patients handle the frustration and anxiety that they may feel.
- Never speak with another sonographer or staff member in front of patients as if they were not there.

Confused or disoriented patients

The sonographer can follow these guidelines:
- Keep talking to confused patients and try to get through to them. Do not label them confused and then ignore them. Confusion may be greater at some times than others; therefore it is important to talk with the patients and to communicate acceptance and security by verbal and nonverbal means.
- Listen and try to understand what patients are trying to communicate.
- Use reality orientation to help patients interact with the world around them. Such techniques are based on sensory stimulation by identifying what is happening around them and clarifying who they are (e.g., time of day, day of the week).
- Keep the environment calm to avoid overwhelming the patient with too many people or too much confusion.
- Talk face-to-face with the patient using short, simple sentences. Ask only one question (or give one direction) at a time, and allow ample time for a response. Try to keep the patient from looking away. Be sure to clarify what is happening.
- Praise and encourage a patient's abilities to cooperate with instruction. Encourage as much independence as possible to help them feel better about themselves.

- Use supportive communication to help patients when they get frustrated, anxious, or depressed. A gentle, caring attitude helps support the patient during periods of extreme confusion.
- Remember that patients in restraints may become confused if they cannot interact with their surroundings.
- Provide the patient with correct information. Do not support patients' confused beliefs or behavior. Correct them gently, however, with supportive communication, and do not argue with patients who continue to be confused.

COMMUNICATION TRIADS

A **communication triad** is a creative technique that can be effective in solving communication problems. This triad involves three people who agree to work together to promote understanding through communication.

Communication triads can be effective in both patient and the employee/employer information exchanges. In employment situations the presence of an employee, a supervisor, and an administrator or another employee can strengthen the power of an individual with unequal resources. The technique is effective to review information, assure understanding, and explain a decision. It is also helpful in supporting or verifying behavior and can actually block manipulation.

In the patient sector, sonographers can invite the participation of a family member to create a triad. This is particularly useful when patients are anxious and need support or when patients do not understand the sonographer's instructions because of language, cognitive, or cultural reasons. The triad is a useful way of providing support and reassurance to the patient because it can involve explaining a complex procedure in two different ways.

In situations in which a language barrier exists, if a family member is unavailable, the third person forming the triad could be an interpreter who speaks the patient's language. The person chosen for this task must be knowledgeable not only about the culture involved but also the sonographic procedure as well. Differences in language, culture, and class must all be considered whenever interpreters are used.

A communication triad should be avoided at times. In the case of the employee/employer situation, the employee's anxiety level may be so high that a one-on-one session is more productive. This is also important when the topic of discussion requires confidentiality.

In the patient/sonographer setting, communication triads are inappropriate if the sonographer has been given information in confidence. Even if the information is critical, the patient should be asked for permission before involving a third party. To clarify, the sonographer might say one of the following:
- "Do you mind if I tell your family member what you have told me?"
- "You might be able to help my patient understand what needs to be done in order to complete this procedure. May I have your help?"
- "You may wish to discuss this privately; however, I am here if you want my help."

In some cases, it may be more important to communicate with the family member in private than to do so in front of the patient. The sonographer should know as much history and clinical information as possible about the patient is important before making this judgment.

Another consideration is the amount of additional time it takes to create and complete a communication triad. If the third party is waiting in the reception area, it is not a problem;

however, if the third party must be summoned from a distance, the benefits of waiting must be weighed carefully.

PROFESSIONAL COMMUNICATION

Health care coworkers

Among the communications that are vital to patient/interdepartmental interaction are the following:
- Participation in team conferences, grand rounds, in-service training, departmental meetings
- Interviewing patients
- Instructing patients and their families
- Reporting the patient's sonographic findings to other members of the health care team
- Recording information in daily logs, charts, and files

Whether a sonographer is hospital-based or office-based, he or she is often asked to communicate by telephone. When doing so, the sonographer should be sure to give his or her name and department identification and ask for the same information from the calling or called party.

Calls should be answered promptly. This is especially important in the health care arena because the next call might be an emergency.

Good telephone etiquette should always be observed. The sonographer should take and deliver messages promptly. He or she should never cover the receiver and continue a conversation with someone else. Callers usually hear what is being said.

When asked to schedule patients, the sonographer should be polite and thoroughly explain any necessary patient preparations. He or she should be fair in awarding the patient the first possible opening and be accommodating if other tests or treatments conflict with the selected appointment time.

Sonographer reports

To contribute to the patient's diagnosis in a professional way, sonographers often are asked to provide written or verbal reports. As trained observers of the interaction of ultrasound transmission and reflection characteristics within the human body, they should be prepared to discuss their technical findings. When properly used, sonographer reports serve as aids to diagnosis by documenting normal measurements and by drawing attention to any unusual findings that might indicate the presence of disease and a need for additional examination.

Sonographer reports should be limited to providing measurements; comments on the echogenicity and location of normal and abnormal structures; and any unusual patient positions, scanning planes, or changes in instrumentation that were required to complete the examination.

The use of written sonographer "impressions" is especially warranted in situations in which the interpretation of the sonographic examinations occurs without the sonographer's presence (e.g., after normal hours or in a distant locale). One of the values of recording these impressions is the availability of written documentation in the event that a case is ever questioned. Sonographer reports also serve a teaching function when follow-up data about the patient's final diagnosis and treatment are obtained and compared with the sonography findings.

Unfortunately, there also are negative aspects regarding sonographer reports. There is a real possibility that these technical impressions may be construed as diagnostic statements. This usually happens when the referring physician demands an instant "diagnosis" or preliminary report instead of waiting for the interpreting physician's findings. The potential for abuse also exists if the sonographer's impressions are used verbatim by physicians with little or no training in the interpretation of sonographic images. In addition, serious ethical and legal implications surround the practice of sonographers communicating their impressions directly to the patient or the patient's family.

To retain the advantages and to minimize the negative aspects of sonographer reports, the ultrasound facility should draw up and publish policies to guide its sonographers in these situations. These policies should establish exactly what type of information (e.g., gender identification, estimated fetal age, number of fetuses, fetal viability) sonographers are permitted to disclose and to whom (referring physicians, patients, or family members) the disclosures may be made. The facility should then alert all house staff members and referring physicians to the new policies and the reasons validating their adoption.

Videotaping obstetric examinations

One of the most controversial sonographic issues is the practice of providing patients with videotapes or Polaroid images of fetal ultrasound examinations or Polaroid images of their fetus. Just as ultrasound has become more technologically sophisticated, so too have the patients in their appreciation and understanding of imaging devices and the content of sonograms.

Proponents of videotaping for parents and family members are quick to point out that this practice enhances fetal bonding, educates both patients and family members, and increases patient acceptance of sonography. Those who oppose providing images for patient use believe that the practice extends scanning time and patient exposure and, more important, that it distracts the sonographer's concentration and teeters on the brink of commercialization.

If videotapes of obstetric examinations are provided to patients in the sonographer's institution, the following recommendations should be considered:

- A written policy should be established for providing patients with hard-copy images of their sonography examination.
- A specific time should be set aside to create a tape for the patient's use. Preferably, this should occur after completion of the diagnostic examination.
- Nothing should appear on the patient's photographs or tape that was not seen on the diagnostic study or survey.
- The supervising physician must be aware of the examination results and should review the patient's photographs or videotape before they are released to the patient. The physician should exercise the right to deny the tape or photographs for patient use if any abnormality is found or suspected.

With the introduction of 3-D and 4-D ultrasound, a growing number of businesses have opened throughout the United States for the sole purpose of providing expectant patients with video and still images of their fetuses. These businesses do not provide a diagnostic service and often use untrained personnel with only several days of "training" to perform the imaging tasks. Furthermore, even when they do hire trained and registered sonographers, the sonograms created are neither prescribed nor read by a licensed physician.

BOX **6-2**   The Society of Diagnostic Medical Sonography's Position on the Nondiagnostic Use of Ultrasound

---

NONDIAGNOSTIC USE OF ULTRASOUND

Diagnostic medical sonography is a medical procedure that is requested by a physician (or a designated health care provider), performed by a sonographer, and interpreted by a physician. It is a diagnostic procedure often used to examine a developing fetus for abnormalities.

A number of private businesses have opened for the sole purpose of providing expectant parents with images of the developing fetus on videocassette or other methods of record. Because the service is provided for entertainment purposes only, it is considered nondiagnostic. The use of 2-D, 3-D, or 4-D ultrasound to only view the fetus, obtain a picture of the fetus, or determine the fetal gender without a medical indication is inappropriate and, in the view of the Society of Diagnostic Medical Sonography (SDMS), contrary to responsible medical practice. Although there are no confirmed biologic effects on patients caused by exposures from present diagnostic ultrasound instruments, the possibility exists that such biologic effects may be identified in the future.

The SDMS recognizes the responsibility it has to its members, the health care community, and patients. Diagnostic medical sonographers are committed to act in the best interest of their patients, to maintain ethical standards to preserve and promote professionalism, and to the use of ultrasound as a diagnostic procedure. Therefore the SDMS opposes the use of ultrasound solely for entertainment purposes.

Approved by SDMS Board of Directors, October 13, 2004.

Modified from Society of Diagnostic Medical Sonography, Plano, Tex, 1999-2005.

The Society of Diagnostic Medical Sonographers and most major professional organizations have issued strong position statements regarding the creation of "keepsake" videotapes using diagnostic medical ultrasound (Box 6-2).

In addition, the U.S. Food and Drug Administration has declared that production of "keepsake" fetal videos is an unapproved use of ultrasound equipment. Also, individuals who promote, sell, or lease the ultrasound equipment may be in violation of state or local laws and regulations for exposing people to ultrasound devices without a physician's order.

THE GRIEVING PROCESS

Everyone knows that eventually they will die. Obviously, people have different views about death based on their backgrounds, past experiences, and religious beliefs. Because the sonographer deals with dying patients or those in danger of losing a pregnancy, it is important to explore personal feelings about death to better understand patients' feelings. The grieving process has been defined as stages of behavior that people experience when a loss occurs. Elisabeth Kubler-Ross, a Swiss-born physician, worked extensively with dying patients and described the following stages of grief as follows:

- Stage 1—denial and isolation
- Stage 2—anger
- Stage 3—bargaining
- Stage 4—depression
- Stage 5—acceptance

The grieving process often takes a considerable period of time, and passage through it may not always go smoothly or in the "proper" order. Some persons do not experience each stage and may skip one, whereas others may go through more than one stage at a time. Some patients move back and forth between the stages, feeling that the pain and stress will never go away. Regardless of the individual patient's reaction, it is important that the sonographer treat each one in a supportive manner, with dignity and compassion.

Denial and isolation

The denial or isolation stage occurs for all patients and is characterized by the *"No, not me— it must be some mistake"* attitude. The person believes that a diagnostic error has been made and seeks other opinions. The refusal to believe this is happening creates a buffer, protecting the individual from shocking news that is too difficult to handle. Denial provides time for people to collect themselves and to prepare their resources.

Some patients may isolate themselves from those who do not allow them to deny the seriousness of their illness, whereas others try to hide their feelings of sadness or fear by assuming a false front or cheerful attitude. Mood swings from high hopes to despair prevail. One reaction is patients' need to talk about and explain what has happened—making up excuses and reasons for their loss or illness—but not really believing it. Sonographers should encourage these patients to talk about their feelings to allow denial of reality and isolation. Encouraging a supportive family member to be present during the patient examinations and transfers is helpful. Because denial or repression is a defense mechanism, the sonographer must be sure that he or she has fully assessed the patient's condition and carefully thought out an approach before engaging the patient in conversation.

Anger

This *"why me?"* stage is difficult for everyone to deal with because of the tendency to displace anger in all directions. Patients at this stage make unreasonable demands or levy unjust criticism at everyone participating in their care. They blame those around them (family, friends, and hospital staff) for their condition and may be dissatisfied with everything a sonographer does. In these ways, patients are able to express their feelings of losing control over their lives. It is essential to remain patient and try to be understanding, by allowing the patient to "act out" feelings. This is not the time to try to divert the patient with humor or cheerfulness. It is a time to carefully explain the nature of the sonographic procedure to avoid patient fear or suspicion. If patients at this stage are given extra attention and a chance to verbalize or act out their anger, they soon become more reasonable and have fewer angry demands.

Another reaction is for patients to display paranoid feelings that staff members are against them or want to hurt them. Not reacting as if the patient is personally attacking the sonographer is important. The sonographer should simply understand that through this behavior patients can unload the intense and often painful feelings they are experiencing.

Bargaining

As patients begin to accept their condition, they may try to bargain with God, attempting to postpone the inevitable. They may want to be rewarded for good behavior by having special favors granted, or they may cling to life until a special event has been experienced. It is in this state of mind that some patients desperately try alternative or "quack" treatments. Sonographers should allow these patients to talk about their bargains with God and share the patient's requests and actions with staff members.

Depression

Depression is encountered when patients finally realize the reality of their loss. Overwhelming sadness and sorrow usually occur, causing patients to cry, lose interest in their surroundings, and become silent and withdrawn.

The sonographer should let these patients express sorrow and feel sad. Encouragement and reassurance do not help patients at this stage, and cheerfulness only distracts them and cuts off their feelings. The sonographer should be willing to sit quietly, encouraging the patient to talk about his or her feelings and expressing his or her own feelings with words of empathy or a simple, caring touch.

Acceptance

With the stage of acceptance, patients are at peace once more and thinking more clearly. Although patients still may not understand the reasons for their condition or believe that they should die, they may want to talk about dying and ask questions.

This is not a joyful stage. It is instead a controlled stage in which intense feelings are absent. Energy and interest decrease, and the patient needs the support and company of family and friends. At this point patients need to be told that it is all right to say nothing, to *"just be."* Appropriate physical touching may replace mere words, so the sonographer should be willing to sit quietly with patients at this stage and hold their hand or stroke their hair.

Throughout all the stages, the belief that things can get better exists. Hope helps maintain patients through their suffering, and patients should be encouraged to have hope even if it seems unrealistic at times.

Working with patients who ask if they are dying is one of the most difficult things for health professionals to handle. Although the sonographer may not know the answer to the question, or even what the patient has been told, he or she must resist the temptation to change the subject or tell the patient not to worry. Answers to questions about dying should be, *"What makes you say that?"* or *"Did your doctor tell you that?"* It is simply not the sonographer's responsibility to tell patients that they are dying or to give them factual information that has been gleaned from their chart or the nursing staff. The sonographer should acknowledge that such fears are upsetting. Then, after providing a chance to talk, the sonographer should ask if the patient would like to speak with his or her physician or nurse because the sonographer has no additional information. He or she should report the patient's concerns and requests. Above all, the sonographer should not leave the patient alone with no one to talk to.

Summary

The accurate communication of information is critical in today's hectic health care environment, whether the communication involves patients or coworkers. In many programs, too little attention to this facet of sonography is given in preparing students to enter the clinical environment.

A great deal of negativity is present in the medical environment; nevertheless, when working among so much illness, good sonographers manage to maintain a warm, genuine smile and an honest, compassionate approach in everything they do. The benefits are many, but most importantly, maintaining such a personality can open the channels of communication and ultimately help patients along their road to recovery.

Positive attitudes are contagious. However, it is difficult to remain positive when a patient is suffering while the sonographer performs his or her examination. The sonographer will experience feelings of helplessness but must remind himself or herself that everything is being done to make this person as comfortable as possible and that this person's needs are being responded to as best as possible at this time. If the patient demonstrates a good sense of humor, the sonographer should "be there" with him or her. If the patient is crying and depressed, the sonographer should try to remain empathetic and, above all, listen.

Interestingly, the common denominator among many elderly patients is that, whether at work or play, they appear happy. They laugh at their personal flaws and accept life the way it is, sometimes even in the face of intractable illness.

Sonographers can have a profound impact on the patients entrusted to their care. By proper communication techniques, sonographers can gain a patient's confidence and cooperation. How sonographers handle their responsibilities can have a direct bearing on the patient's journey to recovery or the patient's lack of progress.

To effectively serve and help patients and colleagues, sonographers must understand that each person has fears, needs, and rights.

At issue are the positive and negative aspects of patient and interdepartmental communications, as well as some of the perplexing issues involving sonographer reports and keepsake videotaping, and possible solutions to those issues.

BIBLIOGRAPHY

Craig M: Family-centered sonography, *J Diagn Med Sonography* 2:96-103, 1986.

Craig M: The challenge of patient interaction, *J Diagn Med Sonography* 3:147-150, 1987.

Craig M: The eternal controversy: sonographer's reports, *J Diagn Med Sonography* 3:244-248, 1987.

Craig M: Baby videos: a boon or a liability? *J Diagn Med Sonography* 4:19-22, 1988.

Craig M: Treating patients with patience, *J Diagn Med Sonography* 1:16-18, 1989.

Craig M: Controversies in obstetric and gynecologic ultrasound. In *Diagnostic medical sonography: a guide to clinical practice, vol 1: obstetrics and gynecology,* edited by Mimi C. Berman, Ph,D., RDMS, Philadelphia, 1991, JB Lippincott.

Food and Drug Administration Consumer Information: *Fetal keepsake videos.* Available at: *http://www.fda.gov/cdrh/consumer/fetalvideos.html.*

Kubler-Ross E: *Death: the final stage of growth,* Englewood Cliffs, N.J., 1975, Prentice-Hall.

Maslow AH: *Motivation and personality,* Upper Saddle River, N.J., 1987, Prentice-Hall.

Clinical Assessments and Sonographic Procedures

Learning Objectives

Students who successfully complete this chapter will be able to do the following:

1. List the major specialty sonographic examinations.
2. Describe and demonstrate the standard patient positions relative to sonographic imaging.
3. Discuss patient preparations for abdominal, obstetric-gynecologic, and cardiac sonography.
4. Describe the basic components of the three major specialty-scanning protocols.
5. Identify the findings and normal values of laboratory tests related to abdominal and obstetric sonography.

Key Terms

alpha fetoprotein assay

amniotic fluid index (AFI)

chorionic villus sampling (CVS)

dobutamine

glutaraldehyde

hormone replacement therapy

human chorionic gonadotropin (HCG)

modified Fowler position

percutaneous umbilical blood sampling

picture archiving and communication systems (PACS)

radiology information systems (RTS)

tamoxifen

transesophageal echocardiography (TEE)

transthoracic echocardiography (TTE)

transvaginal/ endovaginal sonography (TVS/EVS)

Trendelenburg position

Organizing patients into groups such as medical-surgical, obstetric, pediatric, geriatric, or psychiatric is common medical practice. In sonography, it is also common to categorize sonographic examinations by the clinical area or specialty to which they correspond.

Initially, sonographers were expected to perform all of the existing forms of specialty examinations. As the field expanded and sophisticated equipment and techniques were developed, however, this "jack of all trades" concept changed. Today most sonographers choose to specialize in one or more of the following clinically identified examinations:

abdominal sonography

breast sonography

cardiac sonography (adult, pediatric, fetal)

gynecologic sonography

high-resolution sonography (superficial structures, intraoperative techniques)

neurosonography

obstetric sonography

ophthalmologic sonography

vascular sonography

This chapter focuses on the three most widely practiced diagnostic ultrasound specialties: abdominal sonography, obstetric and gynecologic sonography, and cardiac sonography.

Many of these specialty examinations are associated with additional laboratory tests (see Appendix B).

For complete descriptions of sonographic competencies and goals, the SDMS publication *The Sonography Clinical Assessment Notebook (SCAN)* is highly recommended for students, instructors, and working sonographers. Regularly updated, *The SCAN* is a valuable compendium of specialty information that also serves as a logbook documenting sonographers' development and proficiencies. The completed *SCAN* is a record of an individual learner's clinical competency and professionalism (Fig. 7-1).

The SCAN contains specialty-specific master proficiency lists and performance objectives, guidelines, clinical evaluation forms, and logbook forms to document satisfactory mastery of specific scanning objectives.

SCANNING TECHNIQUE

The major goal of sonographers is to master proper sonographic techniques to ensure the production of high-quality diagnostic sonograms and minimal patient discomfort. To acquire proficiency in performing sonographic examinations, it is understood that a sonographer must possess an adequate knowledge of anatomy, disease processes, and sonographic data (Box 7-1).

The evolution of today's high-resolution 2-D, 3-D, and 4-D real-time equipment, however, requires sonographers to bring much more than a systematic approach to scanning if they are to avoid missing or overlooking adjacent or associated pathologic conditions. It is no longer sufficient to simply manipulate transducers, make measurements, and record images. Competent sonographers are also expected to have an excellent understanding of common diseases and to recognize any situation that calls for unusual views or patient preparations. In addition, they are required to skillfully compile clinically relevant data through chart reviews, obtaining additional history and physical data if necessary and communicating (in verbal or written form) their observations of the manner in which ultrasound energy penetrated and reflected back from the patient's tissues.

Clinical Evaluation Form

Student's Name _____ **Evaluation Period (Dates)** _____

Facility's Name _____

Days Absent _____ **Reason(s) for Absence(s)** _____

Number of Days Made Up _____ **Supervising Sonographer** _____

Identify the student's strengths and weaknesses in the following areas:

1. Professional Qualities:

2. Scanning Competencies:

3. Image Evaluation

Sign to indicate discussion of this evaluation:

_____   _____
Student's Signature   Date

_____   _____
Supervising Sonographer's Signature   Date

FIGURE **7-1** *The SCAN* Clinical Evaluation Form.

(*Continued*)

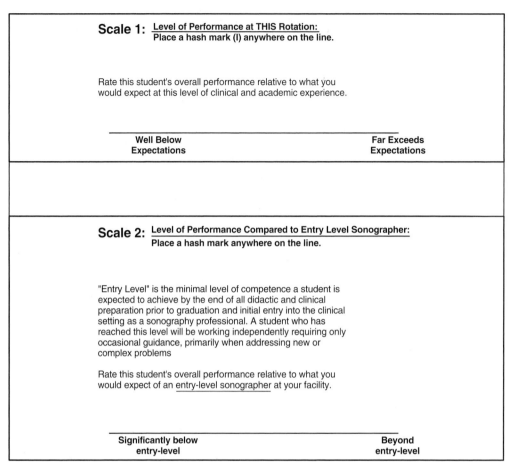

Scale 1: <u>Level of Performance at THIS Rotation:</u>
Place a hash mark (I) anywhere on the line.

Rate this student's overall performance relative to what you would expect at this level of clinical and academic experience.

| Well Below | Far Exceeds |
| Expectations | Expectations |

Scale 2: <u>Level of Performance Compared to Entry Level Sonographer:</u>
Place a hash mark anywhere on the line.

"Entry Level" is the minimal level of competence a student is expected to achieve by the end of all didactic and clinical preparation prior to graduation and initial entry into the clinical setting as a sonography professional. A student who has reached this level will be working independently requiring only occasional guidance, primarily when addressing new or complex problems

Rate this student's overall performance relative to what you would expect of an <u>entry-level sonographer</u> at your facility.

| Significantly below | Beyond |
| entry-level | entry-level |

FIGURE **7-1** Cont'd

BOX **7-1** Routine Duties

The following routine duties are associated with performing any specialty diagnostic ultrasound examinations.
- Confirm that the patient's preparation (fasting or hydrating stomach or bladder) has been carried out.
- Question the patient regarding his or her medical history.
- List present medications.
- Document laboratory data: be aware of and include normal values and the function of any pertinent laboratory tests.
- Review and compare prior ultrasound or other diagnostic tests.

Society of Diagnostic Medical Sonographers Educational Foundation. THE SCAN (Sonography Clinical Notebook). 2003, Educational Foundation. Dallas, Texas.

As a sonographer progresses through training, he or she receives in-depth instructions on how to perform correct sonographic examinations of the many organs and systems of the body. What follows here should be considered a simple introduction to those complex activities, which, along with continuing study and personal experience, will expand the sonographer's potential and value as a respected member of the diagnostic team.

SONOGRAPHIC POSITIONING

An important part of performing sonography examinations involves correctly positioning the patient and knowing when a position change can enhance the visualization of an area of interest. Figure 7-2 depicts the patient positions most commonly used in sonography.

Supine

This position is also referred to as the *dorsal recumbent position.* The patient lies on his or her back with head and upper shoulders slightly elevated to provide comfort and maintain the natural curve of the spine at the neck. A small pillow placed under the knees serves to relieve pressure on the patient's back. The patient's arms should be positioned at the side or across the chest.

For examinations of the upper portion of the abdomen, the patient's right arm is elevated to expand the rib spaces to their fullest. This permits placement of small, narrow-faced transducers within the intercostal spaces and improves both transmission and reflection of the sound beam by eliminating rib artifacts.

Lateral

The patient lies on his or her side with arms positioned in front. The dependent arm may be elevated toward the head, and the other arm crossed over the chest. The dependent leg

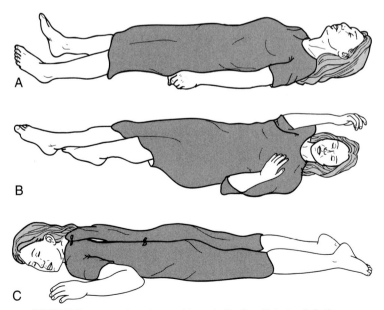

FIGURE **7-2** Primary imaging positions. **A,** Supine. **B,** Lateral. **C,** Prone.

should be straight, and the other leg should cross over so that the knee comes to rest on the tabletop, supporting the patient.

Prone

The patient lies on his or her abdomen, arms flexed at either side or elevated alongside the head to widen the intercostal spaces. A small pad or pillow placed under the patient's head, abdomen, and lower legs serves to relieve pressure. The patient's feet should extend off the scanning table.

Several position variations may be indicated during the course of an examination. These include the upright, modified Fowler, and Trendelenburg positions (Fig. 7-3).

Upright position

The patient sits on the edge of the scanning table, right arm elevated above the head, left arm and hand providing support. This position is helpful in scanning a gallbladder in an extremely high position under the rib cage.

Modified Fowler position

The **modified Fowler position** is useful in advanced pregnancy when elevation of the patient's head and upper portion of the back is necessary to avoid vena caval hypotension. The head of the patient's bed or table is elevated 18 to 20 inches above level; the patient's knees are also elevated.

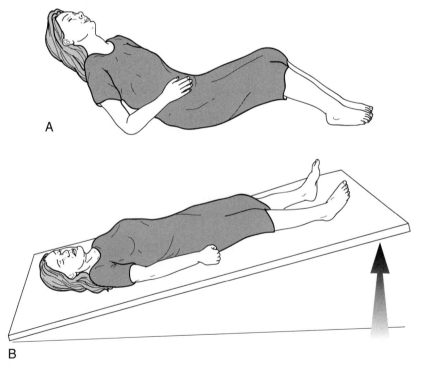

FIGURE **7-3** Secondary imaging positions. **A,** Modified Fowler position: head elevated approximately 25 degrees. Knees slightly flexed. **B,** Trendelenburg position: patient's pelvis positioned higher than her head.

Trendelenburg position

In the **Trendelenburg position**, the head of the patient's table or bed is tilted downward 30 to 40 degrees, and the table or bed is angled beneath the knees to elevate the patient's pelvis. A pelvic elevation of 20% to 30% can be achieved by tilting the lower portion of a scanning table or with the use of pillows or foam bolsters. This position is used whenever fetal parts obscure the lower uterine segment or the fetal lie prevents suitable imaging of the fetal head.

ROUTINE DUTIES

Regardless of what type of ultrasound setting a sonographer works in or what types of examinations are provided, there are regular duties (see Box 7-1) to ensure that the ultrasound laboratory is run smoothly and efficiently:

- Perform quality assurance tests on a regular basis
- Prepare and cleanse all transducers
- Order necessary supplies
- Check the patient schedule daily to obtain any prior ultrasound studies or other diagnostic test results for each scheduled patient
- Record, generate, distribute, and archive appropriate images
- Create/maintain a teaching file

Quality assurance testing

Basic tests of the equipment should be performed on a regular basis and the results recorded in an equipment log or notebook. The areas for testing include instrument sensitivity evaluation, image photography uniformity, and vertical/horizontal measurement accuracy.

Transducer preparation and care

Transducers should be mechanically cleansed with an enzymatic cleanser between patient studies, and before use. They should be cleansed with either a disinfectant or through a sterilization process. When using a disinfecting agent (e.g., alcohol, phenolic solutions), the manufacturer's instructions for dilution, activation, temperature, and contact time should be strictly followed. Following the disinfecting process, the transducer should be thoroughly rinsed with sterile water and dried aseptically.

Strong **glutaraldehyde** solutions are used to disinfectant transducers, but there is growing concern over the potential adverse effects of being exposed to glutaraldehyde liquids and vapors. The sonographer should check with his or her institution's infection control supervisor to be sure that any transducer soaking cups or cleansing stations meet current OSHA and JCAHO requirements. Guidelines for cleaning and preparing endocavitary ultrasound transducers are available at the American Institute of Ultrasound in Medicine website: *http://www.aium.org.*

Supplies

Besides maintaining an adequate supply of linens and coupling gels, each ultrasound room should be equipped with a bedpan; urinal; emesis basin; IV stand; and sterile trays for use in performing paracentesis, thoracentesis, biopsies, aspirations, or amniocentesis procedures.

Schedule review

Whenever possible, the patient schedule should be reviewed so that any charts or previous and pertinent diagnostic or laboratory test results are available before initiating the study.

Image generation, recording, and distribution

To perform and reproduce high-quality ultrasound studies, following current national standards of care guidelines such as those developed by professional specialty organizations (e.g., American College of Radiology (ACR), AIUM, ASE, SDMS, SVU) is important. By periodically checking these organizations' web sites, the sonographer's proficiencies can be kept current as new procedures, clinical applications, and instrumentation are developed. The following information presents an overview of currently accepted procedures in abdominal and retroperitoneal sonography.

The goal of most major hospitals and teaching centers is to create a filmless imaging department. That goal has been achieved by adopting the use of **picture archiving and communication systems (PACS)**, computer-assisted programs that electronically store, manage, distribute, and allow the viewing of images. The ability to share images and data through an institution-wide communication network has a positive impact on clinical/patient outcomes.

Radiology information systems (RIS) are computer-assisted programs designed to streamline scheduling/ordering of appointments, patient registration, work lists, billing, and medical and management reporting. RIS provide an improved turnaround time for the dictation and sending of reports to the referring physicians, patient scheduling, and so on.

Among the additional benefits of filmless PACS and RIS are the savings in time and film costs, patient data tracking, improved dictation and transmission of reports, and validation of procedural codes.

Sonographers are responsible for ensuring that their study images and reports are properly transmitted into PACS or RIS as part of completing each case. If a sonographer works in a setting where such systems are unavailable, he or she is responsible for producing the most pertinent and diagnostic hard copy images of each study and submitting them, along with his or her technical impressions of the study, for interpretation.

Sonographers' technical reports

On completion of the ultrasound study, in many ultrasound departments, sonographers are required to provide a preliminary report of their findings and observations. To avoid litigation, the preliminary report may be referred to as the technical or sonographer's impression and, as such, is subject to reinterpretation. Technical difficulties encountered during the study should also be documented and explained. Any report generated by a sonographer should indicate only essential sonographic findings and not attempt to provide a diagnosis (Box 7-2).

BOX **7-2**   Sonographer's Technical Report

A sonographer's report should describe only what has been documented on film and should include the following information:
- Location of the scan plane
- Normal or abnormal echogenicity, or both, of the organs studied
- Measurements and their locations
- Presence of shadowing or acoustic enhancement
- Presence and location of any masses
- Presence and location of abnormal fluid collections
- Any technical difficulties encountered during the study

Society of Diagnostic Medical Sonographers Educational Foundation. THE SCAN (Sonography Clinical Notebook). 2003, Educational Foundation. Dallas, Texas.

Preparing patients for sonographic examination

Before commencing any ultrasound study, the sonographer must carry out several routine but important tasks. Reviewing the patient's chart to verify the physician's order and evaluate whether the ultrasound examination that has been ordered is appropriate, given the patient's symptoms and clinical diagnosis, is important. The results of any prior diagnostic tests should be included in the patient's workup. After gathering all of this information, sonographers should mentally review the sonographic protocols most likely to provide answers to the clinical question.

The patient should be informed of the purpose of the ultrasound examination, and the sonographer should determine if the patient has followed any preexamination-required preparations.

A brief but pertinent patient history should be obtained (including questions about any possible latex allergies). For some ultrasound examinations, a brief physical examination may be indicated. After instructing the patient on disrobing and then positioning him or her on the scanning table, the sonographer should select the appropriate instrumentation for the examination based on the patient's body habitus and the examination objectives.

ABDOMINAL AND RETROPERITONEAL SONOGRAPHY

As an imaging tool, abdominal and retroperitoneal ultrasound is used to examine the abdominal cavity, liver, spleen, pancreas, gallbladder, kidneys, and major abdominal vessels by using 2-D, 3-D, and Doppler ultrasound techniques.

Clinical indications

- Abdominal, flank, or back pain
- Referred pain from the abdominal or retroperitoneal regions
- Presence of palpable masses or organomegaly
- Abnormal laboratory findings suggestive of pathology
- Evaluation of known or suspected abnormalities
- Exploration for the site of primary or metastatic disease
- Trauma
- Evaluation of known/suspected congenital abnormalities
- Evaluation for pretransplant or posttransplant surgery
- Identification of calculi in the digestive or urinary tracts
- Assessment and evaluation of tumors, cysts, abscesses, or free fluid within the abdomen
- Evaluation of the major abdominal arteries for the presence of an aneurysm
- Evaluation of narrowing of the abdominal arteries
- Guidance during aspiration or biopsy procedures
- Location of a foreign object within the abdominal/retroperitoneal organs/cavities

The presence of bowel gas, barium, or other contrast materials in the intestine can block the ultrasonic viewing of internal organs. Therefore abdominal sonography should be done before other diagnostic imaging tests that require contrast material. Obesity and dehydration also make it more difficult to obtain satisfactory images of the abdominal organs. Depending on examination objectives, patients may be asked to do the following preparations.

DIGESTIVE TRACT EXAMINATIONS

Patients should eat a fat-free meal the evening before the test and avoid eating for 8 to 12 hours before their examination. In some instances, patients may be asked to drink 8 oz of water to fill their stomachs for better visualization of the digestive tract.

ABDOMINAL ARTERY EXAMINATIONS

Patients should avoid eating for 8 to 12 hours before the test.

URINARY TRACT EXAMINATIONS

Patients should drink 4 to 6 glasses of liquid an hour before the test to fill the urinary bladder.

Preliminary abdominal/retroperitoneal examination steps

The sonographer should confirm that the patient's preparation for abdominal studies—fasting or hydrating stomach/bladder—has been carried out.

When taking the patient's history the sonographer should include questions involving pain. The existence of right or left upper quadrant pain, fullness, fever, abdominal pain, nausea, or vomiting should be noted, as well as the presence of midabdominal pain, burning, belching, or regurgitation related to certain types of food (e.g., fatty foods, fried foods). Flank pain or urinary tract symptoms (e.g., hematuria, bacteremia) must also be documented.

The patient's medical history should be reviewed with emphasis on infectious diseases (e.g., mononucleosis, hepatitis), alcohol intake, personal or family history of carcinoma, alcoholism, or blood disorders (e.g., leukemia, anemia, tuberculosis, syphilis).

A list of present medications should be made, with particular emphasis on ulcer medication or antacids, antidepressants, antiarrhythmic agents, or cholesterol-lowering agents.

The findings and normal values of laboratory tests should be documented, specifically aspartate aminotransferase, alanine aminotransferase, alkaline phosphatase, bilirubin, blood urea nitrogen, and urinalysis.

A review of any prior ultrasound or other diagnostic imaging tests should include abdominal radiographs, endoscopic retrograde cholangiopancreatography, CT scans, and MRI.

Transducer selection should be based on the patient's body habitus and the examination objectives. The equipment should be adjusted to operate at the highest clinically appropriate frequency that allows adequate beam penetration and resolution. When examining infants or children, total ultrasound exposure should be kept as low as possible but still provide the necessary information.

The most commonly used acoustic scanning medium is gel; however, on occasion, water or oil may also be used. The recording modalities most commonly used are film, videotape, or computer-generated and archived images.

Abdominal and retroperitoneal examinations employ the use of longitudinal, transverse, coronal, and oblique scanning planes. Depending on examination objectives, a patient may be placed in any of the following positions: supine, lateral decubitus, erect, and prone.

The following organs should be visualized and should demonstrate size, echo texture, and any gross pathology. Any suspected/known pathology must be documented in both longitudinal and transverse sections. Color Doppler images (with or without spectral Doppler) of the major vessels serving the following organs should also be performed:

- Liver
- Gallbladder

- Kidneys
- Pancreas
- Spleen
- Diaphragm
- Aorta
- Common duct

If any fluid collections (abscess, ascites, or hemorrhage) are found, the following areas should also be investigated:

Mid quadrants—transverse images at the level of the umbilicus

Lower quadrants—transverse images at the level of the iliac crests

Pelvis—sagittal midline image

> *NOTE:* Depending on the amount of fluid and patient body habitus, sagittal or decubitus scans, or both, may be helpful.

A standard protocol for a right and left upper quadrant sonogram should include longitudinal (sagittal) views of the following:

- Aorta and distal aorta if patient is older than 55 years of age
- Right and left liver lobe and caudate lobe
- Inferior vena cava
- Main lobar fissure and gallbladder
- Head of the pancreas
- Right and left kidneys
- Lateral aspects of the liver to view diaphragms and pleural spaces
- Spleen
- Adrenal glands

Color Doppler images (with or without spectral Doppler) of the main portal vein should be performed to demonstrate blood flow direction. Transverse views should include the following:

- Levels of the hepatic and portal veins
- Porta hepatis: to demonstrate common duct and hepatic artery
- Caudate lobe
- Gallbladder region: to demonstrate the neck, body, and fundus of the gallbladder
- Pancreatic region: to demonstrate the head, body, tail, and, when possible, the uncinate process of the pancreas
- Right and left kidneys
- Inferior aspect of the liver
- Spleen
- Adrenal glands

Color Doppler images (with or without spectral Doppler) of the splenic vein and artery and renal veins and arteries should be used to demonstrate blood flow direction and patency.

Left lateral decubitus (right side up) views should include the following:

Longitudinal views through the gallbladder

Longitudinal view through the common duct

Transverse views of the gallbladder at the level of the neck, body, and fundus

Upright scans are valuable in revealing the presence of gallbladder sludge/stones, while prone scans are helpful in visualizing the kidneys, especially when moderate to severe gas in the bowel compromises the examination.

> *NOTE:* Examination of the bowel, adrenal glands, spleen, and urinary bladder is not typically included in abdominal scans, unless specifically requested. An adrenal examination is usually performed in newborns or young infants, or in any age patient with suspected adrenal pathology.

Interventional procedures

Real-time ultrasonic guidance may be requested for several invasive procedures:
- Ultrasonically localizing a lesion to be punctured, and puncturing large superficial cysts or fluid collections. However, depending on the location of large heterogeneous lesions or smaller and more deeply located lesions, other imaging techniques may be indicated.
- Puncturing lesions using a "free-hand" technique in which the transducer and the needle are not connected. Providing that the needle penetrates tissues in the imaging plane, its advance may be followed on the viewing monitor. This technique is suitable for puncturing superficial lesions.
- Puncturing lesions by using a needle guide firmly connected to the transducer. The needle guide keeps the needle in the imaging plane, and its pathway can be indicated on the viewing monitor by means of electronic guidelines.

OBSTETRIC SONOGRAPHY GUIDELINES

Pregnancy is divided into three unequal segments: first trimester, second trimester, and third trimester. Although the standard ultrasound study during each of these periods is similar, each trimester also requires additional views, measurements, and observations. In addition to the standard protocols for first, second, and third trimester examinations, a limited examination may be ordered. The limited study is typically used in emergencies or as a follow-up to a prior (and recorded) complete examination. When an abnormality is suspected, or unexpectedly found, an even more meticulous and specialized examination may be indicated—one that might include biophysical profiles, fetal Doppler examination, or fetal echocardiography.

Clinical indications
- Confirm/deny intrauterine pregnancy
- Detect extrauterine pregnancy
- Estimate fetal age, size, and position
- Document fetal number
- Monitor fetal well-being (e.g., biophysical profile)
- Determine abnormal fetal growth patterns
- Evaluate possible fetal abnormalities
- Identify fetal gender (in suspected sex-linked fetal abnormalities)
- Evaluate placental location
- Evaluate placenta/fetal blood flow patterns
- Evaluate amniotic fluid index (AFI), a method of estimating the second and third trimester volume of amniotic fluid

- Guide amniocentesis or chorionic villus sampling (CVS), a prenatal diagnostic procedure to determine genetic abnormalities in the fetus
- Evaluate cervical length for possible signs of preterm labor
- Advanced maternal age concerns
- Confirm/deny intrauterine fetal death

Preliminary obstetric examination steps

The sonographer should ensure that any patient preparation (full/empty bladder) has been carried out before taking the patient's history. He or she should also establish the patient's parity and date of last menstrual period (LMP) or estimated date of confinement, or both. A history of miscarriage, abortion, infertility, multiple births, prior surgery, or congenital anomalies should be queried. The medical history should list the patient's past or current history regarding the following:

- Hypertension
- Sequelae
- Diabetes
- Rh isoimmunization
- Thyroid abnormality
- Heart disorders
- Hepatitis
- Herpes type II
- AIDS
- Drug use
- Cigarette smoking
- Alcohol use
- Latex allergies

Any medications the patient is taking should be listed. Any prior sonograms or diagnostically related tests should be reviewed and documented (see Appendix B). This includes pertinent laboratory tests:

Human chorionic gonadotropin (HCG): Quantitative HCG measurements can predict pregnancy and the age of a fetus. Abnormally elevated HCG levels are an indication of possible trophoblastic disease.

Amniotic fluid analysis

CVS

Alpha fetoprotein assay: An alpha fetoprotein test, along with the examination of amniotic fluid, can help detect fetal defects and diagnose or monitor fetal distress or fetal abnormalities. The test is usually performed at 16 weeks' gestation.

Percutaneous umbilical blood sampling: The prenatal sampling of fetal cord blood. The procedure is generally performed after the eighteenth week of gestation; however, the timing depends on the reason the test is being done (e.g., for certain high-risk situations such as fetal blood typing, anemia, infection).

Estrogen and progesterone levels

Based on the patient's body size, uterine contents, and the examination objectives, a transvaginal or transabdominal transducer, or both, should be selected. When examining gravid patients, total ultrasound exposure should be kept as low as possible, and the frequency selected should be limited to that which will provide adequate penetration and resolution.

The most commonly used acoustic medium is gel, which should be warmed before application to the patient's body.

The most commonly used recording modalities are film, videotape, or computer-generated and archived images.

Routine obstetric sonography may employ the use of longitudinal, transverse, coronal, and oblique scanning planes. Depending on the gestational age, a patient may be scanned in the supine, lateral decubitus, or erect positions.

First trimester (standard examination)

Transvaginal/endovaginal sonography (TVS/EVS) is an intracavitary ultrasound imaging technique that employs the insertion of a specialized transducer into the vaginal canal. TVS/EVS provides the best resolution during the first trimester. Before proceeding with a transvaginal examination, the patient should be questioned about any known latex allergies. If there is a negative history, a clean vaginal probe should be sheathed with a protective cover. Sterile gel should be applied, and the transducer should be inserted into the anterior fornix of the vagina. Depending on institutional policies, either the sonographer, patient, or physician may perform the insertion. When evaluating the adnexa, the probe should be moved into the lateral fornix for improved visualization. The following structures and procedures should be recorded:

- Location of gestational sac (measurement of any gestational sac younger than 8 weeks)
- Identification of embryo, yolk sac, and measurement of crown-rump length
- Measurement of nuchal translucency (from 11 to 14 weeks' gestation)
- Documentation of positive fetal heart motion (preferably with M-Mode)
- Documentation of fetal number
- Evaluation of uterus and ovaries
- Documentation of location, echo characteristics, and size of any uterine masses
- Documentation of location, echo characteristics, and size of any ovarian or adnexal masses

Second and third trimesters (standard examination)

All second and third trimester obstetric ultrasound examinations should start with an initial survey performed in a transverse scanning plane. The examination should begin in the lower left quadrant of the pelvis, scanning superiorly to the uterine fundus, then across the fundus to the right, and down the right side of the patient. This allows a rapid overview of the uterine contents to include the following:

- Number of fetuses
- Presence of fetal heart motion with M-Mode
- Fetal lie
- Fetal organ situs
- Placental location and relationship to the internal cervical os
- Presence of any uterine masses
- Location and appearance of maternal ovaries

Once the survey scanning has been completed, the following measurements/calculations should be made to assess gestational age:

Biparietal diameter (BPD)

Head circumference (HC)

Transcerebellar diameter

Outer orbital diameter (OOD)

Abdominal circumference (AC)
Femur length (FL)*
Fetal weight and growth assessment

NOTE*: In some ultrasound practices the humerus, tibia/fibula, ulna, and radius are
also routinely measured.

A detailed fetal anatomic survey should also be performed including the following
structures and measurements:
- Head
- Examination of brain parenchyma
- Integrity of cranial vault
- Lateral ventricles
- Measurement of the posterior horn of the lateral ventricle (normal limits: ≤10 mm)
- Measurement and documentation of the third and fourth ventricles if abnormal
- Cerebellum—measurement and evaluation of the integrity of the vermis and cerebellar lobes
- Cisterna magna measurement (normal limits: ≤10 mm)
- Nuchal skin fold measurement (from 15 to 21 weeks)
- Face
- Upper lip integrity
- Facial profile
- Measurement of nasal bone
- Orbital sizes and separation
- Measurement of OOD to check for hypertelorism/hypotelorism
- Thorax
- Evaluation of the appearance of lung parenchyma
- Evaluation of the integrity of the right and left diaphragms
- Evaluation for the presence of masses
- Evaluation for the presence of pleural effusion
- Heart
- Determination of the cardiac location and axis
- Documentation of a four-chamber view and cardiac outflow tracts
- Abdomen
- Evaluation of bowel size and echogenicity
- Location of the abdominal cord insertion site. If abnormal, documentation of the location,
  size, and contents of the abdominal wall defect
- Evaluation of the size and location of the stomach
- Documentation of the umbilical arteries lateral to the bladder (preferably with power Doppler)
- Evaluation of the location and size of the gallbladder, liver, and spleen
- Evaluation of the location, size, and echogenicity of kidneys
- Evaluation for any abnormal intraperitoneal fluid collections, masses, or calcifications
- Genitalia
- Determination of gender if parents want to know the sex of their child or if there is any
  concern for sex-linked abnormalities
- Limbs

- Documentation of the number, size, and architecture
- Evaluation of the anatomy and position of hands
- Evaluation of the anatomy and position of feet
- Spine
- Long and short axis views to evaluate symmetry and paraspinous muscles
- Placenta and cord
- Documentation of placental cord insertion site (color or power Doppler preferable)
- Assessment of placental echogenicity, grade, and thickness
- Evaluation of the size, thickness, and location of intrauterine membranes and the presence/absence of associated fetal entrapment or entanglement
- Documentation of the number of cord vessels (cross-sectional view)
- Evaluation of the placenta for the presence of any masses
- Amniotic fluid
- Subjective evaluation of the amniotic fluid volume and calculation of the AFI when appropriate

Second trimester (follow-up examination)

Quite often, patients are referred for serial ultrasound examinations throughout their pregnancies. Once a complete study has been done and a baseline established, repeat examinations may be limited in scope, and only the following fetal components evaluated:
- Fetal number and presentation
- Fetal gestational age assessment by multiple measurements including BPD, HC, AC, FL
- In pregnancies of less than 32 weeks' gestation, a four-chamber view of the heart and cardiac outflow tracts using M-Mode tracings
- In pregnancies of more than 32 weeks' gestation, a four-chamber view of the heart using M-Mode tracings
- Cerebral ventricles—measurement of the posterior
- Documentation of the placental location and the presence of a three-vessel cord
- Documentation of the number, location, and size of the kidneys
- Documentation of the fetal face
- Subjective evaluation of amniotic fluid unless the volume is abnormal, in which case AFI should be performed

Third trimester (follow-up examination)

From approximately 35 weeks to term, a limited examination may be performed and should include the following fetal components:
- Fetal number and presentation
- Fetal gestational age assessment by multiple measurements including BPD, HC, AC, FL
- Documentation of placental location and presence of a three-vessel cord
- Calculation of estimated fetal weight and BPD/AC, FL/AC ratios
- Calculation of AFI
- A cord Doppler study of the umbilical artery

   If the fetus appears to be large for gestational age, the sonographer may want to obtain the following additional scans/measurements:
- Humeral soft tissue thickness
- Optional facial cheek-to-cheek measurement (if fetus is in an optimal position)

Limited second and third trimester examination for cervical length

Transvaginal ultrasound is performed with an *empty* maternal bladder. Using a sheathed transducer and sterile gel, the transducer is inserted into the anterior fornix of the vagina.

Once the cervix is visualized, the probe is retracted so that undue pressure is not applied to the cervix. The sonographer should do the following:

- Obtain a true long axis view of the cervix
- Record and measure cervical length (from internal os to external os) on three images
- Select and record the shortest cervical measurement obtained
- Apply suprapubic or fundal pressure, or both, to evaluate the cervix for funneling
- Request the patient to perform a Valsalva maneuver in order to evaluate the cervix for funneling

Interventional procedures

Amniocentesis or CVS is the most common obstetric interventional procedure performed in the ultrasound department. Localization, puncture, and needle or catheter placement is done under ultrasound guidance.

The sonographer's role in amniocentesis is to do the following:

- Confirm fetal life and gestational age
- Localize a suitable pocket of amniotic fluid that is free of uterine, placental, or fetal vessels; umbilical cord; or fetal parts
- Monitor the advance of the amnio needle, once the site is chosen
- Perform a posttap study 15 to 30 minutes following the procedure to verify fetal well-being and to rule out the possibility of fetal or maternal hemorrhage

For CVS, after fetal viability has been established, the sonographer should do the following:

- Localize an area of chorion frondosum that will not risk perforation of the gestational sac
- Monitor the method of aspiration (either by catheter, transcervically, or by needle puncture, transabdominally)
- Perform a postprocedural study 15 to 30 minutes afterward to verify viability and rule out fetal or maternal hemorrhage

Intrauterine fetal transfusions for Rh incompatibility, fetal paracentesis, thoracentesis, or selective terminations are also ultrasound-assisted interventional procedures. However, these procedures are generally performed in the obstetric/surgical departments.

GYNECOLOGIC SONOGRAPHY GUIDELINES

Pelvic sonography is used to evaluate the organs of the female reproductive system: the uterus, ovaries, fallopian tubes, cervix, vaginal canal, and adnexal regions of the pelvis.

Clinical indications

Pelvic ultrasound is often requested to demonstrate the following:

- Pelvic pain
- Unexplained vaginal bleeding
- Presence of pelvic inflammatory disease
- Location of a misplaced intrauterine contraceptive device
- Evaluation of the size and structure of the uterus and ovaries
- Monitoring of the ovarian size/cycle during infertility treatments

- Confirmation of the presence of an intra- or extrauterine pregnancy
- Evaluation of palpable pelvic masses
- Evaluation of the presence of uterine fibroids
- Assistance at ovarian follicle harvesting for in vitro fertility procedures
- Demonstration of any congenital anomalies of the female reproductive organs
- Assessment of the endometrium for normal/abnormal appearance relative to the stage of the patient's cycle
- Examination of the adnexa for the presence of any free fluid or masses

Patient examination preparations

Patients may need to fill their urinary bladder before the ultrasound examination depending on body habitus, the transducer selected, and examination objectives.

Preliminary steps

The sonographer should do the following:
- Check that any patient preparation (full/empty bladder) has been carried out
- Establish parity and date of LMP
- Obtain history of contraception, miscarriage, abortion, infertility, multiple births, ectopic pregnancy, prior surgery, congenital anomalies, or hysterectomy
- Query the patient about general physical status and past or current history regarding:
  Pelvic pain
  Irregular bleeding
  Heavy discharge
  Irregularity in bladder or bowel function
Ask the patient to list current medications:
  Hormone replacement therapy: Combined estrogen and progestin therapy used for relief of menopausal symptoms
  Oral contraceptives
  Tamoxifen: An estrogen antagonist used to treat breast cancer
Document any pertinent laboratory or diagnostic tests including the following:
  CA125
  CA 15-3
  CBC
  AIDS
  Hepatitis C
  Mammography
  Pap smears
  Sexually transmitted diseases
  Examinations of the female pelvis may include longitudinal, transverse, and oblique scanning planes. Depending on the examination objectives, a patient may be scanned in the supine or lateral decubitus positions, or both.
  During the standard gynecologic ultrasound examination, the following organs should be visualized, measured when necessary, and documented:
- Uterus
- Fundus, corpus, and cervix

- Endometrium
- Ovaries (right and left)
- Fallopian tubes (if enlarged)
- Adnexal regions (right and left)
- Cul-de-sac
- Vaginal canal/fornix

On the basis of the patient's body size, uterine contents, and examination objectives, a transvaginal or transabdominal transducer, or both, should be selected. The frequency selected should be limited to that which provides adequate penetration and resolution.

The most commonly used acoustic scanning medium is acoustic gel (which should be warmed).

Film, videotape, or computer-generated and archived images are the methods used to record the diagnostic images.

Scanning options

Gynecologic sonography may require the use of one or more of these techniques: transvaginal, transabdominal, or transrectal examination approaches.

TRANSVAGINAL/ENDOVAGINAL SONOGRAPHY

The initial examination is performed with an empty maternal bladder. However, if the patient has had a hysterectomy, a fluid-filled bladder is preferred to help move the bowel out of the true pelvis and serve as a visual landmark.

The properly prepared vaginal transducer is placed into the anterior fornix of the vagina in the longitudinal scanning plane to do the following:
Demonstrate the cervix, body, and fundus of the uterus
Measure the anteroposterior dimension of the endometrial lining
- Document the appearance of the endometrial lining with respect to its menstrual, proliferative, periovulatory, or secretory phase
- Document the presence of any endometrial masses
- Measure any uterine myomas in three dimensions and demonstrate whether the myoma is intramural, submucosal, subserosal, or pedunculated
- Investigate the cul-de-sac for the presence of free fluid or masses
- Evaluate the urinary bladder and urethra

The transducer should then be rotated to evaluate the uterus in the transverse scanning plane. By placing the transducer in the lateral fornix of the vagina, the adnexal area can be evaluated to document the position of the ovaries and measure them in both longitudinal and transverse scanning planes.

If any ovarian masses are present, they should be measured, and their fluid-filled, solid, or complex nature should be documented. Adnexal masses, if present, should be measured, and their fluid-filled, solid, or complex nature should be documented. If the fallopian tubes are dilated, they also should be measured.

Performing manual compression of the lower abdomen may help to bring structures of interest into the field of view. This technique can also be used to move overlying bowel, which frequently obscures the ovaries. In some instances, this technique can be used to demonstrate the degree of organ mobility.

TRANSABDOMINAL SONOGRAPHY

Transabdominal sonography (TAS) is generally performed after a TVS/EVS examination. Therefore a distended urinary bladder *may not* be required. The TAS technique is used to better evaluate the endometrial lining, obtain uterine measurements, and visualize ovaries that are positioned outside the field of view of a vaginal probe.

The uterus, if anteverted, can be visualized to obtain more accurate measurements.

Ovaries that were not visualized with TVS/EVS, especially in obese patients or patients with an enlarged myomatous uterus, can be better visualized using the TAS technique.

Documentation of which technique was used to evaluate the ovaries should be noted on the preliminary report as an aid for follow-up ultrasound examinations.

The maternal kidneys should be evaluated for possible hydronephrosis if uterine, ovarian, or adnexal masses are present.

TRANSRECTAL SONOGRAPHY

These studies are optional techniques for performing studies on young virginal patients, or postmenopausal patients with a stenotic introitus. A physician should insert the properly prepared transducer into the rectum. The uterus and ovaries should be evaluated and measured. A TAS examination should then be conducted.

> *NOTE:* In some institutions the practices of transperineal or translabial scans are preferred to transrectal scans.

Doppler examination

Color flow and duplex Doppler studies are performed to help characterize the adnexa or any uterine masses. Color Doppler is also used to identify and differentiate vascular structures from nonvascular entities.

Interventional procedures

Biopsy or aspiration procedures may be indicated in patients being treated for infertility or in those with masses or free fluid. Paracentesis may be performed for patients with severe abdominal/pelvic ascites.

ADULT ECHOCARDIOGRAPHY

Ultrasonic investigation of the heart can be performed on adult, pediatric, or fetal patients. Echocardiographers are required to have knowledge of cardiac anatomy, physiology, and pathology, as well as valvular disease, ventricular wall movement, and congenital heart abnormalities. However, for our purposes, the following guidelines are limited to adult echocardiography.

One of two major cardiac ultrasound procedures is **transthoracic echocardiography (TTE),** which is a noninvasive, 2-D, real-time imaging technique used to evaluate cardiac structure and function. TTE is the more commonly used cardiac ultrasound procedure. The second method, **transesophageal echocardiography (TEE),** is an invasive, 2-D, real-time cardiac imaging technique that employs the placement of a specialized transducer within the esophagus.

The sonographic modalities most commonly used in echocardiography are 2-D and 3-D imaging, M-Mode tracings, Doppler flow studies, and tissue Doppler-imaging techniques.

Additionally, interventional procedures such as stress (exercise) testing or the use of injected contrast agents may also be employed. These techniques require specialized training and equipment.

Clinical indications

The following is a list of patient symptoms and conditions that can be evaluated with echocardiography:

- Shortness of breath
- Chest pain
- Evaluation of abnormal heart sounds
- Investigation of cardiac arrhythmias
- Evaluation of cardiac performance (evaluate cardiac valves and chambers, estimate cardiac ejection fractions)
- Investigation of heart injury or heart failure
- Detection of cardiomyopathy
- Identification of pericardial effusion
- Detection of endocarditis
- Detection of cardiac thrombi or tumors
- Evaluation of coronary arteries
- Evaluation of known congenital heart defects
- Evaluation of prosthetic heart valve function
- Detection of aortic dissection
- Detection of ischemia related to stress exercise or medication

Patient preparation

The sonographer should ensure that any necessary patient preparation, with respect to the specific type of study, has been carried out.

TTE

The sonographer should ask the patient to remove any jewelry and clothing above the waist and prepare him or her for electrocardiography (ECG).

TEE

The patient should do the following:

- Be NPO 6 hours before TEE
- Remove any dentures/dental prostheses
- Remove any jewelry and clothing above the waist
- Arrange for transportation home after the study, as patients are sedated and unable to drive for at least 12 hours after the procedure
- Sign a patient consent form before the test
- The sonographer should assemble supplies (e.g., IV apparatus, pulse oximeter, medication, contrast, sterile tray)

STRESS TESTS (EXERCISE ECHOCARDIOGRAPHY OR DOBUTAMINE STRESS ECHO TESTING)

The patient should do the following:

- Be NPO for several hours before testing
- Wear loose, lightweight, two-piece clothing and flat, comfortable shoes with good support

• Sign a patient consent form before the test

The sonographer should prepare the patient for ECG and IV medications.

Preliminary cardiac examination steps

After confirming that the patient has followed any necessary examination preparations, the sonographer should obtain a patient history. The patient should be questioned about the history of his or her current chief complaint (onset, duration, precipitating condition).

The sonographer should list the patient's cardiac symptoms, which may include the following:

• Chest pain
• Dyspnea
• Orthopnea
• Fatigue
• Cough
• Edema
• Syncope
• Dizziness
• Palpitations
• Fever
• Cyanosis
• Ascites

The patient should be questioned about any previous medical conditions such as hypertension, myocardial infarction, rheumatic fever, diabetes, heart murmur, endocarditis, pericarditis, cardiomyopathy, and pulmonary disease. He or she should also be questioned about previous cardiac surgery such as coronary artery bypass graft, or valve replacement (mitral, aortic, tricuspid, or pulmonic).

A list of current medications should be documented, with specific attention to antihypertensives, antiarrhythmics, and anticoagulants.

The sonographer should obtain information about the use of cigarettes, alcohol, or drugs (e.g., cocaine, other narcotics) and list any known allergy to medications such as digitalis, nitrates, beta-blockers, or diuretics.

If indicated, the sonographer should perform a brief physical examination of the patient to do the following:

• Obtain blood pressure readings in both arms while the patient is in the supine, sitting, and standing positions
• Auscultate lung fields (optional)
• Determine heart sounds: systolic and early/late diastolic filling sounds; low-pitched sounds; midsystolic clicks; pericardial rubs; coarse systolic murmurs; and high-pitched, blowing murmurs
• Determine other diastolic sounds and murmurs

Transthoracic examination

Echographic examinations of the heart may be carried out using long and short axis scan planes, as well as a four-chamber view. The transducer is typically positioned suprasternally, subcostally, apically, and parasternally.

Depending on the examination objectives, the patient may be scanned in the supine, lateral, or erect positions, and a transthoracic or transesophageal transducer should be selected. The frequency selected should consider the patient's body size and provide adequate penetration and resolution. An index mark should be placed on the side of each 2-D transducer to indicate the edge of the imaging plane. The image inversion switch should be turned "on" for four-chamber imaging.

The most commonly used acoustic scanning medium is acoustic gel, which should be warmed before application.

The recording modalities commonly used are film, M-Mode tracings, videotape/ cine-loop, or computer-generated and archived images.

The following cardiac structures should be imaged and evaluated, and appropriate measurements should be taken:
- Cardiac chambers
- Atria (right and left)
- Ventricles (right and left, left posterior wall, right and left ventricular outflow tracts)
- Septum (interatrial and interventricular)
- Valves
- Mitral
- Aortic
- Pulmonic
- Tricuspid
- Papillary muscles
- Pericardium
- Coronary sinus
- Arteries
- Aortic (aortic arch; ascending, transverse, and descending aorta)
- Pulmonary (right and left)
- Common carotid
- Subclavian artery
- Innominate artery
- Veins
- Inferior/superior vena cava
- Pulmonary veins
- Hepatic veins

Transesophageal examination

The TEE examination differs from the TTE in terms of increased resolution because of the less attenuating transesophageal window and the ability to view additional cardiac structures. Additionally, many "off-axis" imaging planes can be achieved depending on the type of TEE probe used. TEE examinations are only performed when clinically relevant questions cannot be answered by the TTE examination.

A qualified physician performs TEE, inserting the transducer (attached to an endotracheal tube) through the mouth and into the esophagus. TEE permits closer monitoring of cardiac function during surgery and allows better visualization of the posterior structures and of prosthetic valves that may not be seen well on TTE. Echocardiographers are tasked with patient support duties and operating system controls.

Many protocols are available for performing a TEE. The following information is intended only as a general guideline.

The examination room setup should include adequate examining room space (~250 sq ft) and a separate location for TEE transducer disinfecting or sterilization.

Equipment required consists of the following:
- TEE-capable ultrasound unit with video recorder
- TEE transducer
- Patient monitoring equipment (oximeter, suction, blood pressure devices, emergency cardiac life support equipment)
- Medication lock boxes and appropriate drugs
- IV setup and normal saline solution (500 cc)
- TEE tray

Stress (exercise) echocardiography

Exercise echocardiography is highly sensitive, specific, and of predictive value when evaluating the following:
- Coronary artery disease
- Patients who are scheduled for surgical or percutaneous revascularization
- Patients who have undergone surgical or percutaneous revascularization
- Patients who have had a myocardial infarction
- Regional wall motion both at rest and after exercise
- Left ventricular size and ejection fraction

The echocardiography procedure is performed during or immediately after an exercise stress test or after injection of **dobutamine**, a potent cardiac stimulant that produces a stress on the heart similar to exercise.

Contraindications to stress echocardiography are patients with *recent* myocardial infarction, unstable angina, serious cardiac dysrhythmias, acute pericarditis, severe hypertension, or acute pulmonary embolism.

The procedure is performed with the patient in the left lateral decubitus position, preferably on a customized scanning bed (with a drop leaf) to provide comfortable patient support and easy transducer access to the apical imaging windows.

Resting or baseline images are produced using the parasternal long and short axis and apical four- and two-chamber views. Next, the patient performs maximal, symptom-limited exercise. This may be achieved using upright or supine bicycle exercise or treadmill equipment. Conventional monitoring of blood pressure, ECG, and any symptoms is carried out. Immediately following the test, the patient returns to the examination table and the four previously described views are repeated as rapidly as possible.

Some patients, unable to perform an adequate exercise test, may require the use of drugs instead of exercise to provoke ischemia. These patients suffer from the following:
- Peripheral vascular disease
- Musculoskeletal disorders
- Neurologic disorders
- Pulmonary disease
- Obesity

The drug most favored for clinical use in these situations is dobutamine, which is infused with a calibrated infusion pump. Continuous monitoring of electrocardiograms, blood pressure, and heart rate is performed during the infusion. Echocardiographic images are obtained at rest, at each infusion level, and during recovery. Once a target heart rate has been obtained or when adverse symptoms occur or the regional wall motion abnormalities have been clearly demonstrated, dobutamine stress is terminated.

Contrast echocardiography

The use of injected contrast agents has increased dramatically because of better contrast agents, improved technology, and increased safety. Microbubbles of contrast are used as reflectors to enhance the visualization of cardiac structures and Doppler signals. Contrast procedures are employed to evaluate the following:

- Left and right heart structures
- Pulmonary artery pressures
- Mitral regurgitation
- Aortic stenosis
- Left ventricular function (with or without stress echocardiographic procedures)
- Presence or degree of patent foramen and other shunts
- Coronary artery stenosis and perfusion

Summary

Obviously, the roles that sonographers or echocardiographers play are more complex than simply taking pictures and being minor functionaries on a diagnostic team. As valued and respected members of the diagnostic team, sonographers work toward mastering the technical skills demanded of them while doing all that they can to maintain or restore the patient's health. This is their ultimate goal.

BIBLIOGRAPHY

Allen MN: *Diagnostic medical sonography. A guide to clinical practice. Echocardiography,* ed 2, Philadelphia, 1999, JB Lippincott.

American Institute of Ultrasound in Medicine: *Guidelines for cleaning and preparing endocavitary ultrasound transducers between patients.* Available at: *http://www.aium.org/provider/statements.*

Berman MC, Cohen H: *Diagnostic medical sonography. A guide to clinical practice. Obstetrics and gynecology,* ed 2, Philadelphia, 1997, JB Lippincott.

Curry RA, Tempkin BB: *Exercises in ultrasonography: introduction to normal structure and function,* ed 2, St Louis, 2003, Elsevier Science.

Gould BE: *Pathophysiology for the health professions,* Philadelphia, 2000, WB Saunders.

Hagen-Ansert SL: *Textbook of diagnostic ultrasonography,* ed 5, St Louis, 2000, Elsevier Science.

Kawamura DM: *Diagnostic medical sonography. A guide to clinical practice. Abdomen and superficial structures,* ed 2, Philadelphia, 1997, JB Lippincott.

Perry ARG, Potter PA: *Clinical nursing skills techniques,* ed 5, St Louis, 2004, Mosby.

Society of Diagnostic Medical Sonographers Educational Foundation: *The SCAN (Sonography Clinical Assessment Notebook),* Dallas, 2003, SDMS Educational Foundation.

Medico-Legal Aspects of Sonography

Learning Objectives

Students who successfully complete this chapter will be able to do the following:

1. Define the term tort and cite examples that might involve sonographers.
2. Explain the standard of care expected of a reasonably prudent sonographer.
3. Explain the role of institutional policies in legal decision making.
4. Identify the factors that contribute to a suit being instituted against a sonographer.
5. Discuss the steps sonographers should take to protect themselves against malpractice suits.
6. Explain the various aspects of giving a deposition and testifying for a legal proceeding.

Key Terms

accountability	defamation	medical malpractice
assault	duty	negligence
battery	informed consent	rights
breach of duty	invasion of privacy	statutory laws
cause	laws	subpoena
common law	liability	tort

We live in an era that strongly emphasizes the legal rights of patients and health care professionals. The threat of legal consequences has highlighted the need for professional accountability. **Accountability** is defined as responsibility for events for which one may have to give a judicial explanation of events. Therefore this chapter has been written to provide an overview of the legal issues sonographers are most likely to encounter in their work. Understanding and following the dual obligations of legal and ethical constraints are essential to the practice of sonography. Sonographers must be aware of their responsibilities and understand to whom they are responsible for their actions.

DEFINING THE LAW

Laws are the rules of conduct enforced by a controlling authority. Laws may be recognized by custom or formal enactment that a community considers binding on its members. Medical law deals with a particular sphere of human activity—the care of the patient. The goal of medical law is to protect people, correct injustice, and compensate for injury. Along with the permission to practice medicine, society demands that health care professionals conduct their practices according to accepted standards. Any failure to adequately meet these codes of conduct leaves all health care professionals open to civil actions.

Sonographers should follow their professional scope of practice but also understand the concepts and mechanisms of law and the legal restrictions placed on health care (Box 8-1). A basic knowledge of the law and how it works can help sonographers avoid litigation and allow them to practice their profession confidently.

The underpinnings of the law follow:
• Concern for justice and fairness
• Need for laws to be pliable
• Similar standards of performance
• Individual rights and responsibilities

The primary method of managing the complex social actions that occur within a society concerns for justice and fairness. Obviously, laws must be pliable enough to change in order to reflect ongoing technologic and societal advances. Because individuals with similar education, experience, and background are expected to act similarly, a sonographer's actions are judged by universally accepted standards of what a prudent and reasonable sonographer with similar education and training would do in a similar situation. The final factor to remember is that although each person possesses inherent rights, the more rights a person claims, the greater are his or her responsibilities.

FORMS OF LAW

All law is ultimately based on natural law—the inherent human desire to do good and avoid evil. The four basic forms of law follow:
• The Constitution
• Statutory law
• Administrative law
• Common law

Statutory laws are enacted and enforced by federal or state legislators to help maintain the governmental right to uphold social order and protect the rights of individuals.

BOX **8-1**   Scope of Practice for the Diagnostic Ultrasound Professional

PREAMBLE

The purpose of this document is to define the scope of practice for diagnostic ultrasound professionals and to specify their roles as members of the health care team, acting in the best interest of the patient. This scope of practice is a "living" document that will evolve as the technology expands.

Definition of the Profession

The diagnostic ultrasound profession is a multispecialty field composed of diagnostic medical sonography (with subspecialties in abdominal, neurologic, obstetric/gynecologic, and ophthalmic ultrasound), diagnostic cardiac sonography (with subspecialties in adult and pediatric echocardiography), vascular technology, and other emerging fields. These diverse specialties are distinguished by their use of diagnostic medical ultrasound as a primary technology in their daily work. Certification* is considered the standard of practice in ultrasound. Individuals who are not yet certified should reference the scope as a professional model and strive to become certified.

Scope of Practice of the Profession

The diagnostic ultrasound professional is an individual qualified by professional credentialing† and academic and clinical experience to provide diagnostic patient care services using ultrasound and related diagnostic procedures. The scope of practice of the diagnostic ultrasound professional includes those procedures, acts, and processes permitted by law for which the individual has received education and clinical experience and in which he or she has demonstrated competency.

Diagnostic ultrasound professionals do the following:

• Perform patient assessments
• Acquire and analyze data obtained using ultrasound and related diagnostic technologies
• Provide a summary of findings to the physician to aid in patient diagnosis and management
• Use independent judgment and systematic problem-solving methods to produce high-quality diagnostic information and optimize patient care

*Examples of credentials: RDMS (registered diagnostic medical sonographer), RDCS (registered diagnostic cardiac sonographer), RVT (registered vascular technologist); awarded by the American Registry of Diagnostic Medical Sonographers, a certifying body with National Commission for Certifying Agencies (NCCA) Category "A" membership.

†Credentials should be awarded by an agency certified by the NCCA.

Endorsed by:

Society of Diagnostic Medical Sonography

American Institute of Ultrasound Medicine

American Society of Echocardiography*

Canadian Society of Diagnostic Medical Sonographers

Society for Vascular Sonography

*Qualified endorsement

Modified from the Society of Diagnostic Medical Sonography, Plano, Tex., 1999-2005.

Rights can be defined as entitlements that one deserves according to just claims, legal guarantees, or moral principles. The three categories of rights are (1) freedom of choice, (2) legal rights, and (3) moral rights. Statutory laws include rules and regulations established by governmental agencies. In states requiring licensure of sonographers, the regulations formulated by the state agency are examples of statutory law.

Administrative law is a form of law made by administrative agencies appointed by the President or Governor. Such agencies make rules under authority established by acts of the legislature. One example that directly involves the practice of sonography is that of the federal Occupational Safety and Health Administration.

Common law, on the other hand, is court-made law based on custom and usage. In fact, most malpractice laws are court-made laws. For example, no statutory law dictates that sonographers cannot leave any seriously ill patients until they have assured that someone else will care for them, yet it is a customary and common practice. Failing to meet such a standard would be considered a violation of common law. Of the two, statutory law carries more respect. However, the final decision involving either statutory or common lawsuits rests with the court.

Torts

A **tort** is a wrongful act resulting in injury to another's person, property, or reputation—independent of a contract—for which the injured party is entitled to seek compensation. Torts are of two types: those that result from intentional action and those that result from unintentional action.

The following are examples of situations in which tort action can be taken against health care professionals because of their deliberate actions.

Intentional torts (misconduct) can include the following:
- Assault
- Battery
- Invasion of privacy
- False imprisonment

ASSAULT
Threatening or unsuccessfully attempting to inflict physical injury on another through force or violence and producing fear of immediate harm are considered **assault**. Any sonographer who causes a patient to be apprehensive of injury could be held liable or responsible to provide financial compensation to the patient for damages that may have resulted from the apprehension. The sonographer who says to an unruly or uncooperative patient "If you do not stop moving and start cooperating during this examination, I will have to restrain you" is one such example.

BATTERY
Battery is the unlawful touching of another person (directly or with an object) without that person's consent, with or without resultant injury. Assault and battery often are charged together because of a successful attempt to injure. For example, if a patient consents to a vaginal examination but changes her mind halfway through the study, any sonographer who argues, cajoles, or intimidates her and continues the examination would be liable for battery.

Sonographers cannot touch patients for any reason unless there is a valid consent by the patient to receive medical care. With or without bodily harm, the potential for liability against the sonographer exists.

Informed consent

Three categories of rights exist: freedom of choice, legal rights, and moral rights.

The patient has the right to consent to or refuse any service of a hospital or other medical setting. **Informed consent** requires that permission be obtained from the patient to have a test or procedure performed after the patient has been fully informed about the test or procedure.

The consent may or may not be in writing, but a written consent provides better legal protection for the health care professional. Such consent can be written, oral, or implied and is valid only if the patient is characterized by the following:

• Is of legal age
• Is mentally competent
• Gives consent voluntarily
• Is adequately informed about the medical care being recommended (i.e., understands the type of care and potential risks)

Sonographers should be aware that written consent is favored because it is easier to prove. One exception is that of *implied* consent, which is usually used when an unconscious patient is at risk. Implied consent assumes that the patient would want consent extended in order to secure care. Patients can revoke consent at any time, whether or not the patient gave previous verbal, written, or implied consent. At no time can that patient be denied the right to withdraw or revoke consent.

Invasion of privacy

Confidentiality and the right to privacy, with respect to one's personal life, are basic concerns in our society. The growing use of computerization in health care has made easier retrieval and cross-referencing of patient information available from various sources. Consequently, the public has become increasingly concerned about the potential for **invasion of privacy**, which is the wrongful intrusion into a person's private life, including publication of private facts.

The law of privacy is composed of the following:

• Intrusion on the patient's physical and mental solitude or seclusion
• Public disclosure of private facts
• Publicity that places the patient in a false light in the public eye
• Appropriation for the defendant's benefit or advantage of the patient's name or likeness

All information regarding a patient belongs to the patient. Any sonographer who gives out patient information without authorization can be held liable. Only professionals involved in a patient's care and with a need to know about the patient can be allowed access to the patient's records. The sonographer must be cautious about what information he or she shares verbally and with whom. The sonographer who discusses privileged and confidential information obtained from the attending physician or the patient's medical record can be sued for invasion of privacy.

An employer's policy and procedure manual should provide specific guidelines about what can be revealed without violating confidentiality. The recent Health Insurance Portability and Accountability Act (HIPAA) legislation has caused most hospitals, clinics, and physician offices to create or revise policies and procedures related to patient information (see Chapter 5). Privacy standards became mandatory for all hospitals, clinics, office practices, and other organizations on April 14, 2003.

On April 20, 2005 HIPAA security standards became effective. Complete information can be obtained online at the following website: http://www.hhs.gov/ocr/hipaa

Sonography educators, lecturers, and writers are also held to the privacy law when they reproduce, distribute, or display images of patient examinations without removing patient identification from those images.

False imprisonment

The illegal detention of a person without his or her consent constitutes false imprisonment. Sonographers could be charged with false imprisonment if they unnecessarily confine or restrain a patient without obtaining permission from the patient to be so restricted. In hospital settings, applying restraints requires that a physician's order be documented in the patient's medical record. Forcing a patient to stay by the use of verbal means (e.g., threats) also constitutes false imprisonment. All patients have the right to make decisions for themselves, regardless of the consequences. Sonographers should be careful what they say to try to convince a patient who refused an examination to change his or her mind. Sonographers protect themselves by recording their efforts and reporting the behavior to a supervisor and the referring physician.

Intentional misconduct

Any communication that holds a person up to contempt, hatred, ridicule, or scorn or lowers the reputation of a person constitutes **defamation**. This includes spoken (slander) or written (libel) defamation. Sonographers should avoid confrontations with patients, family members, or other staff, as these situations place them at the most risk. If reasonable attempts to resolve a conflict are not working, it may be more prudent to ask a supervisor or department head to intervene.

Unintentional misconduct

The following represent the most common forms of unintentional misconduct:
• Negligence
• Duty
• Breach

NEGLIGENCE
Negligence is deviation from the accepted standard of care that a reasonable person would use in a particular set of circumstances. Any sonographer who unintentionally causes injury to a patient may be accused of committing a negligent act. A tort action could be brought by either the patient or the employer if a sonographer, who intended to help, actually caused damage by failure to perform. To establish negligence and culpability for damages in court, the civil proceedings must address the issues of duty, breach, cause, and injury.

DUTY
Duty relates to the standard of care. A sonographer, as an employee of the institution who provides patient care, is obliged under law to perform services for a patient that meet current national standards of practice.

BREACH
Breach of duty occurs when a standard of care has not been met and results in patient injury. Breach of duty could be interpreted to include the failure of the sonographer to produce a scan with adequate diagnostic information.

Cause
In the health care setting, **medical malpractice** is the term used for the specific negligence of a specially trained or educated person in the performance of his or her duties that results in injury, loss, or damage.

   Cause or causation refers to any damage caused by a breach of duty that a specially trained or educated person is expected to perform.

Legal doctrines
Negligence is based on four doctrines: (1) liability: master–servant, (2) the twin doctrines of borrowed servant and captain of the ship, (3) ostensible agency, and (4) res ipsa loquitur. **Liability** is defined as a legal responsibility for one's actions.

MASTER–SERVANT DOCTRINE
The master–servant doctrine (*respondeat superior*—"let the master answer") states that an employer, along with an employee, is liable for the employee's negligence on the job. Although hospital or physician employers may automatically be held jointly liable, sonographers are not necessarily immune from damage suits or in any way relieved of personal responsibility for breach of duty. Because all persons are responsible for their own injurious conduct, the employer may opt to sue the sonographer.

BORROWED SERVANT AND CAPTAIN OF THE SHIP DOCTRINE
The borrowed servant and captain of the ship doctrine can be interpreted as follows: A sonographer is employed by a hospital as a temporary servant or agent of the physician. The physician is an independent contractor directly supervising the sonographer. Therefore the physician and the sonographer are liable for the sonographer's negligence, but the hospital is not.

OSTENSIBLE AGENCY DOCTRINE
According to the ostensible agency doctrine, a hospital or other health care agency may be held liable for the negligence of a nonemployee (such as an independent agent or contractor) if (1) either the person or the agency has represented or implied to the public that the person was an employee and (2) the patient relied on that fact when seeking care at the agency.

RES IPSA LOQUITUR DOCTRINE
The doctrine of *res ipsa loquitur* ("let the thing speak for itself") refers to the fact that in some cases of negligence, defendants are required to prove innocence. The defendant must demonstrate that injury could not have occurred if there had been no negligence and that the defendant was in no way responsible for the negligent act. This doctrine might be invoked when a patient was in surgery, sedated, or otherwise unconscious during the performance of the ultrasound examination.

   Malpractice can also involve professional misconduct such as unreasonable lack of skill or fidelity in professional duties, evil practices, or illegal or immoral conduct. A serious example is that of the sexual assault of a patient by a sonographer entrusted with his or her care.

PROTECTION AGAINST LAWSUITS

Currently, less than 15% of sonographers are males. Nevertheless, the number is sufficient to address the need for female chaperones to be present when male sonographers are scanning female patients. Most of these issues arise in the areas of cardiac, obstetric, or gynecologic sonography. It is prudent to check the policy and procedure manuals when students are rotating through their clinical assignments to determine when the use of a chaperone is indicated.

Although sonographers generally work under the direction of a physician, they are still personally liable for any harm a patient suffers as a result of their own acts. Many health care professionals protect themselves from possible legal actions by carrying malpractice insurance obtained through private insurance companies or through professional organizations. However, there is a possible downside to carrying insurance. Some health care professionals feel that lawyers target individuals with coverage.

Sonographers have a right to expect malpractice insurance to cover any charges brought against them, providing they have practiced within the limits of their job description, level of training, and professional scope of practice (Box 8-1). Such policies should cover legal fees and judgment expenses in the event that the sonographer is sued for malpractice.

In selecting malpractice insurance, sonographers should be aware than an *occurrence* policy provides more coverage than a *claims-made* policy because it protects the insured not only for incidents that occurred during the policy period, but also those that may not have been reported until after the policy had expired. The term of coverage is especially critical for obstetric sonographers who may be later sued by individuals who were fetal patients at the time of the alleged negligence or malpractice. Sonographers should understand that even if they are innocent of charges, it will still cost them money to prepare a defense, as well as lost wages because of time spent in court.

Uninsured or underinsured sonographers presume that the risk of being sued and found guilty is insufficient to justify the premium price of personal malpractice insurance. In assuming personal responsibility for financial damages awarded to a patient, such sonographers risk losing personal assets, property, and wages.

The sonographer who seeks to make himself or herself "lawsuit proof" should do the following:

- Always perform procedures as taught or outlined in the procedure manual of the sonographer's laboratory or health care facility. If such policies are outmoded or incorrect, the sonographer should work through proper channels to improve them.
- Remember that every individual is responsible for his or her own behavior. Therefore the sonographer should refuse to perform procedures for which he or she has not been prepared. Ignorance is not a legal defense, any more than lack of sleep or overwork are acceptable legal reasons for carelessness or mistakes.
- Ask for assistance if he or she is unsure how to perform a procedure. The sonographer should not assume responsibilities beyond his or her level of knowledge. It would be better to admit that he or she does not know how to do something than to attempt to do it and harm the patient.
- Keep exact records of all procedures performed (technical impressions, as well as the physicians' findings). Record any unusual patient behavior or incidents that might have occurred while the patient was in the sonographer's care. Records of studies involving pregnancy and

fetuses must be kept for longer periods (until the fetal patient reaches the age of majority) than other types of patient studies.

- Learn what legal protection is provided by his or her employer, as well as the terms of employment in relation to duties and salary.
- Determine if the state in which he or she practices has any licensing laws. Because malpractice laws vary from state to state, also review the medical malpractice laws in effect in the state of employment.
- Determine if any work practices place him or her in violation of those laws.

ALTERNATIVES TO MALPRACTICE LITIGATION

As one way to prevent malpractice claims from being brought, many institutions have developed risk management programs. The duties vary by institution. Identifying risks is the first step in any successful program, followed by evaluation and "treatment" of the risks. Because risks may be tangible, as well as theoretic, one component of such a program is the implementation of quality assurance testing to ensure that the ultrasound equipment functions correctly and safely and is not a factor in any litigation.

To handle the increasing number of claims, many states have developed arbitration panels to screen malpractice cases so that nuisance claims are dismissed.

BEING CALLED AS A WITNESS

Sonographers who are involved in a lawsuit may be served with a **subpoena**, a court document that requires a witness to appear and testify, or to produce documents or papers pertinent to a pending controversy, under penalty. When subpoenaed to testify at a malpractice trial, the sonographer is wise to always consult an attorney before talking to anyone about the matter. Believing that counsel is not needed, even if the sonographer has done nothing wrong, is foolish. Making unwise statements could jeopardize the sonographer's institution or his or her professional future. The possibility exists that the person suing may amend his or her original complaint to involve new defendants, including the sonographer.

A sonographer who has professional liability insurance should advise his or her insurance company, and an attorney will be assigned to talk to him or her. If a sonographer is covered by an employer's policy, he or she should consult with the legal/risk management department immediately to obtain counsel.

When asked to testify as a witness in a personal injury suit, the attorney who asked the sonographer to testify should provide him or her with all of the information needed for the testimony. The sonographer should find out what his or her role is in the case and in which area his or her testimony is expected.

As a witness, the sonographer is required to give a deposition, and at the trial, to take an oath to tell the *entire* truth and to answer any questions asked, to the best of his or her ability. The sonographer is not required to provide an answer that would incriminate himself or herself or to answer a question for which he or she does not remember or know the answer. It is permissible to say, *"I do not remember."* The sonographer should be brief and direct and not introduce additional information that has not been asked for by the client's attorney. The attorney's job is to ask questions that will produce the facts or information that he or she wants from the sonographer's testimony. On cross-examination, the opposing attorney will ask the sonographer additional questions that he or she believes are necessary to enhance the case. During cross-examination it is extremely important for the sonographer to be direct and succinct in his or her answers and not introduce any additional information.

Expert witnesses

As an expert witness, the sonographer will work closely with the client's attorney. The testimony of an expert witness usually requires giving explanations or opinions about highly technical skills or information. Those opinions or responses are usually given to answer hypothetical questions. A sonographer serving as an expert witness should be able to analyze the facts presented and draw inferences from those facts.

When a sonographer is a defendant, the ideal expert witness is another sonographer with a similar level of education and experience.

Summary

The expanding role of diagnostic ultrasound has had a profound effect on medicine and has resulted in many revolutionary changes in patient evaluation and treatment. It has also raised some ethical questions.

The purpose of this chapter is to show how the law affects the practice of sonography. The examples used were chosen to illustrate a specific concept. In reality, there are many more factors to consider than could be included in a brief chapter. The interaction of all factors and their interpretation by judges or juries determine the outcome of a legal case.

Sonographers who are concerned about a specific problem encountered in their practice should check with their institution's legal counsel, risk management officer, or private counsel who can be recommended by the local bar association.

The best testimonial sonographers can offer their profession is found in daily interactions that result in a patient who has been served well, treated fairly, and received the sonographer's personal best. A sonographer who wants to reach these goals must apply his or her knowledge and training in sonography to perform in the following manner.

Do:
- Thoroughly explain the procedure and what is expected of the patient
- Work with extreme care to avoid injuring the patient
- Question any abnormal instructions
- Maintain records and documents of the procedures performed in the event one is asked to provide information later
- Use common sense and judgment and practice within the limits of one's abilities and as one was taught

Do not:
- Perform sonography procedures that the sonographer has not been taught
- Fail to meet the established standards for the safe care of patients
- Fail to prevent injury to co-workers, other hospital employees, or visitors because this may subsequently result in a lawsuit.

The best protection against legal jeopardy is to practice sonography in a safe, ethical, and competent manner.

BIBLIOGRAPHY

Aiken TD: *Legal and ethical issues in health occupations*, Philadelphia, 2002, WB Saunders.

Brent NJ: *Nurses and the law: a guide to principles and applications*, ed 2, Philadelphia, 2000, WB Saunders.

Craig M: Treating patients with patience, *J Diagn Med Sonography* 1:16-18, 1989.

Lecca PJ, Valentine PA, Lyons KJ: *Allied health: practice issues and trends in the new millennium*, Binghamton, N.Y., 2003, Haworth Press.

Obergfell AM: *Law and ethics in diagnostic imaging and therapeutic radiology*, Philadelphia, 1995, WB Saunders.

Uribe CG: *The health care provider's guide to facing the malpractice deposition*, Routledge, N.Y., 1999, CRC Press.

Office for Civil Rights—HIPAA. Available at: *http://www.hhs.gov/ocr/hipaa*

Wilson BG: *Ethics and basic law for medical imaging professionals*, ed 1, Philadelphia, 1997, FA Davis Publishing.

Chapter 9

Ethics and Professionalism

Learning Objectives

Students who successfully complete this chapter will be able to do the following:

1. Describe ethical theories that may be used when working on ethical problems.
2. Explain how socio-cultural factors affect ethical decision making.
3. Identify the recent trends in health care and society that have affected current ethical and legal issues.
4. Describe the sonographer's role in relation to medical ethics.
5. Discuss the importance of professional confidentiality.
6. Explain how patients, peers, and other health care professionals interact in a considerate and professional manner.

Key Terms

autonomy	deontology	professionalism
code of conduct	ethical decision making	teleology
dehumanization	ethics	values

In general terms, **ethics** are systems of valued behaviors and beliefs that govern proper conduct and character to ensure protection of individuals' rights.

The concern about right and wrong and good and evil has existed since the beginning of mankind. Each generation has grappled with the issues of its times and formulated codes of behavior, and even laws, to address social problems. Looking back, we may find it difficult to understand those views. One example was the belief that it was wrong to alleviate the pain of childbirth because some Biblical interpretations stated that pain was meant to be a part of childbearing. With the benefit of advanced education and scientific knowledge, we can no longer agree with this viewpoint. We will not be immune from being cast in a similar light because hundreds of years from now, other generations may find it hard to believe the ethical positions that were taken in the twentieth and twenty-first centuries.

Medical ethics grew out of the patient-physician relationship and mandated that physicians know what is in the best interest of their patients and, above all, that they *do no harm.*

Sonographers, acting under the direction of physicians, share these ethical obligations to protect and promote the best interests of their patients. Working together, sonologists and sonographers cooperatively seek a correct diagnosis through their use of high-frequency ultrasound imaging.

Currently, the ethics of sonography can only be analyzed in terms of the sonographer's role as a member of the health care team because sonography is not yet a fully autonomous profession. In 1991 Chervenak and McCullough cited social workers as an example of health care professionals who had achieved autonomy by developing patient-client categories (e.g., the dysfunctional family, the victims of child abuse). At present, sonography still lacks any method of establishing reliable diagnostic categories and nomenclature that is independent of physicians. Thus until sonographers possess full autonomy, they will be limited to performing as agents of the physician.

The Society for Diagnostic Medical Sonography has taken the initiative to move in that direction by developing the guidelines of a new sonographic career category, that of the *ultrasound practitioner* (Box 9-1).

Everyone must determine his or her own basis for arriving at ethical decisions. Some rely on formal religious or philosophic beliefs that define matters in relation to truth or good and evil. Others weigh their decisions on what the greatest good would be for the greatest number. Many reach decisions on the basis of their personal experience or the experience of

BOX **9-1**   The Ultrasound Practitioner

DEVELOPMENT OF A MIDDLE CARE PROVIDER IN ULTRASOUND IMAGING

The Ultrasound Practitioner Commission recently published a proposal in the *Journal of Diagnostic Medical Sonography (JDMS):*

The Ultrasound Practitioner is a health care professional who autonomously performs and interprets ultrasound procedures in primary or specialty care settings. As part of the interdisciplinary team, the Ultrasound Practitioner will provide services based on clinical competency obtained by advanced education and clinical experience.

View/Print JDMS article on Ultrasound Practitioner (July/August 1999)

View/Print JDMS article on Ultrasound Practitioner (May/June 2001)

From the Society of Diagnostic Medical Sonography, Plano, Tex., 1999-2005 .

a parent or other loved one. As a result of these differing methods, it is not surprising that people confronted with the same difficult ethical questions often arrive at different conclusions.

In some instances the sonographer can accept the decisions of others; however, eventually there comes a time when one's own position causes one to disagree and oppose their actions. When such a conflict occurs, the sonographer must follow his or her conscience, but it should be done constructively, not destructively. **Values** are concepts, goals, ideals, and behaviors. They are produced and instilled in people by family, friends, culture, environment, education, and their own life experiences. However, it is important to remember that establishing values is a lifelong process and the strongly held opinions of today may change as one moves through life.

BASIC ETHICAL CONCEPTS

Most health care professionals are guided by the principles of kindness, good works, avoidance of harmful behavior, autonomy, justice, truth, and faithfulness to duty. From Hippocrates to Florence Nightingale, health care professionals have been exhorted to *"do no harm"* to their patients. Modern sonographers are taught to respect a patient's right to make his or her own decisions. They are taught to deal justly with patients so that age, ethnicity, gender, language, and insurance status are left outside the door of the ultrasound examining room. Sonographers pledge fidelity to their profession, employer, coworkers, and patients to faithfully perform their duties. They avoid lying to patients to preserve their trust in them as caregivers, but also because they realize that the anxieties and lost opportunities to deal with personal concerns associated with not knowing the truth far outweigh any perceived advantages of lying to patients.

The two most prominent ethical theories in play in our culture are the teleologic and deontologic theories. **Deontology** is the study of duty, moral obligation, and right action. **Teleology** is the study of evidence of the design and purpose of nature. Teleologic theory states that an act is right if it is useful in bringing about a good outcome, while the deontologic theory states that one must do his or her duty regardless of the outcome. Most sonographers find themselves straddling both of these theorems as they face ethical decisions in their practices.

Ethical decision making

All around, the world is experiencing change. Yesterday's "truths" are being challenged by today's realities and by new problems that have not been faced before . . . and that includes the field of sonography. **Ethical decision making** requires dealing with concrete judgments in situations in which action must be taken, despite uncertainty.

Since the second half of the twentieth century, patients have formulated their own ideas about their best interests and have developed the capacity to express and carry out value-based preferences. They have achieved patient autonomy and, in doing so, have obligated health care professionals to acknowledge their values and beliefs and to avoid interfering with their expression or implementation. The switch from the term *medical care,* which focused on the physician, to *health care,* illustrates the concerns for patients' rights.

These concerns have increased dramatically since the inception of managed care and its reforms. More than anything else in the past century, the effects of managed care on health care delivery have given rise to the most basic ethical questions and concerns. Medicine and society once shared a special bond of mutual interest and trust because the best interest of the patient was their guiding force. The health care environment of today is different. What originally inspired many people to enter the field were their deep values. Today, as they confront the definite realities of a changed system, it is powerful and helpful for health care professionals to remember the motives that brought them to their careers and to continue to believe in the intrinsic good of what they do. This is what will keep all health care professionals on track, oriented to what really matters—not only staying current with medical and technologic advances but continuing to focus on the human values as well. In the managed care environment, allocation of care and the goal of increasing profits have become the barometers for treatment. Consequently, health care professionals are more frequently required to make judgments in situations in which action must be taken despite uncertainties.

Faced with ethical decisions, health care professionals hope to find the right answers. However, often there is no right answer to satisfy everyone or for every situation. The following recommendations provide a basic framework that allows one to look beyond one's feelings in making good decisions.

- Identify the problem
- Gather pertinent data and information
- Identify options and solutions
- Think the problem through and evaluate the short- and long-term consequences for each solution
- Make a decision
- Act
- Review and evaluate the results

Ethical dilemmas

Recent technologic advances and increasingly complex patient-related issues require sonographers to be aware of and sensitive to ethical dilemmas. Religious, social, and cultural influences sometimes can create ethical dilemmas as well.

Obstetrics, more than any other sonographic specialty, has produced various ethical questions and dilemmas. Serving two patients, an expectant mother and her fetus, carries an obligation to both parties, although at times they may seem at cross purposes.

In pregnancies that progress to term, sonographers are expected to provide clinical protection and promotion of fetal interests because fetuses are not autonomous. Through their imaging skills, sonographers contribute to the prevention of premature death, disease, handicapping conditions, and unnecessary pain and suffering. These same obligations, however, do not extend to previable fetuses that are electively scheduled to be aborted.

ABORTION

The U.S. Supreme Court has recognized a woman's **autonomy**: the right to make her own decisions and to be independent and self-governing. The court has acknowledged her right to privacy and to be the final arbitrator in matters of her own body. However, the Supreme Court has also recognized the interest of the State in protecting potential life and has placed certain limits on a woman's rights in relationship to that of an unborn child.

Although the states are virtually powerless to restrict or regulate abortion procedures in the first trimester of pregnancy, they may, during the second trimester, stipulate medical conditions under which the procedure can be performed. During the third trimester, because of the interest in protecting the rights of the unborn, the State may justify stringent regulations and prohibition of abortion. That said, society's failure to achieve emotional resolution and political clarity regarding the sanctity of life has created the tenuous legal, ethical, and moral climate in which sonographers must perform.

Ethically, the abortion issue revolves around the definition of human life and when a fetus should be considered a human being. Consequently, sonographers must be aware of the assertion of fetal rights and should be particularly aware that they are legally responsible for their actions and their images *until the fetal patient reaches its age of majority.*

SELECTIVE TERMINATION

In cases of multifetal pregnancy, if serious complications occur or if serious anomalies are detected, the obstetrician may offer the expectant parents the option of selective termination. This step is taken only if it will improve the outcome for the remaining embryos or fetuses. Terminations are indicated when the following exist:

- Only one twin shows signs of a serious chromosomal or congenital anomaly
- The number of embryos or fetuses presents a threat to a successful perinatal outcome

Some sonographers may have moral objections to abortion or selective termination. If so, they should approach the request for their services by avoiding moral judgment of the pregnant woman and respecting her autonomy. They must respect the fact that the patient and her physician have considered her problems and have based their decision on multiple factors that may be unknown to the sonographer. Regardless of personal beliefs, it is not the province of sonographers to attempt to dissuade, encourage, or punish their patients. Should they do so, they would be operating outside of their scope of practice by expressing their personal feelings and beliefs in an attempt to influence a patient's decision. Instead, sonographers should take a personal inventory of their feelings and beliefs regarding abortion and medical intervention procedures. Those unable to accept the current laws and the medical practices regarding them must express their convictions to their supervisors and request to be relieved of the duty of working with patients destined to undergo such procedures. The sonographer's beliefs also must be respected, and there should be no fear of professional or economic reprisals. Once a sonographer accepts responsibility toward a patient, however, he or she must never refuse to carry out or complete a procedure.

VIDEOTAPING OBSTETRIC EXAMINATIONS

Just as ultrasound has become more technologically sophisticated, so too have the patients in their appreciation and understanding of imaging devices and the content of sonograms. One controversial sonographic issue involves the practice of providing patients with videotapes or hard copy images of fetal ultrasound examination.

Proponents of videotaping are quick to point out that this practice (1) enhances fetal bonding, (2) educates both patients and family members, (3) increases the patient's resolve to follow doctor's orders during their pregnancy, thereby ensuring the health of their fetus, and (4) increases the patient's acceptance of sonography. Those opposed to providing images for patient use believe that the practice (1) extends scanning time and patient exposure, (2) distracts the sonographer's concentration, and (3) teeters on the brink of commercialization.

The institution in which the sonographer works should maintain a policy and procedure manual clearly stating how to handle patient requests for fetal images. If videotapes or Polaroid images of obstetric examinations are provided to patients in an institution, the following recommendations should be considered:

- A written policy should be established for providing patients with hard copy images of their sonography examination.
- A specific time should be set aside to create a tape for the patient's use. Preferably, this should take place after completion of the diagnostic examination.
- Nothing should appear on the patient's photographs or tape that was not seen on the diagnostic study or survey.

The supervising physician must be aware of the examination results and should review the patient's photographs or tape before they are released to the patient. The physician should exercise the right to deny the tape or photographs for patient use if any abnormality is found or suspected.

Nondiagnostic use of ultrasound

In the mid-1990s, many imaging departments were abandoning the decades-old practice of providing obstetric patients with keepsakes of their sonogram experience. They feared potential lawsuits over missed diagnoses and were influenced by the desire to increase profits. To no one's surprise, expectant parents clamored for a return to this practice. Some enterprising physicians and sonographers recognized that this controversy had created a niche for nondiagnostic fetal imaging. Denied their previous fetal keepsakes, patients turned to the trendy ultrasound portrait studios, with catchy names like *Womb with a View, Sneak Peek,* or *Fetal Fotos* to satisfy their desires. There, in comfortable nonclinical environments, emotion-filled videotaping sessions were carried out and turned into family affairs. In some instances, the entrepreneurs promoted their establishments as the choice location for baby showers.

As far as the expectant mothers were concerned, these taping sessions were no different than the ultrasound examinations they had in the clinical setting, except that the costs were not covered by insurance and must be paid for out of pocket. Exposure time, power settings, the skill and knowledge of the operators, and the possibility that the happy experience might turn cold with the discovery of fetal abnormalities never entered their minds.

Those factors, however, greatly concerned the ultrasound community, and their concerns were relayed to the Food and Drug Administration (FDA) for investigation. The FDA began a nationwide effort to identify companies using ultrasound in an unapproved manner. In several instances, FDA inspections of fetal portrait studios resulted in the confiscation of equipment and closure of several sonographer-owned businesses. Physician-owned businesses, however, were not targeted, and with time, the issue slipped from the headlines.

A decade later, the availability of high-resolution (and higher-power) 3-D and 4-D imaging equipment saw the reemergence of fetal portrait studios. Lucrative franchising spread them across the country. The FDA and professional medical organizations again raised the concern about using ultrasound imaging to obtain fetal images when there is no medical need. In 2004 the FDA advised parents against using ultrasound to obtain keepsake images. Organizations such as the American Institute of Ultrasound in Medicine, Society of Diagnostic Medical Sonography, and European Committee for Medical Ultrasound issued position papers warning against the practice (see Box 6-2).

As of this writing, the fetal imaging fad continues to proliferate. Clever marketing offers "packages" that provide 2-D, 3-D, or 4-D tapes or CDs complete with background music and color portraits and prints at prices ranging from $150 to $400. As one of the fastest growing franchises in the United States, franchisers recommend that their franchisees keep overhead low and profits high by employing nonmedical personnel who can be "trained" by the franchiser in 4 days to 4 weeks.

A safe alternative to this problem may be one that uses a different approach to satisfying patient demands. A Massachusetts company has developed a way for specific ultrasound images to be recorded separately, during a patient's regular diagnostic examination. This allows the mother to have a video without any unnecessary scanning. Although these videos may lack slick packaging and background music, they answer the patients' requests and provide safety in the form of limited exposure and performance by a medical professional.

As the ultrasound community waits for the FDA to develop and consistently and fairly enforce guidelines or regulations, we are again faced with the ethical dilemma to either support the closure of all of these practices or not oppose them at all.

Confidentiality

One of the most basic concerns of society is that of confidentiality and the right to privacy. Patients' rights have been strengthened by the Health Insurance Portability and Accountability Act regulations that emphasize the patient's expectation of confidentiality in relation to their health care. Sonographers, physicians, and patients comprise the three personal elements of medical sonography examinations. Diagnostic information about a patient, therefore, can be justifiably disclosed to outside parties only with the patient's approval and explicit permission. However, not only diagnostic information but personal information as well should be considered. For example, a sonographer is ready to take a brief medical history of a pregnant patient who is accompanied by her mother-in-law. To protect the patient's right to confidentiality and to ensure that the sonographer is given a complete and truthful history, questioning of the patient should always be conducted in private.

As discussed in Chapter 8, disclosure of confidential information may subject a sonographer to liability. Sonographers carry a unique burden of responsibility because patients may share many personal and intimate details during their examinations. The time will come when it may be necessary to balance the duty to disclose certain information against the right to confidentiality. Specifically, if a disclosure would prevent injury to the patient or others (e.g., knowledge of contagious diseases, child abuse), the sonographer has a duty to report it.

Competency

Sonographers have an ethical obligation to perform a competent examination and provide physicians and patients with accurate and reliable information. Doing so requires continuing education in addition to preparatory training to ensure that a general level of competence in sonography is maintained. A serious breach of ethics results whenever sonographers lag behind the advances made in their field. By performing inaccurate or incomplete examinations or reporting the results of such examinations to patients, such sonographers seriously undermine the patient's and the physician's trust and future reliance on sonography and harm the reputation of the profession.

Professional disclosure

If sonographers discover errors based on faulty equipment, technique, or interpretation, they have a duty to bring such errors to the attention of the interpreting physician.

BOX **9-2**   Characteristics of Drug and Alcohol Impairment

The following behaviors are observed in the health care professional who is impaired by either alcohol* or drugs.
- Increased absenteeism
- Inability to meet schedules
- Tendency to back away from new and challenging assignments
- Changes in personality and mental status (mood swings)
- Changes in behavior
- Illogical and sloppy work
- Excessive errors
- Unkempt appearance
- Inability to concentrate
- Poor/inaccurate recall

*Alcohol impairment is associated with alcohol on the breath, a flushed face, slurred speech and an unsteady gait.

Sonographers can be placed in an adverse position if the errors are not corrected or communicated by the interpreting physician to the referring physician. As patient advocates, sonographers must then express their concerns to the risk management or quality improvement departments of their institution or directly to the referring physician.

Being asked to perform a task outside of a sonographer's legal scope of practice requires speaking to the department director or administrator first. If the situation is not resolved, the sonographer should seek the advice of the hospital risk manager.

Knowledge that a physician, supervisor, or fellow sonographer's practice has deteriorated because of chemical dependence legally obligates the sonographer to report this information by going through the channels established by the place of employment (Box 9-2).

Before moving forward, the sonographer should gather any relevant data that is vital to his or her claim and keep a journal to record the events. He or she should not dwell on being considered a "whistle blower." The bottom line in these situations is that a professional sonographer should never ignore unethical behavior.

PROFESSIONALISM

Considerable overlap exists in the topics of ethics and professionalism and many individuals believe the terms are synonymous. **Professionalism** means being involved in and worthy of the high standards of a profession. In health care, professionalism is based on integrity, honesty, and compassion. The ethics of the profession demand that conduct toward patients be totally devoid of any self-interest. For this reason, in addition to developing technical knowledge and skills, sonographers must also learn about patient behaviors, patient interaction, and the standards of conduct that are expected of them.

For many years, the health care profession was governed by rigid, no-nonsense rules that discouraged any emotional or personal involvement with patients, and it demanded unquestioning obedience to authority figures. The training of health care practitioners in the past was limited to specialized classes devoted to the recognition of normal and abnormal body structure and functions and rudimentary techniques for meeting the physiologic needs of such patients. Classroom theories were reinforced by countless hours of practical, voluntary, on-the-job training.

As the various health care professions evolved during the second half of this century, academic programs were incorporated into the training process and concern for the psychosocial aspects of health care began to emerge. Courses in the behavioral sciences of psychology and sociology were added to curricula in the hope that knowledge of theory in these areas would improve graduates' ability to understand and cope with the personal problems of their patients.

Little effort, however, was made to relate these new curriculum components to the practical rules that governed the conduct and performance of the health care professional. Therefore the two varieties of professional instructions coexisted without any basic integration.

For the past 4 decades the arbitrary rules that governed the professions have been challenged and, in some cases, rejected. Studies in the behavioral sciences have been expanded, but, more importantly, the health care specialties have begun to build bridges between theory and patient interaction.

Formerly rigid professional-role behaviors have become more sensible and flexible. An integrated focus of helping patients get well, as well as tolerate and reduce the psychologic discomfort of their illnesses, has elevated the patient from being a "case" to being a person. In this discovery process, health care professionals have begun to analyze their own psychosocial conditions as they strive to become the best they can be. The goal of this chapter is to explore these needs, as well as the aspirations of all people, as a means to improving the quality of life.

Interactions with patients

The primary attribute of health care professionals is their inseparable identification with human suffering. Their concern carries with it feelings of responsibility for patients and a willingness to serve all of the sick and helpless entrusted to their care.

Patients usually come to the sonographer for diagnostic assistance because of the presence of some symptom (e.g., pain, disability, questions involving pregnancy). In most instances the patient-sonographer relationship is over when the examination is completed and the patient leaves the sonography department. During the time patients are with sonographers, however, they may need reassurance about their physical problems and understanding and guidance to help them adjust to their new situation.

The sonographer must consider carefully not only what to say to patients but also how to deliver the information. He or she should keep in mind that patients often do not fully understand what is said, or they may misunderstand or take statements out of context. Some patients hear only what they want to hear! Nevertheless, these factors should not deter the sonographer from communicating with patients because such communication can be one of the most rewarding experiences available. Instead, he or she should work toward preparing patients psychologically for their examinations by explaining the procedure and establishing realistic expectations.

AVOIDING DEHUMANIZATION
Dehumanization can be defined as depriving one of human qualities or attributes such as pity, kindness, and individuality. Each patient brings some degree of anxiety to his or her ultrasound examination. Each one of them is concerned with how his or her possible or known

illness will affect daily life, loved ones, and activities. Too often, health care practitioners think of patients in the abstract terms of their condition. The sonographer must avoid that kind of trap and always accord patients respect for their individuality, as well as their physical condition.

EXPECTATION OF COMPETENCE

Patients arrive at their sonography examination with clear expectations of the person who will be conducting their examination, and they respond according to the treatment they receive. For instance, some patients may refuse to submit to an examination by a "student" simply because they perceive a student as someone who is not yet fully trained or competent. Observing the interaction of sonographers with their coworkers and other health care professionals can also influence a patient's perceptions of professionalism. Patients have little confidence in sonographers who exhibit overly casual or immature behavior.

In addition to expectations of professional conduct, patients expect sonographers to project a professional image. Specific standards of dress and grooming must be met because patients' first impressions are strongly influenced by personal appearance. The dress and grooming of the entire staff and the appearance of the sonography section and the institution that houses it can influence patient opinions. Neatness, cleanliness, and friendly efficiency are essential to inspire patient confidence.

Although social attitudes, dress, and grooming have become more casual, nothing changes the fact that a casual attitude does not epitomize the professional image of health care personnel that has been perpetuated in the mind of the public for many years. Each hospital, clinic, or ultrasound practice establishes appropriate dress and grooming codes to reflect its professionalism. Sonographers must adhere to these guidelines or regulations regardless of their own personal taste.

RECOGNIZING TRANSFERENCE

The act of shifting one's feelings about a person in the past to another person is called *transference*. Both negative and positive reactions can be stimulated such as feelings of hostility, cooperation, and confidence. Thus sonographers must conduct themselves properly during all patient interactions, communicating concern yet maintaining a professional distance. They must respect and give service with equal care and dedication to all patients regardless of sex, race, creed, color, or economic background.

PROTECTING PATIENT MODESTY

One particularly sensitive area of interaction is consideration for the patient's modesty. By observing the rules of draping and covering the patient to the greatest extent possible during an examination, sonographers can reduce patient anxiety. Providing privacy when patients disrobe or perform bodily functions will be appreciated by most patients and will obtain their grateful cooperation. When examinations require patients to be exposed or to assume positions that are potentially embarrassing, sonographers must use considerable tact to preserve the patient's modesty and personal dignity, even if it means stepping aside in favor of a sonographer who is of the same sex as the patient.

INTERACTING WITH DIFFICULT PATIENTS

Professionals learn to master verbal communication, facial expression, and other facets of body language. They learn to converse intelligently, pleasantly, and courteously with patients.

If a patient is under stress or is unpleasant to deal with, a professional is able to maintain emotional control and attempts to alleviate the patient's apprehension and determine what is causing the unpleasant behavior.

During their initial contact with patients, sonographers are expected to determine the most appropriate manner in which to deal with a particular patient. They should communicate their interest in the patient at all times and provide assurance at the end of the examination that they have given their best services.

CONFIDENTIALITY

Professional confidentiality imposes a major restriction on the health care professional. Because medical and personal patient information must always be held in strict confidence, revealing such data to patients, family, or others outside the department cannot occur without the direct consent of the patient's physician. Failure to respect the patient's rights in this regard can result in legal problems.

Interacting with other health care professionals

As a student and ultimately as a graduate, the sonographer is required to interact with many different health care professionals. Initially his or her time is spent with instructors. Often these are professional sonographers who have developed the teaching skills necessary to prepare one academically and technically for the role of sonographer. Instructors can also offer the benefit of their personal experience to ease their students' entry into the patient setting and help them develop professional judgment.

Although most physicians, nurses, and other health care workers are friendly and cooperative, some may seem distant, preoccupied, or indifferent. In many instances this negative behavior is the result of an ongoing and wide gap in professional standing between the medical and technical fields. Rather than becoming part of such a problem, a professional finds ways to break the cycle. By asking for guidance or information from physicians or by expressing an interest in how other departments function and what ideas they might have for improving interdepartmental cooperation, effective bridges can be created to span such gaps.

Obligations toward the sonography profession

The sonographer's first obligation to sonography is to recognize that it is more than just a job. This realization should motivate one to not only become proficient but continue to grow with the field to avoid becoming "second rate."

In addition to pursuing continuing education, the sonographer should participate in and support the activities of professional organizations. Many offer student membership categories and special services that can help master the skills one desires. The universal benefits of membership in such groups include resources that provide the following advantages:
- Helping maintain high educational and performance standards
- Advancing professional stature
- Providing a training ground for leadership applicable to the laboratory, the institution, and the profession

The sonographer's ultimate obligation to his or her profession is to pursue excellence and superior performance. Through the efforts of the Society of Diagnostic Medical Sonography, a **code of conduct**, which guides the members of the profession in the proper conduct of their duties and obligations, has been developed (Box 9-3).

BOX **9-3**   Code of Ethics for the Profession of Diagnostic Medical Sonography

PREAMBLE

The goal of this code of ethics is to promote excellence in patient care by fostering responsibility and accountability among diagnostic medical sonographers. In so doing, the integrity of the profession of diagnostic medical sonography will be maintained.

OBJECTIVES

To create and encourage an environment where professional and ethical issues are discussed and addressed. To help the individual practitioner identify ethical issues. To provide guidelines for individual practitioners regarding ethical behavior.

PRINCIPLES

Principle I: In order to promote patient well-being, the diagnostic medical sonographer shall do the following:
A. Provide information to the patient about the purpose, risks, and benefits of the ultrasound procedure and respond to the patient's questions and concerns.
B. Respect the patient's autonomy and the right to refuse the procedure.
C. Recognize the patient's individuality and provide care in a nonjudgmental and nondiscriminatory manner.
D. Promote the privacy, dignity, and comfort of the patient (relatives and significant others) by thoroughly explaining procedure protocols and implementing proper draping techniques.
E. Protect confidentiality of acquired patient information.
F. Strive to ensure patient safety.

Principle II: To promote the highest level of competent practice, diagnostic medical sonographers shall do the following:
A. Obtain appropriate ultrasound education and clinical skills to ensure competence.
B. Achieve and maintain specialty-specific ultrasound credentials. Ultrasound credentials must be awarded by a national sonography credentialing body recognized by the Society of Diagnostic Medical Sonography (SDMS) Board of Directors.
C. Uphold professional standards by adhering to defined technical protocols and diagnostic criteria established by peer review.
D. Acknowledge personal and legal limits, practice within the defined scope of practice, and assume responsibility for his or her actions.
E. Maintain continued competence through continuing education or recertification, or both.
F. Perform only medically indicated studies, ordered by a physician or designated health care provider.
G. Protect patients or study subjects, or both, by adhering to oversight and approval of investigational procedures including documented informed consent.
H. Refrain from the use of any substances that may alter judgment or skill and thereby compromise patient care.
I. Be accountable and participate in regular assessment and review of equipment, procedures, protocols, and results.

Principle III: To promote professional integrity and public trust, the diagnostic medical sonographer shall do the following:
A. Be truthful and promote appropriate and timely communications with patients, colleagues, and the public.
B. Respect the rights of patients, colleagues, the public, and oneself.
C. Avoid conflicts of interest and situations that exploit others or misrepresent information.
D. Accurately represent his or her level of competence, education, and certification.
E. Promote equitable care.
F. Collaborate with professional colleagues to create an environment that promotes communication and respect.

BOX **9-3** Code of Ethics for the Profession of Diagnostic Medical Sonography—cont'd

G. Recognize that well-intentioned health care providers can find themselves in ethical dilemmas; communicate and collaborate with others in resolving ethical practice. Report deviations from the SDMS Code of Ethics for the Profession of Diagnostic Medical Sonography to supervisors so that they may be addressed according to local policy and procedures.

H. Engage in ethical billing practices.

I. Engage only in legal arrangements in the medical industry.

Approved by SDMS Board of Directors, September 29, 2004.
From the SDMS, Plano, Tex., 1999-2005.

Summary

Although sonographers have serious ethical obligations, they do not enjoy unlimited freedom because their roles are derived from the patient-physician relationship. This factor, in addition to sonography's evolutionary quality, creates some degree of difficulty in practicing ethical distinctions. Nevertheless, these distinctions are crucial to provide an understanding of the sonographer's proper role in the health care team. Toward that goal, it is extremely important that internal policies and procedures reflecting the ethical concerns raised in this chapter should be defined, drafted, and implemented by sonographers and their supervising physicians. Only in this way can sonographers discharge their duties without evading their responsibilities or breaking the patient's trust.

A professional is a person who does something with great skill and who meets the high standards of his or her profession. The key to developing professionalism is understanding. Professional sonographers are sonographers who understand what their jobs are, which enables them to direct their energies toward performing those jobs. The "pros" understand the roles of other people in their profession—patients, physicians, and various health care specialists—and have acquired the ability to deal with each other in terms of reasonable expectations. Only through experience can the sonographer gain this understanding; however, experience takes time.

If a sonographer wants to be thought of as a professional, he or she must be willing to ask for information and guidance, seek explanations of terms and jargon, become skillful at interacting with patients, and learn how clinicians think in order to develop a dialogue with them and their agents. A sonographer also needs to understand and inform those within his or her professional sphere not only about the strengths but also about the limitations of sonography and its purveyors.

The expanding role of diagnostic ultrasound has had a profound impact on medicine and has resulted in many revolutionary changes in patient evaluation and treatment. It has also simultaneously raised some ethical questions.

The best testimonial sonographers can offer their profession is found in daily interactions that result in a patient who has been served well, treated fairly, and received the sonographer's personal best. The sonographer who wants to reach the goal of doing the best for the patient and the profession must perform in the following manner.

Do:

• Thoroughly explain the procedure and what is expected of the patient

• Work with extreme care to avoid causing the patient injury

- Question any abnormal instructions
- Maintain records and documents of the procedures performed in the event the information is requested later
- Use common sense and judgment, and practice within the limits of the sonographer's abilities and as taught

Do not:

- Perform sonography procedures that the sonographer has not been taught
- Fail to meet the established standards for the safe care of patients
- Fail to prevent injury to coworkers, other hospital employees, or visitors because this may result in a lawsuit

BIBLIOGRAPHY

Chervenak FA, McCullough LB: Ethical issues in obstetric sonography. In Herman M, editor: *Diagnostic medical sonography: a guide to clinical practice, vol 1: obstetrics and gynecology,* Philadelphia, 1991, JB Lippincott.

Craig M: Treating patients with patience, *J Diagn Med Sonography* 1:16-18, 1989.

Craig M: Controversies in obstetric and gynecologic ultrasound. In Herman M, editor: *Diagnostic medical sonography: a guide to clinical practice, vol 1: obstetrics and gynecology,* Philadelphia, 1991, JB Lippincott.

Lea JH: Psychosocial progression through normal pregnancy. A model for sonographer-patient interaction, *J Diagn Med Ultrasound* 1:55-58, 1985.

Maslow AH: *Motivation and personality,* ed 2, New York, 1987, Harper & Row.

Society of Diagnostic Medical Sonography website. Available at: *http://www.sdms.org.*

U.S. Food and Drug Administration: *FDA cautions against ultrasound 'keepsake' images, FDA Consumer Magazine,* Jan/Feb 2004. Available at: *http://www.fda.gov/fdac/default.htm.*

U.S. Food and Drug Administration: *FDA statement on fetal keepsake videos.* Available at: *http://www.fda.gov/cdrh/consumer/fetalvideos.html.*

Chapter 10

Sound Futures

Learning Objectives

Students who successfully complete this chapter will be able to do the following:

1. Compare and contrast the roles and functions of hospitals and clinics.
2. List common nonhospital sonography settings.
3. Identify major job search strategies.
4. Name the common types of resumes.
5. Discuss the importance of first impressions at job interviews.
6. Identify the factors necessary to produce a salary-negotiating strategy.
7. List the most credible individuals to use as references.

Key Terms

attitude	functional resumes	work ethics
chronologic resumes	resumes	

As sonographers near the end of the training experience, they engage in looking for that first job as a sonographer. Some graduate sonographers choose to specialize in a single branch of medical sonography, whereas others who want broader exposure look for a setting in which they can practice and increase their specialty skills. Hospitals, clinics, office practices, and mobile services are the most common settings for graduate sonographers to begin their careers, but there are others. This chapter explores those settings and their hierarchies and acquaints the reader with the planning and implementation of a successful job search.

INSTITUTIONAL SETTINGS

According to the U.S. Department of Labor, Bureau of Labor Statistics (BLS), more than half of all sonographers work in hospitals and most of the remainder work in physicians' offices or diagnostic laboratories. The job forecast for sonographers is excellent due to the growth and aging of the American population. Faster-than-average growth has been predicted through the year 2012.

Additional information about working conditions, training, qualifications, and more is available at the BLS website: *http://www.bls.gov/oco/ocos273.htm.* The Society of Diagnostic Medical Sonography also offers a "model job description" in the career section of its website: *http://www.sdms.org* that is helpful in formulating postgraduation plans (Box 10-1).

BOX **10-1** Society of Diagnostic Medical Sonography Model Job Description:
Diagnostic Medical Sonographer

The U.S. Department of Labor, Bureau of Labor Statistics' (BLS) most recent edition of the *Occupational Outlook Handbook* lists the diagnostic medical sonographer as an occupation that is separate and distinct from the radiology technologist.

The following is a recommended MODEL job description for the position of diagnostic medical sonographer. This model job description is basic and may be used as is or modified as necessary to meet other specific requirements of employment.

For additional related information, see the *Scope of Practice for the Diagnostic Ultrasound Professional (http://www.sdms.org/positions/scope.asp)* and the *Diagnostic Ultrasound Clinical Practice Standards (http://www.sdms.org/positions/clinicalpractice.asp).*

JOB TITLE

Diagnostic medical sonographer

JOB DESCRIPTION

A diagnostic medical sonographer is a diagnostic ultrasound professional who is qualified by professional credentialing and academic and clinical experience to provide diagnostic patient care services using ultrasound and related diagnostic procedures. The scope of practice of the diagnostic medical sonographer includes those procedures, acts, and processes permitted by law for which the individual has received education and clinical experience; has demonstrated competency; and has completed the appropriate American Registry of Diagnostic Medical Sonographers (ARDMS) certification, which is the standard of practice in ultrasound.

ORGANIZATIONAL REPORTING RELATIONSHIP

- Administrative supervisor: chief sonographer*
- Medical supervisor: attending or supervising physician*

BOX **10-1**   Society of Diagnostic Medical Sonography Model Job Description: Diagnostic Medical Sonographer—Cont'd

JOB SUMMARY

- The diagnostic medical sonographer is responsible for the independent operation of sonographic equipment and for performing and communicating results of diagnostic examinations using sonography.
- The diagnostic medical sonographer is responsible for daily operations of the sonographic laboratory, patient schedule, equipment maintenance, the report of equipment failures, and quality assessment. The sonographer maintains a high standard of medical ethics at all times and is self-motivated to increase level of understanding and knowledge of the field, disease, and new procedures as they evolve.

ESSENTIAL FUNCTIONS

- Performs clinical assessment and diagnostic sonography examinations
- Uses cognitive sonographic skills to identify, record, and adapt procedures as appropriate to anatomic, pathologic, diagnostic information and images
- Uses independent judgment during the sonographic examination to accurately differentiate between normal and pathologic findings
- Analyzes sonograms, synthesizes sonographic information and medical history, and communicates findings to the appropriate physician
- Coordinates work schedule with departmental director or scheduling desk, or both, to assure workload coverage
- Assumes responsibility for the safety and mental and physical comfort of patients while they are in the sonographer's care
- Assists with the daily operations of the sonographic laboratory
- Maintains a daily log of patients seen and completes examination billing forms
- Maintains ultrasound equipment, work area, and adequate supplies
- Participates in the maintenance of laboratory accreditation
- Establishes and maintains ethical working relationships and good rapport with all interrelating hospitals and referral or commercial agencies
- Performs other work-related duties as assigned

EXAMPLES OF DUTIES AND RESPONSIBILITIES

- Performs all requested sonographic examinations as ordered by the attending physician
- Prepares preliminary reports and contacts referring physicians when required, according to established procedures
- Coordinates with other staff to assure appropriate patient care is provided
- Addresses problems of patient care as they arise and makes decisions to appropriately resolve the problems
- Organizes daily work schedule and performs related clerical duties as required
- Assumes responsibility for the safety and well-being of all patients in the sonographic area/department
- Reports equipment failures to the appropriate supervisor or staff member
- Provides in-service education team on requirements of sonographic procedures as requested by other members of the health care team
- Performs other related duties as assigned

Continued

BOX **10-1** Society of Diagnostic Medical Sonography Model Job Description: Diagnostic Medical Sonographer—Cont'd

QUALIFICATIONS

Education

- Graduating from a formal diagnostic medical sonography program or cardiovascular technology program that is accredited by the Commission on Accreditation of Allied Health Education Programs (CAAHEP) is required
- Bachelor of science degree in diagnostic medical sonography is desirable

Required Licenses/Certifications

- Active certification by ARDMS in the specialty or specialties as appropriate
- Current compliance with continuing medical education requirements for the specialty or specialties as appropriate

Experience

- As defined by the institution

Demonstration of Skills and Abilities

- Ability to effectively operate sonographic equipment.
- Ability to evaluate sonograms in order to acquire appropriate diagnostic information.
- Ability to integrate diagnostic sonograms, laboratory results, patient history and medical records, and adapt sonographic examination as necessary.
- Ability to use independent judgment to acquire the optimum diagnostic sonographic information in each examination performed.
- Ability to evaluate, synthesize, and communicate diagnostic information to the attending physician.
- Ability to communicate effectively with the patient and the health care team, recognizing the special nature of sonographic examinations and patient's needs.
- Ability to establish and maintain effective working relationships with the public and health care team.
- Ability to follow established departmental procedures.
- Ability to work efficiently and cope with emergency situations.

PHYSICAL REQUIREMENTS

The employee must be physically capable of carrying out all assigned duties:
- Emotional and physical health sufficient to meet the demands of the position
- Strength sufficient to lift some patients, move heavy equipment on wheels (up to approximately 500 lb), and move patients in wheelchairs and stretchers
- Ability to maintain prolonged arm positions necessary for scanning

RISK OF EXPOSURE TO BLOOD-BORNE PATHOGENS

- Category I—tasks involve exposure to blood, body fluids, or tissues

SALARY/BENEFITS

- As defined by the institution

NOTE: Salary should be competitive for geographic location, practice setting, and practice specialty. Refer to the latest edition of the *Society of Diagnostic Medical Sonography (SDMS) Annual Income Report* for specific information.
From the SDMS, Plano, Tex., 1999-2005.

Hospitals

Hospitals are the largest and most common locations of medical imaging services. With a mission to provide treatment and diagnosis to both inpatients and outpatients, a hospital requires the services of many skilled and unskilled individuals. A newly employed sonographer must become acquainted with and work cooperatively with many of them.

The term *hospital* describes an institution for the reception, medical treatment, and care of the sick or wounded. The original definition of the word derived from the term *hospes*, or *guest*, and referred to an inn offering hospitality to those in need of shelter and maintenance.

Through the years, hospitals generally have been nonprofit, charitable institutions, often operated by religious groups and generally administered by retired physicians. Today's hospitals still provide for the care of the sick and the wounded, but most are operated as businesses rather than charitable organizations.

ADMINISTRATION

At the top of the chain of command, overseeing all of the hospital activities, is the administrator, or chief executive officer (CEO). Surrounding this individual is a large support staff whose task is to administer the daily business affairs of the institution. The sonographer's first experience with this administrative staff is likely with the human resources department. He or she also makes use of the services of the accounting department, which issues payroll checks, and if the sonographer requires personal medical services at any time, he or she may interact with the insurance and accounts-payable division. The purchasing department of the hospital also falls within the administrative services, and the sonographer may work with these employees when requesting or evaluating diagnostic ultrasound equipment. As the sonographer becomes a contributing employee of the sonography field of service, he or she may also consult or be consulted by the risk management, quality improvement, or corporate compliance representatives of the hospital to review or develop policies and procedures for a department.

OPERATIONS

This category encompasses all the services necessary to keep the physical plant running such as maintenance, laundry, central supply, housekeeping, food services, mail room, and communication services. A sonographer should visit each of these areas during new-employee orientation. He or she will learn firsthand that without the services of these employees, there would be no working environment would exist.

MEDICAL STAFF

The physician component of the medical staff includes the chief physician, staff physicians, residents, fellows, and interns. A sonographer is called on frequently to communicate with referring physicians and their staff members. Whether scheduling patients or relaying the results of their examinations, the sonographer must be knowledgeable, articulate, precise, cooperative, and courteous. He or she is expected to follow the department's policies regarding scheduling and the transmission of examination results. The sonographer may also be required to assist staff members or referring physicians with procedures such as biopsies, aspirations, amniocentesis, and catheterizations.

NURSING STAFF

The nursing service administrator usually oversees the operation of the nursing staff, head/charge nurses, and staff nurses. Both registered nurses (RNs) and licensed vocational or practical nurses (LVNs/LPNs) usually constitute the nursing staff. Nurse aides, orderlies, and ward clerks also report to nursing services.

Hospitals are composed of many specialty departments such as pharmacy, surgery, nursery, labor and delivery, and emergency. All, including the imaging department, are organized and operated under a similar chain of command. Sonography services may be part of the radiology department, the nuclear medicine department, the noninvasive imaging department, or an adjunct to other departments such as cardiology and obstetrics (Fig. 10-1).

Clinics

A clinic is a smaller version of the hospital, with the exception that it usually does not provide 24-hour or inpatient services. It has many, but not all, of the professional services offered in a hospital setting. Sonography services may be centralized in an imaging department, with the sonography staff expected to perform a broad spectrum of sonography studies. A chain of command, similar to that found in the hospital setting, exists in a clinic setting.

NONHOSPITAL SETTINGS

Office practices

It was inevitable that technologic advances would be incorporated into physicians' clinical practices. The only limitations were cost and difficulty of operation. Consequently, sonographers found requests for their services in private office settings. Just as the clinic evolved as a smaller version of the hospital, so also does the office practice mirror the clinic in miniature form.

Working as a sonographer in an office practice allows for clinical specialization and the promise of a unique and personalized learning experience. It also offers a relatively low-stress environment compared with the sometimes-intense environment of a hospital, and of course—not having to be on call.

Depending on the structure of the office hierarchy, the sonographer may work independently or be expected to conform to office policies and procedures. The operational, clinical, and personal inventories are much smaller, and activities are limited to examining ambulatory office patients referred by a select group of physicians.

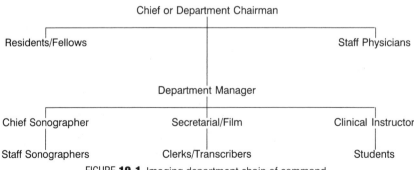

FIGURE **10-1** Imaging department chain of command.

Mobile ultrasound services

The most obvious difference between a mobile setting and the more traditional hospital-based or clinic-based laboratory is that the sonographer and equipment must be absolutely self sufficient.

Mobile ultrasound services may operate in metropolitan city medical practices, nursing homes, rural hospitals, and clinics or within the confines of the mobile transport vehicle itself. Many large mobile ultrasound companies provide specially adapted and equipped company-owned vans to each sonographer. In addition to performing patient examinations, mobile sonographers may be responsible for the following:

- Equipment and vehicle maintenance (e.g., gasoline, repairs, and administrative tasks such as keeping track of insurance/warranty policies and telephone pagers)
- Billing clients
- Maintaining their own time cards
- Delivering and transmitting their diagnostic images for interpretation if their client hospitals have no qualified physician interpreters on staff

With the introduction of smaller, portable ultrasound units, some companies have dispensed with the vans and either provide automobiles to employees or reimburse them for gas, mileage, and maintenance for using their own vehicles.

Mobile sonographers must be exceptionally experienced and particularly independent. Typically, they have no one to consult on questions while out in the field, so their clinical and administrative judgment must be excellent. They also must be physically fit to transport equipment in and out of the vans or automobiles at each stop. Importantly, they must be skilled drivers, experienced in all-weather driving conditions.

Logistics is one of the most important elements of a mobile service. For smooth functioning, the mobile sonographer requires the help of a competent coordinator to log scheduling calls, chart sonographer assignments, and handle calls from the field.

Freelancing

Because medical sonography is so technically demanding, a skilled sonographer is often recruited to perform after-hours scanning in private practices or operate full time as an independent agent. In some instances the sonographer also must provide the ultrasound instrument and arrange for its transportation and upkeep. Malpractice and liability insurance coverage is highly recommended.

The freelance sonographer shares many of the same obligations and benefits of the mobile sonographer. In addition to being well trained, extremely experienced, and independent, he or she must also possess an entrepreneurial spirit and good business and public relations skills.

Traveling

Sonographers who sign on with temporary staffing agencies must be able to readily adapt to many different types of equipment and to interact with many different departments and coworkers.

As a rule, "travelers" are paid higher salaries to compensate for having to travel, staying in hotels or apartments, eating out, and being away from family and friends.

Many staffing companies may not be willing to hire a new graduate without several years' experience. However, in a high-demand-low-supply employment cycle, a graduate sonographer should investigate this type of career. He or she may find a company that can provide the first assignment, and the experience gained would be invaluable.

The best way to start researching is to make a list of staffing companies that advertise in medical journals, in professional organization newsletters, or on the Internet. By calling many companies, one can begin to narrow the list on the basis of personal needs. The following checklist suggests questions a sonographer should ask a staffing agency recruiter:

- How long has this company been in the staffing business?
- Where are most assignments located?
- What type of salaries and benefits are offered?
- How long must one work before receiving benefits?
- What types of accommodations are provided (single/roommate, housing in apartments or motels)?
- What is the daily food allowance?
- What transportation allowances are offered: airfare, rental car, and so on?
- What experience level does this company require (e.g., years of experience, formal education, registry credentials)?
- Is the name of a traveling sonographer available in order to ask him or her questions about this type of job?

For someone who likes variety and the opportunities to travel to new places, meet new people, and be in control of one's own schedule, the traveling sonographer's job may be a good fit.

Commercial ultrasound: applications specialist and sales

The commercial world of ultrasound may be the best of all worlds because it offers sonographers a chance to use their ultrasound skills and education as they speak to and instruct physicians and other sonographers. The expanding use of contrast agents in some clinical studies has opened a new career option for sonographers in the pharmaceutical industries. However, the two most common jobs are those of commercial applications specialist or sales. Both of these are usually the *next* step for sonographers who feel they have reached the "ceiling" in clinical work. Nevertheless, depending on the sonographer's education and previous work experience, as well as the demands of the marketplace, a recent graduate might be hired.

Both sales staff and applications specialists get the opportunity to see and use the latest technology and possibly play a part in the design of new-generation equipment. Candidates for either job need good communication and presentation skills. Not only is it important to be articulate, but more importantly, they must also be excellent listeners. Commercial ultrasound requires asking customers open-ended questions (*why, what, when*), listening closely to their issues and concerns, and trying to find solutions among the company's products.

A sense of humor, great stamina, and the ability to work under pressure are necessary to meet the extensive travel demands of both jobs. In the commercial world, performance is measured by productivity (i.e., quotas), rather than patients scanned.

The transition from clinical to commercial ultrasound presents a steep learning curve and requires developing attitude and personality. Many sonographers begin their commercial careers as applications specialists, but those who stay with commercial ultrasound often move next into developing customer education programs or sales. From sales, the career ladder can eventually lead to management and marketing.

Research

One of the most interesting and least talked about nonclinical careers in sonography is that of *research sonographer.* The rapid technologic advances in sonography and its widening scope of clinical and commercial application have increased the demand for sonographers in the research arena.

The research sonographer's role is often varied and may involve clinical scanning of humans/animals for part of the day and the remainder involved in actual research activities. Among those activities are the ability to develop research and grant proposals, daily data entry and analysis, writing scientific abstracts and articles, traveling, and giving presentations.

Those selected for research positions are usually sonographers with at least 5 years' clinical experience. Often, they are selected from academic institutions where research and teaching are highly prized.

If a research position is among a sonographer's long-term goals, he or she should consider the following traits that embody the research sonographer:
• Intellectual curiosity
• Passion for ultrasound
• Objectivity when working with and studying animals
• Knowledgable and perceptive with data and statistics
• Skillful in time management
• Flexibility
• Good communication skills
• Willingness to travel

Valuable resources for the research-oriented sonographer are available at the National Institutes of Health website, *http://www.nih.gov,* and at *http://www.studentjobs.gov.* These resources offer information on assessing one's skills and interests to match potential career opportunities and how to build a resume, post a resume online, or receive automated job alerts.

JOB SEARCH STRATEGIES

The versatility, portability, and affordability of diagnostic ultrasound have made it one of the most popular of all imaging modalities, and the career opportunities for sonographers extend far beyond the traditional hospital, clinic, or physician practices. The aim of this chapter is to offer information and recommendations on choosing and successfully landing one's first sonography position. No magical formulas for getting a job exist; it takes much thought, planning, and action (Box 10-2).

First, the graduate sonographer must consider the following:
• What kind of job is desired
• What location is of interest
• What hours, wages, and benefits the sonographer wants

Graduate sonographers should check out the jobs currently available in their area of choice to see if they qualify and if the jobs meet their needs.

Resumes

Most people view **resumes** as simply summaries of a job applicant's previous employment, experience, and education. A resume is actually nothing more than an advertisement.

BOX **10-2** Job Search Questionnaire

Getting a job requires much thought and planning. The following questionnaire is designed to help the graduate sonographer organize his or her efforts.

STRATEGIC PLAN
- What would be the ideal job for me?
- What are my long-term goals?
- What are my short-term goals?
- What compensation do I need? (e.g., salary, wages, benefits, perquisites)
- Where do I want to work?
- Would I accept less compensation to live in the location I prefer?
- What working conditions do I expect? (e.g., work schedule flexibility, environmental safety issues, job sharing)
- What compromises am I willing to make?
- What will I not accept?

TACTICAL PLAN
- What resources will I use? (e.g., resumes, employment agencies, newspapers and journals, the Internet)
- Whom will I tell about my job search? (Instructors, fellow students or coworkers, family, friends)

OPERATIONAL PLAN
- How much time will I dedicate to searching?
- How much am I willing to budget for a job search? (e.g., resume preparation, postage, travel to interviews, wardrobe)

The sonographer is selling him or herself. Nevertheless, a resume is the *first* impression one gives to an employer, so it should be good so that it is not the *last*.

Many styles of resumes exist, and graduate sonographers are encouraged to study them. Here are some practical thoughts about creating a resume:
- The document should be easy to convert—it should be created on a computer so that it is easy to correct, print, or send as an e-mail attachment.
- The resume should be readable, with the font size between 8 and 12 points. Standard fonts like Times New Roman and Arial should be used.
- Contact information should be included—one's name, address, phone number, and e-mail address should be positioned at the beginning of the resume so that it is easy for an employer to contact the applicant.
- The resume should be concise and focused. The words *I* or *me* should be avoided. The skills and personal traits that relate to the particular job should be offered. Biographic information and hobbies should be near the end of the resume. In some instances, unless specifically asked in the employment ad to provide references, one may want to have them ready at the job interview rather than incorporating them into the resume.
- Because the graduate sonographer is just starting out on a new career, perhaps he or she does not have many job experiences to list. Instead, he or she can indicate how many hours of clinical experience have been logged or give an approximate estimate of the number and types of patients who have been scanned.

- Background and reference checks are standard in today's workplaces. One should not lie about dates, education, salaries, accomplishments, or references.
- Objectives and goals should be included. To gain the reader's attention, in the first part of the resume the sonographer needs to tell the employer who he or she is and what he or she hopes to achieve.
- The sonographer should proofread the resume several times and eliminate any typos or grammatical mistakes.
- Several others should review the resume. Another pair of eyes can shed light on the resume's strengths and weaknesses, so a friend, family member, or instructor should read the resume and offer opinions.
- Resumes and cover letters should be mailed, and each resume should be followed up with a telephone call to check on the status of its review and to schedule an interview if possible.

Two basic types of resumes exist: functional and chronologic. **Chronologic resumes** list qualifications and past employment in reverse chronologic order. They are best suited for those with a fair amount of experience. **Functional resumes** highlight one's abilities rather than work history and work well for people just entering (or reentering) the work force. They are also suited to those who are transitioning to a new job or who have frequently changed jobs.

If this is a sonographer's first job, he or she can emphasize education and clinical experience to date. Any prior employment history should be listed at the bottom of the page and should be limited to company names, job titles, skills, and responsibility. With a little work and attention to details, a graduate sonographer can produce a resume that places him or her at the top of the list of candidates.

Cover letters

For a resume to stand out, the candidate must write a targeted, personalized letter that will make a positive impact.

Sonographers should not resort to using a form letter; instead, they should write an easy-to-read letter that makes the reader want to learn more about the candidate. Here are some tips to get started:

- *The candidate should focus on what the employer needs.* He or she should research each potential employer and find out how to help him or her.
- *The candidate should write to the right person.* This requires finding out the name of the person with hiring authority. Although this person is not usually a human resources staff member, he or she should be sent a copy of the letter.
- *The letter should be focused and to the point.* It should answer these simple questions:
  - What the candidate can do for the employer
  - What the candidate's current situation is
  - Why he or she wants to work for the employer
  - Why he or she is qualified for this position

The cardinal rules of writing a successful cover letter follow:

- *Keep it short.* A few paragraphs with short, direct sentences are adequate. Follow a traditional business letter format.
- *Write in one's own words.* Keep it conversational and do not use overly formal or stilted language (e.g., *pursuant, commensurate*).

- *Communicate positive energy and personality.* Let glimpses of one's personality come through. Skills are not the only consideration of employers. They are also interested in the sonographer's *likeability* and how well he or she sonographer's would *fit in* with their environment.
- *Follow up.* The "Golden Rule of Cover Letters" is to follow up. Otherwise, save everyone's time and oneself the postage!
- *Do not restate the resume.* Use the cover letter to summarize, explain, expand, or reposition one's skills. The employer should be reassured that one has a career plan and that the employer fits into it.
- *Eliminate excessive use of "I" or "me."* Put more variety and detail in the writing. For example, change "I scanned 1200 patients during my program" to "With 1200 patient scanning experiences, you will get an employee with a variety of scanning skills and knowledge."

Interviewing

Conducting interviews with job candidates enables an employer to evaluate the candidate, test his or her own expectations, and find the "best fit" to meet the hiring goals. Here are a few essential points to consider about job interviewing:

- The description of job duties provides a road map for the content of the interview.
- The candidate should listen to the interviewer and answer the questions asked in a straightforward, concise manner.
- He or she should maintain eye contact without staring.
- The candidate should be prepared to ask a few solid questions to demonstrate his or her knowledge and comfort level with the prospect of the job.
- The candidate should show that he or she prepared for the interview by learning something about the institution, even if only mentioning a visit to the institution's website!
- The candidate should ask for the job!
- He or she should follow up with a quick e-mail or thank you note for the chance to interview.

An important part of interviewing for a job is **attitude**, a manner of acting or thinking that shows one's disposition, opinions, and reactions. Attitudes are the outward signs of the values and character traits that people develop early in childhood. What interests employers the most are candidates' **work ethics**—how well they will adapt to the environment and what qualities they will bring to the job (Box 10-3).

Interviewers also look for confidence, a desirable trait. However, there is a fine line between confidence and arrogance, which is not desirable. Those with a realistic understanding of their skills are confident; those who attempt to convey skills or experience they do not have are often viewed as arrogant. The converse situation exists when job seekers underestimate their skills and experience. They are often seen as lacking self-confidence. Employers also like candidates who show humility (e.g., describing the input of other team members as being equally as usable as their own).

Many job candidates attempt to use humor to relieve the tension of an interview. That kind of humor, unfortunately, is often perceived as insincerity. Humor can be used effectively in an interview when describing something positive, like the teamwork previously mentioned. When humor is used in relation to a problem or challenge, it may be seen as diminishing the significance of the event. Sincerity is highly valued by employers. They want employees who understand when to be serious and when to be humorous.

Flexibility is also highly prized, and some interviewers test a job seeker on this issue. Applicants may be asked to interview at inconvenient times and places. For instance,

BOX **10-3**   Work Ethics Checklist

Listed below are the qualities and skills that demonstrate the meaning of the term *work ethics.*

Concerned: Cares for those entrusted to the sonographer's care. Willing to do whatever is necessary to make patients more comfortable or the task less painful.

Conscientious: Follows instructions carefully and exactly, giving the best effort to every task.

Considerate: Respects patients' and coworkers' physical and emotional feelings. Kind and caring.

Cooperative: Willing to help and work with others and pitch in during especially busy times.

Courteous: Polite to patients and staff and always addressing them by name or title, or both. Says *please* and *thank you* whenever appropriate. Answers patients' questions and is willing to explain what is going to happen so that patients know what they can expect.

Dependable: Reporting to work on time and completing all assigned tasks.

Enthusiasm: Being interested and excited by work as a sonographer.

Honest: Truthful and accurate in reporting on cases and acknowledging any personal errors.

Pleasant: Cheerful when greeting and talking to patients and staff.

Respectful: Careful to treat patients and staff with respect and dignity at all times.

Trustworthy: Inspires confidence of patients and staff by following through on all promises and by keeping patient or staff information in confidence.

Understanding: Sees things from another's point of view and appreciates how a patient feels.

someone who is in school or working during the day may be asked to come for a 10 AM interview. The object of this test is to see how flexible and honest the applicant is in solving the potential problem.

Body language, voice inflections, and gestures often speak louder than words, so the candidate should be mindful of what his or her nonverbal communication indicates.

First impressions

During a job interview, a first impression is made within the first 30 seconds. If a candidate is too formal in appearance, he or she might be perceived as being rigid or stuffy. Conversely, too casual an appearance might send the signal that he or she is insincere or lazy.

As part of making a good first impression, a candidate should do the following:

- Choose clothing that gives a professional impression. Avoid wearing clothes that are trendy, and dress simply and conservatively.
- Be clean and well groomed. Hairdos should be neat and well-maintained, and men should have well-trimmed head and facial hair.
- Refrain from strong perfumes or aftershaves, as many people are allergic. Due to nervousness, using an unscented antiperspirant is advisable.
- Cover any tattoos, avoid gaudy jewelry, and limit pierced jewelry to the ears only.
- Wear shoes that are clean, polished, and in good repair.
- Ensure that nails are clean and trimmed. Ladies' nails should not be too long or polished with garish colors. Artificial nails are not permitted in most health delivery settings because they pose an increased risk of infection.

Even after a sonographer is successful in getting a job, he or she should continue to follow these suggestions because the impression left on the job at the end of each day will be considered, along with one's performance, when the time comes for advancement or a raise.

Salary negotiations

Salary issues arise at different points of an interview. For some, the issue of money comes after one receives an offer. For others, it is discussed early on to ensure that neither the candidate nor the interviewer is wasting one another's time.

When the topic of pay arises, the sonographer should have a salary negotiation ready. The first thing to do is find out the salary range for a similar position in one's area. Sometimes this information is available from job listings, friends, employment agencies, professional journals, the Bureau of Labor Statistics, or online salary surveys. Once the sonographer possesses these numbers, he or she should determine how much money is necessary to maintain his or her cost of living:

- Rent/mortgage
- Food
- Clothing/uniforms
- Utilities
- Car/transportation
- Education
- Loans
- Insurance
- Disposable income for things like gifts, vacation, and entertainment

After making these calculations, the sonographer can decide what salary is really necessary and what salary he or she is willing to take.

When discussing money, the sonographer should let the interviewer state the salary range first. How much salary is negotiable depends on factors such as the position, the hospital or company, the number of available applicants, the sonographer's potential value to the employer, and his or her experience. Most entry-level salaries are not up for much negotiation, but midlevel ranges can fluctuate as much as 10% to 20%. Employers negotiate within that range but seldom exceed it, except in special circumstances. Written backup is a good way to justify a salary request. The sonographer should bring in any statistics that may have been found, as well as performance evaluations, letters of recommendation, or other proof of the candidate's worth.

After the sonographer states a salary request, the employer may disagree with the number and make a counter offer instead. The sonographer should take at least 24 hours to do some figuring and be certain that this offer will really work for him or herself. Factors like vacation, insurance, retirement plans, and continuing education stipends should be considered as important as income. Money should not be the main factor in choosing a particular job or career. Although education and experience may earn the right to higher pay, working at a job one loves is priceless.

Nevertheless, the sonographer should get the final offer in writing so that there are no surprises in the first paycheck.

Talking about wages is new to most graduates or first-time job seekers, so they should practice their "pitch" in advance with a friend or family member. Showing professionalism and enthusiasm will help sell the applicant in a positive manner.

Once the sonographer has started the new job, he or she should close the loop by writing to or calling everyone involved (family, friends, references, and those who have given interviews) to thank them for their input and participation.

References

The purpose of providing references is to help future employers understand the applicant's assets and potential growth areas. The following list presents the most credible references:
- Managers or supervisors with whom the sonographer has worked directly
- Managers and supervisors with whom the sonographer has worked indirectly
- Experienced coworkers who are familiar with his or her work
- Professional instructors and peers who are familiar with his or her abilities

After making a list, the sonographer should talk to each possible reference to do the following:
- Get advice regarding the sonographer's job search
- Learn how they perceive his or her strengths and areas of future growth
- Clear up any misconceptions the reference may have so that both parties give accurate information to the job interviewer
- Get permission to use the person as a reference in his or her job search
- Ask each person that agrees to notify the sonographer after he or she has been contacted

After speaking with all potential references, the candidate should identify the three people who will serve as the most positive and accurate references. This will provide him or her with the best references possible; however, it is wise to remember that just as there are no perfect people, there are no perfect references. To identify possible problems, when they call to say they were contacted by a potential employer, one should ask them about their conversation. What questions were asked? How did they respond? This information will help the candidate address any concerns a job interviewer may have about him or her.

Summary

Although the hospital is the most complex of the health care organizations, it also provides the broadest benefits. The opportunities to work with both inpatients and outpatients; interact with the multiple subdivisions of medical care; and be involved in teaching or research activities, or both, are incomparable. However, other strong career desires such as autonomy or specialization, relief from being on call, heavy workloads, or being in a dead-end job may motivate some sonographers to select employment in an alternative area.

Regardless of the type of job chosen, the common denominator is delivery of high-quality patient care. One common method is necessary to reach that goal: teamwork. Even the freelance sonographer must be a team player.

No matter what the job is, if someone wakes up *dreading* to go to work, he or she will not be motivated and the chances of success will be slim. Sonographers are members of one of the most popular occupations in health care and, as such, need to recognize the valuable contributions of each fellow health care professional and work cooperatively with all of them to achieve their mission.

BIBLIOGRAPHY

Craig M: Have skills. Will travel, *J Diagn Med Sonography* 13:313-314, 1997.
Craig M: Climbing the sonography career ladder, *J Diagn Med Sonography* 15:120, 1999.

Craig M: Travelers: the pros and cons, *J Diagn Med Sonography* 18:252, 2002.

National Institutes of Health: *Student Jobs.* Available at: *http://www.jobs.nih.gov/student.asp*

U.S. Department of Labor, Bureau of Labor Statistics: *Occupational outlook.* Available at: *http://www.bls.gov/home.htm*

U.S. Office of Personnel Management and the U.S. Department of Education's Student Financial Assistance office: *Career interests center.* Available at: *http://www.studentjobs.gov*

Chapter 11

Professional Development and Leadership

Learning Objectives

Students who successfully complete this chapter will be able to do the following:

1. Describe the functional skills expected of a diagnostic medical sonographer.
2. Discuss the need for continuing education and the role played by the American Registry for Diagnostic Medical Sonography.
3. Describe the operational, interpretive, and administrative duties, as well as the ongoing activities of a staff sonographer.
4. List and describe nonhospital careers.

Key Terms

Agency for Healthcare Research and Quality (AHRQ)

Centers for Medicare and Medicaid Services (CMS)

Current Procedural Terminology (CPT) codes

As the completion of education and training as a sonographer comes to a close, it is time to turn attention to how to become the best sonographer possible one can be and how to contribute to the profession. The didactic and clinical practice sessions will soon be exchanged for front-line work with patients in the "real world." Rather than studying theory and scanning techniques, the sonographer's attention must now focus on not only getting a good job, and on how sonography relates to society and how society affects sonography. The sonographer needs to be concerned with the legal, ethical, legislative, and political issues that will affect him or her. He or she needs to find resources to deal with the challenges of practicing sonography in one or more work settings. Hopefully the sonographer will begin to see how the field needs strong, committed, and visionary leaders to keep it moving along successfully.

BIRTH OF AN OCCUPATION

The practice of sonography, as with any relatively new endeavor, has attracted people from many backgrounds, who entered the field through any of several avenues. Although sonography has grown in experience, technologic advances, and popularity, it has struggled to create enough accredited educational facilities to meet the workplace demand. This is partially due to the fact that in the first few decades, much sonographer training occurred through short courses and on-the-job training. Additionally, it was nonphysicians, neurologists, obstetricians, and cardiologists—as much or more than the imaging specialties—who nurtured and promoted the technique until it began to achieve clinical recognition. Therefore diagnostic ultrasound became an adjunct of many existing specialties rather than becoming aligned with and the responsibility of a single medical specialty group.

The early years were devoted more to research than the delivery of health care, as physicians and their "technicians" worked in concert to explore the clinical possibilities and dream of what the future might hold. The American Institute of Ultrasound in Medicine (AIUM), one of the first organizations devoted exclusively to diagnostic ultrasound, began to address the issue of training. The AIUM encouraged the formation of a technical branch, the American Society of Ultrasound Technical Specialists (ASUTS), so that it could concentrate on the issue of physician training. Both organizations have had a tremendous effect on the field of diagnostic ultrasound, not only in the United States but globally as well.

The ASUTS developed the first guidelines and requirements for the training of sonographers. Realizing how imperative it was to create a new and separate occupation, with the help of AIUM President Gilbert Baum, the ASUTS applied to the Manpower Division of the American Medical Association (AMA) to create a new occupation. In 1973 the field now known as *diagnostic medical sonography* was created.

The ensuing years were devoted to working with many multidisciplinary groups to develop a *Document of Essentials for Education* and to help form the American Registry of Diagnostic Medical Sonographers (ARDMS) as a means to evaluate sonographer competency. Efforts also led to the Joint Review Committee for Diagnostic Medical Sonography (JRCDMS) accrediting sonography educational programs.

During this period, the ASUTS replaced the term *ultrasound specialist* with *diagnostic medical sonographer* and became the Society of Diagnostic Medical Sonography (SDMS). One of the society's continuing missions is to elevate the occupation of sonographer to that of a professional.

PROFESSION VERSUS OCCUPATION

The popular opinion of a profession depends on the approach he or she has to an occupation.

Most *professionals* are serious about striving for excellence in their work and demonstrating their responsibility and ethical concerns. Their work is more than an occupation. They do not consider their occupation simply as a way to support themselves or as a stepping stone to other career opportunities. To them, there is positive value in being recognized as professionals and they consider being referred to as *technicians* or *nonprofessionals* as being unfavorable and a negative description of their positions, status, and motivation.

Many patients' views of a professional focus on conduct, attitude, and dress, but those reflect the personal values or stereotypes of the viewer. To achieve true and recognized professional status will require advanced education and autonomy in all areas of sonographic practice.

Some of the best arguments for recognizing sonographers as professionals are that they are characterized by the following characteristics:

- Engaged in predominantly intellectual and varied work as opposed to routine, manual, mental, mechanical, or physical jobs
- Required to consistently exercise judgment and discretion
- Produce work that cannot be standardized in relation to a given period of time
- Require advanced knowledge of a scientific field that can only be acquired by prolonged intellectual instruction and study at an institution of higher learning

The debate over using the terms *profession* and *professional* is restrictive if confined to the legal and sociologic definitions. Only those within the field, or closely involved in it, can appreciate the impact of a sonographer's role.

A graduate sonographer must decide whether he or she wants to be part of an occupation, in which the basic requirement is to show up and do a job reasonably well in exchange for a paycheck, or to challenge himself or herself with the continuing education, personal standards, and goals that separate professionals from "9 to 5" employees.

BECOMING AN OUTSTANDING SONOGRAPHER

Once a sonographer-student overcomes the obvious educational and training hurdles that face all sonographer-students, he or she becomes aware of other equally important facets of being a good sonographer—those that are more attitudinal than tangible and are acquired only through patience and experience. The goal of this chapter is to instill an understanding of what is expected of the sonographer and the confidence to take him or her from the familiar, protected world of the student into a professional career.

Role models

If graduate sonographers were to think for a minute of the instructors and the clinical sonographers who have assisted them in the goal of becoming a sonographer, beyond the memory of their technical abilities, what desirable personal qualities come to mind? As sonographer-students learn what is expected of them after graduation, they should be able to match these early role models with the qualities and abilities they hope to acquire and perfect—qualities such as integrity, accountability, and an obvious concern for maintaining high professional standards. Like their early role models, graduate sonographers, too, are expected to uphold and promote quality education, protect and enhance the professional status of sonographers, and demonstrate leadership to advance wider recognition of sonographers within the medical profession and among the public.

Attitudinal qualities

Emotional maturity is expected of graduate sonographers. This quality may be revealed through the use of initiative and independent judgment whenever necessary while always remaining within departmental guidelines, whether working with or without supervision. Acting in a diligent and responsible manner; recognizing and respecting the boundaries of professional closeness to patients; and demonstrating discretion, as well as empathy and understanding with regard to patients, also are expressions of maturity.

Patience and tenacity are two important attributes that help sonographers see each patient examination to full completion. Recognizing the need to expand some studies to other anatomic areas also is important in the quest to answer clinical questions.

Most students eagerly await the day they can put aside their textbooks and actually do the things they have studied and worked so hard to perfect. As a sonographer enters the sonography work environment, however, he or she becomes acutely aware of how much more knowledge is necessary. The sonographer needs motivation to advance beyond basic skills.

Graduates are expected to maintain competency and to engage in continuing education to remain current with advances in the field. Toward that end, most sonographers seek certification by the ARDMS in one or more of the following specialties:

- Abdomen
- Breast
- Cardiac (Adult/Pediatric)
- Fetal echocardiography
- Neurosonology
- Obstetrics and gynecology
- Ophthalmology
- Vascular

Although earning certification or registry credentials is not mandatory, it is an excellent means of assuring the medical and lay communities that a sonographer is competent to perform quality diagnostic examinations. A sonographer should keep in mind, however, that simply acquiring credentials does not mean that all of his or her goals have been satisfied.

In addition to developing technical skills, a sonographer should bring imagination and artistry to his or her scanning activities. Each examination should become a personal challenge as the sonographer questions and confronts his or her fund of knowledge. Graduate sonographers must develop interpersonal skills and a willingness to involve others in their growth. Above all, they must be team players and not soloists!

Functional skills

Full-fledged sonographers should come into the profession with a high degree of technical ability and in-depth knowledge of anatomy and physiology, as well as the basic aspects of clinical medicine. Obviously, knowledge of ultrasound scanning protocols should be thorough. The number of procedures a sonographer knows depends on his or her background, training, and particular interests.

Although some sonographers decide to focus on a single specialty, many choose positions that require skill in each of the major sonography specialties. These general sonographers should have current knowledge of neurologic, cardiac, vascular, abdominal, obstetric, and gynecologic applications. Like their specialist counterparts, they must be capable of dealing effectively with patients and acting quickly in an emergency.

Both groups must have a complete understanding of the complex instrumentation required to ensure its high-quality performance. They must also be capable of deviating from normal techniques whenever necessary, as well as resourceful enough to develop new and better techniques to keep their departments up to date.

Sonographer-students have only limited opportunities to establish and maintain effective working relationships with patients, employees, physicians, and the general public. The realities of constantly changing and short clinical rotations shield students from the experience of carrying those relationships over longer periods—or to conclusion. Some graduates may find themselves thrust into situations in which they must supervise the work activities of backup sonographers and ancillary personnel.

A graduate sonographer is expected to complete more patient examinations than he or she did as a student. In whatever work situation the sonographer encounters, he or she must learn to organize the work so well that each patient is provided with a quality examination that is complete and that assists the diagnosis. Time management skills are required to meet this challenge. Expertise will develop with experience, but in the beginning, the sonographer should not hesitate to ask for and follow the advice of a supervisor and coworkers. The following are several commonsense guides for a new graduate to remember:

- *Ask* . . . whenever in doubt about a scanning procedure or patient care techniques
- *Know* . . . when and to whom to report significant patient symptoms
- *Acquaint oneself* . . . with the department and how it functions: hours, duties, supplies, resources, and intradepartmental, as well as interdepartmental, conduct
- *Become knowledgeable* . . . about the institution's emergency, fire, and disaster regulations and procedures

Because a sonographer's interpretive decisions play a crucial role in patient diagnosis, he or she must possess the writing and verbal skills necessary to communicate effectively with physicians, other health care workers, and patients.

Full-time sonographers are often required to work shifts or in an on-call capacity. This may mean working with less supervision and working at times when the usual staff or institutional resources are not available. Although the sonographer is more "on his or her own" in these instances, again, he or she should not hesitate to seek assistance whenever questions arise. One negative aspect of being on call is the possibility that one will have a busy night on call and get insufficient sleep to meet the demands of the next day's work.

In time, the sonographer may want to develop additional skills in other specialties. For each specialty area he or she wants to master, a broad appreciation of the anatomy, physiology, pathophysiology, and imaging skills particular to that area is required. Once sufficient clinical experience has been achieved, the sonographer should take on the challenge of passing the registry or certifying examinations governing that specialty.

In the preceding chapter, an overview of the various careers in sonography was presented. In this chapter, each of those career categories is expanded.

HOSPITAL-BASED CAREER OPPORTUNITIES

Staff sonographer

In large departments the level of experience usually classifies staff sonographers. Novice staff sonographers are expected to perform the most basic functions, whereas those with more experience are given additional responsibility and autonomy.

OPERATIONS

The following operational duties are expected of hospital-based sonographers:

- Check requisitions for completeness and procedure requested; refer any questions to the supervising sonologist before beginning the sonography procedure.
- Obtain any previous ultrasound studies and review the patient's chart to obtain pertinent clinical history; correlate laboratory data and other diagnostic test results. If necessary, consult with referring physicians regarding a patient's medical history or the clinical questions that prompted the sonography request, or both.
- Determine if any patient preparations have been properly carried out.
- Position patients correctly for the requested examination; explain the procedure to the patient and give necessary instructions for its completion.
- Perform or assist with interventional or emergency examinations (either in the department or at the bedside) with physician supervision.

INSTRUMENTATION

The sonographer is also expected to do the following:

- Knowledgeably operate all necessary diagnostic ultrasound equipment (A-Mode, M-Mode, B-Mode, and Doppler techniques)
- Select appropriate transducers (e.g., choosing type, frequency, diameter) for performance of the examination
- Use ancillary devices (e.g., oscilloscopes, cameras, recorders, strip-charts, computerized PAC systems) to permanently record the diagnostic images
- Conduct quality-control checks of ultrasound and recording equipment and record results in an equipment log; calibrate ultrasound and recording equipment as needed

INTERPRETATION

The sonographer has the following responsibilities:

- Recognize the significance of all visualized structures and be able to differentiate artifacts from anatomic or pathologic structures. If any equipment limitations are encountered, the sonographer should apprise the supervising sonologist of the situation.
- Recognize a diagnostic scan and appreciate the possible need to expand the scope of the study to include other anatomic areas or the use of other sonographic techniques, or both.
- Write a technical report on his or her examination findings that will accompany the images taken.
- With proper authorization, to render the supervising sonologist's initial interpretations to the referring physician if a "stat" report is required.

ADMINISTRATION

The hospital-based sonographer also has the following duties:

- Develop or maintain a departmental procedure manual
- Maintain cleanliness of all equipment and of the scanning area; maintain supplies for the unit or assigned room
- Fill out all forms such as a chronologic log; **current procedural terminology (CPT) codes** (five-digit numeric codes used to describe medical procedures); enter PAC systems; and, if no PAC system is available, create filing materials (film jackets/file folders) for each patient study

- Record and make copies of teaching- or research-quality examinations for the department's teaching file
- Keep records on all equipment, recording technical problems (including a photograph of the problem if possible), service calls, and any resulting repairs in an equipment log
- Establish and maintain good working relationships and rapport with referring physicians, hospital staff, patients, and commercial representatives

ONGOING SONOGRAPHIC RESPONSIBILITIES
Hospital-based sonographers have the following ongoing responsibilities:
- Evaluate new products and equipment as requested
- Demonstrate or teach sonographic techniques and clinical applications to students, visiting sonographers, nurses, interns, residents, fellows, and physicians
- Provide impromptu demonstrations or explanations, or both, to patients, family, visitors
- Review pathology, surgery, and delivery reports concerning previously scanned patients for follow-up; use these data to evaluate the accuracy of the sonography studies performed in the sonographer's facility
- Maintain currency by reading journals and attending local study groups, annual conventions, seminars, and symposia
- Contribute to departmental or institutional in-service education programs, or both

Technical director or lead sonographer

In addition to performing all of the tasks of the staff sonographer, the lead sonographer should be able to do the following:
- Work without supervision but within guidelines established in the departmental policies and procedures manual.
- Gain knowledge of all department equipment, accessories, and operating procedures; develop the ability to diagnose basic equipment malfunctions and communicate them to service personnel.
- Maintain records of revenues and expenditures and so on; review monthly budgets for accuracy and report any discrepancies.
- Secure supplies for the sonography section.
- Recognize and recommend action (as needed) for improvement of department functions.
- Coordinate activities of staff sonographers; mediate problems regarding staffing, scheduling, salary reviews and adjustments, discipline, morale, and so on. Provide input as requested on hiring, promoting, or terminating employees.
- Take responsibility for patient flow and patient care within the sonography department.
- Conduct inspections of the facility to ensure patient and sonographer safety.
- Prepare/assist in the applications for Ultrasound Practice Accreditation.

Department manager

Ideally, the manager of a sonography department should be a sonographer with management training or experience. A combination of skills is important because this individual must serve as the conduit (and sometimes the buffer) among administration, physicians, sonographers and other employees, and patients.

Courses such as health care administration, management principles, introduction to data processing, statistics, industrial relations or personnel management, financial accounting, health planning, and the legal aspects of health services administration are offered at many colleges and universities. If local institutions do not offer degrees in health administration, a course in business administration should be considered (accounting, economics, finance, law, management, marketing, and personnel management and labor relations).

Some of the major responsibilities of a department manager are as follows:

- Supervising (1) the professional and support staff and (2) the scheduling activities of the department (patients and staff)
- Assuming responsibility for the communication and practice of departmental and institutional policies, procedures, regulations, and information
- Handling personnel affairs (e.g., evaluations, promotions, raises, dismissals) and union negotiations
- Preparing or assisting in developing a budget, controlling inventory, and coordinating departmental purchasing (final decisions and authorizations)
- Overseeing quality assurance testing
- Participating in decision making and planning of the immediate, intermediate, and long-term goals of the department
- Preparing/assisting in the applications for Ultrasound Practice Accreditation

NONHOSPITAL CAREERS

Chapter 10 described various nonhospital settings in which sonographers perform patient examinations. This chapter continues exploring career opportunities that are not primarily hospital based or directly related to patient services.

Teaching

Along with the dynamic growth and acceptance of diagnostic ultrasound and sonography techniques came the critical need for educators skilled in sonography. Initial "teaching" occurred informally in a show-and-tell fashion. Over time, sonographers (the individuals usually drafted to perform early teaching chores) realized that they would need additional formal training in teaching techniques. The demands for sonography services increased, and produced a corresponding demand for the development of educational and training programs inside and outside the hospital environment. Sonography instructors may be active in didactic or clinical settings, or both. One of their primary duties is to develop a course curriculum and operational plans. Classroom instructional techniques may be gained through educational degree programs at the college or university level, as well as from seminars, symposia, and textbooks.

Sonographer-educators are also called on to supervise and evaluate student progress, maintain student records, schedule student assignments, and counsel students in both didactic and clinical settings. One of the biggest and most important responsibilities of a program director is the application for Commission on Accreditation of Allied Health Education Programs (CAAHEP) accreditation. The first hurdle is the preparation of documentation; the second is undergoing an accreditation site visit.

The rewards of teaching are immeasurable, but to be effective, candidates for this profession also must possess a love of working with students and the highest professional standards befitting a role model.

Research

Sonographers who thrive on intellectual stimulation and who are not content until they discover the "whys and wherefores" possess the basic traits of researchers. Along with the excitement of discovery, however, goes the task of performing detailed investigations and recording large amounts of data. Developing research grants, writing papers, educating new employees, and lecturing at scientific meetings are also important tasks expected of a research sonographer.

Research positions exist within universities, hospitals, or commercial manufacturing facilities. Sonography experience and a strong science background are important assets; in addition, some positions may require an advanced science degree. Communication skills, both verbal and written, are essential, as are precision and tenacity.

Commercial/corporate

Excellent opportunities exist in commercial manufacturing companies, manufacturers of related ultrasound products, and pharmaceutical companies that market ultrasound contrast agents. Typically, the most common entryway into the field of commercial ultrasound is as an applications specialist. This position involves providing customer training and support, as well as a great deal of travel and consulting with research and development engineers.

Applications specialists are expected to have an excellent grasp of the physical principles of diagnostic ultrasound and of all types of ultrasound instrumentation manufactured by their employers. They must be prepared to perform didactic and clinical demonstrations, conduct patient examinations, consult with physicians regarding interpretation, plan and implement customer courses, and represent their company as exhibitors at medical meetings. Their opinions and evaluations are also sought by research and development colleagues, and they may be expected to write procedural manuals, develop teaching slides and tapes, and contribute to advertising brochures.

The nature of the applications specialist's job requires him or her to work without direct supervision most of the time and therefore demands an extensive knowledge of sonographic technique and interpretation, pertinent clinical medicine, equipment operation and basic repairs, and professional conduct.

The second most common commercial career opportunity is in ultrasound equipment or accessories sales. Again, the sonographer-salesperson must possess all the requisite skills of a sonographer and have, or be willing to develop, sales skills and an understanding of business and finance. Extensive travel is required, along with the ability to coordinate both the shipping and installation of equipment and the services of applications specialists and service engineers.

Sales representatives are expected to interact with engineers, other salespersons, and each of the major functionaries in a commercial ultrasound setting (e.g., advertising, education, finance). They are also required to deal directly with physicians, department managers, sonographers, and purchasing agents. Like the applications specialists, salespersons are required to handle company exhibits at medical conventions and shows. Because of their wide exposure to both the commercial and scientific areas of medical sonography, they should be willing to serve as resources of information. As a result, they must continuously strive to keep abreast of all aspects of the field.

Communications

The need for disseminating diagnostic medical ultrasound information has steadily increased. The communications aspects of medical sonography include various endeavors such as writing, lecturing, and audiovisual production.

Communication skills, orientation to details, and the abilities to write and speak effectively and meet deadlines are only a few important attributes. Sonographers who also possess experience or degrees in journalism, public speaking, photography, art, or film production are the strongest candidates for such positions.

Law

The steady rise in ultrasound-related lawsuits has focused attention on the need for expert witnesses and attorneys with knowledge of sonography. A small number of sonographers have entered law school with the goal of becoming advocates for sonography personnel or patients, or both. It is still too early to define the complete dimensions or requirements of this developing career opportunity, but it will undoubtedly present an interesting career option.

The sonographer hired as an expert witness is usually one with years of experience in diagnostic ultrasound and national/international recognition of his or her expertise. Sometimes, all that is required of the sonographer expert witness is to review films and comment on the technical aspects and whether or not the films meet accepted standards. In other instances, the sonographer may be required to testify similarly, but under oath, in the courtroom. In the courtroom appearance the sonographer must try to simplify his or her answers about complex issues so that the judge and jury can understand both the questions asked and answered.

Additional opportunities exist in the areas of risk management and quality improvement for sonographers with experience, education, and interest in the corporate aspects of hospital administration.

INTERACTION WITH GOVERNMENTAL AGENCIES

Because of the current managed care climate, sonographers who work in hospitals, clinics, and office practices should familiarize themselves with various insurance billing codes and governmental agencies involved in health insurance and patient affairs.

Agency for Healthcare Research and Quality

The **Agency for Healthcare Research and Quality (AHRQ)** is charged with "improving the quality, safety, efficiency, and effectiveness of health care for all Americans." The agency's website, *http://www.ahrq.gov,* offers many publications, press releases, and clinical and consumer health items of interest. Additionally, the agency provides access to grant funding opportunities, research findings, and the Freedom of Information Act Reading Room.

Centers for Medicare and Medicaid Services

Formerly known as the Health Care Financing Administration (HCFA), **Centers for Medicare and Medicaid Services (CMS)** is the federal agency within the Department of Health and Human Services that is responsible for the national administration of Medicaid, Medicare, and State Children's Health Insurance Program (SCHIP), as well as the Health Insurance Portability and Accountability Act. CMS offers a wide range of information including manuals; forums; demonstrations; and lists of initiatives, regulations, statistics, and data. The CMS website is *http://www.cms.hhs.gov.*

Current procedural terminology codes

As mentioned earlier, CPT codes are used to describe medical procedures performed by physicians and other health care providers. HCFA developed CPT codes to assist in the assignment of reimbursement amounts to providers by Medicare carriers. The AMA publishes CPT codes and updates on their website at *http://www.ama.org.* Regularly visiting the site for information about coming additions or changes is important.

Summary

The roles and functions of a sonographer are multiple, varied, and still evolving. At first glance, performing sonography examinations appears deceptively simple because the basic operational concept is not difficult to understand. On closer inspection, it becomes apparent that the person wielding the ultrasound transducer has a profound effect on the quality of the examination and requires in-depth education and training if the greatest possible diagnostic benefits are to be realized.

The prerequisites for a sonographer candidate are many. They include intellectual curiosity, emotional maturity, the ability to conceptualize images in three dimensions, paramedical background, demonstrated psychomotor skills, and the ability to interact skillfully with people (physicians, patients, and other health care professionals).

Sonographers perform sonographic studies of patients to gather diagnostic data. Although such studies may be performed in various settings, they should always be carried out under the direct or indirect supervision and responsibility of a qualified physician.

The independent judgment of sonographers is critical because of the need to tailor sonographic examinations to each particular patient's disease process and body habitus. This judgment can be refined only by the sonographer's knowledge of anatomy, physiology, pathophysiology, and relevant clinical medicine and laboratory findings. Differential diagnosis is also an integral part of any sonography study in which pathologic conditions are found, and it is in this regard that sonographers have often been compared with physician assistants.

Sonographers must master the intricacies of ultrasound instrumentation if they expect to routinely produce diagnostic quality studies and overcome any scanning difficulties that might arise.

Interpersonal skills are required because sonographers are expected to discuss procedures with sonologists, referring physicians, other health care professionals, and patients. Each type of discussion requires a different approach and intent.

The dramatic advances in technology and the drastic changes in the delivery of health care have added new responsibilities for today's sonographers. However, with the added challenges come more opportunities to advance not only in the field of sonography but beyond.

The modern sonographer is usually cast in the role of teacher to students, staff members, and patients. Therefore as members of a fluid and continually evolving specialty and as seekers of professional autonomy, sonographers must mold every thought, word, and deed toward maintaining the highest of professional standards.

Sonography is many things. It is clinically valuable, exciting, and seemingly limited only by the sonographer's imagination. On behalf of all sonographers, past and present,

I encourage graduate sonographers to remember that their sonography education is a valuable and powerful tool that will help them get somewhere in life. Once "there," however, they must make the most of each day.

BIBLIOGRAPHY

Agency for Healthcare Research and Quality: *Quality research for quality health care.* Available at: *http://www.ahcpr.gov/about/qr4qhc/qr4qhc-1.htm.*

American College of Radiology: Ultrasound accreditation program. Available at: *http://www.acr.org.*

American Institute of Ultrasound in Medicine: The accreditation of ultrasound practices—impact on compliance with minimum performance guidelines. Available at: *http://www.aium.org.*

American Medical Association: *Current procedural terminology.* Available at: *http://www.ama-assn.org/ama/pub/category/3113.html.*

Baker JP: The history of sonographers, *J Ultrasound Med* 24:1-14, 2005.

Centers for Medicare and Medicaid Services (CMS): *About CMS.* Available at: *http://www.cms.hhs.gov.*

Joint Commission on Accreditation of Healthcare Organizations: *The HIPAA privacy regulation.* Available at: *http://www.jcaho.org.*

Makely S: *Professionalism in health care: a primer for career success,* ed 2, Upper Saddle River, N.J., 2004, Prentice-Hall.

Metcalf ZW: *Career planning guide for the allied health professions,* Philadelphia, 1997, Williams & Wilkins.

Society of Diagnostic Medical Sonography: *Professional risk management for sonographers.* Available at: http://www.sdms.org.

Patient Care Partnership: Understanding Expectations, Rights, and Responsibilities

WHAT TO EXPECT DURING YOUR HOSPITAL STAY

Understanding expectations, rights, and responsibilities

When you need hospital care, your doctor and the nurses and other professionals at our hospital are committed to working with you and your family to meet your health care needs. Our dedicated doctors and staff serve the community in all its ethnic, religious, and economic diversity. Our goal is for you and your family to have the same care and attention we would want for our families and ourselves.

The following sections explain some of the basics about how you can expect to be treated during your hospital stay. They also cover what we will need from you to care for you better. If you have questions at any time, please ask them. Unasked or unanswered questions can add to the stress of being in the hospital. Your comfort and confidence in your care are important to us.

High-quality hospital care

Our first priority is to provide you the care you need, when you need it, with skill, compassion, and respect. Tell your caregivers if you have concerns about your care or if you have pain. You have the right to know the identity of doctors, nurses, and others involved in your care, and you have the right to know when they are students, residents, or other trainees.

A clean and safe environment

Our hospital works hard to keep you safe. We use special policies and procedures to avoid mistakes in your care and keep you free from abuse or neglect. If anything unexpected and significant happens during your hospital stay, you will be told what happened, and any resulting changes in your care will be discussed with you.

Involvement in your care

You and your doctor often make decisions about your care before you go to the hospital. Other times, especially in emergencies, those decisions are made during your hospital stay. When decision making takes place, it should include the following:

DISCUSSING YOUR MEDICAL CONDITION AND INFORMATION ABOUT MEDICALLY APPROPRIATE TREATMENT CHOICES

To make informed decisions with your doctor, you need to understand the following:

- The benefits and risks of each treatment
- Whether your treatment is experimental or part of a research study
- What you can reasonably expect from your treatment and any long-term effects it might have on your quality of life
- What you and your family will need to do after you leave the hospital
- The financial consequences of using uncovered services or out-of-network providers Please tell your caregivers if you need more information about treatment choices.

DISCUSSING YOUR TREATMENT PLAN

When you enter the hospital, you sign a general consent to treatment. In some cases, such as surgery or experimental treatment, you may be asked to confirm in writing that you understand what is planned and agree to it. This process protects your right to consent to or refuse a treatment. Your doctor will explain the medical consequences of refusing recommended treatment. It also protects your right to decide if you want to participate in a research study.

GETTING INFORMATION FROM YOU

Your caregivers need complete and correct information about your health and coverage so that they can make good decisions about your care. That includes the following:

- Past illnesses, surgeries, or hospital stays
- Past allergic reactions
- Any medicines or dietary supplements (such as vitamins and herbs) that you are taking
- Any network or admission requirements under your health plan

UNDERSTANDING YOUR HEALTH CARE GOALS AND VALUES

You may have health care goals and values or spiritual beliefs that are important to your well-being. They will be taken into account as much as possible throughout your hospital stay. Make sure your doctor, family, and care team know your wishes.

UNDERSTANDING WHO SHOULD MAKE DECISIONS WHEN YOU CANNOT

If you have signed a health care power of attorney stating who should speak for you if you become unable to make health care decisions for yourself, or a "living will" or "advance directive" that states your wishes about end-of-life care, give copies to your doctor, family, and care team. If you or your family need help making difficult decisions, counselors, chaplains, and others are available to help.

Protection of your privacy

We respect the confidentiality of your relationship with your doctor and other caregivers and the sensitive information about your health and health care that are part of that relationship. State and federal laws and hospital operating policies protect the privacy of your medical information. You will receive a "Notice of Privacy Practices" that describes the ways that we use, disclose, and safeguard patient information and that explains how you can obtain a copy of information from our records about your care.

Preparing you and your family for when you leave the hospital

Your doctor works with hospital staff and professionals in your community. You and your family also play an important role in your care. The success of your treatment often depends on your efforts to follow medication, diet, and therapy plans. Your family may need to help care for you at home.

You can expect us to help you identify sources of follow-up care and to let you know if our hospital has a financial interest in any referrals. As long as you agree that we can share information about your care with them, we will coordinate our activities with your caregivers outside the hospital. You can also expect to receive information and, where possible, training about the self-care you will need when you go home.

Help with your bill and filing insurance claims

Our staff will file claims for you with health care insurers or other programs such as Medicare and Medicaid. They also will help your doctor with needed documentation. Hospital bills and insurance coverage are often confusing. If you have questions about your bill, contact our business office. If you need help understanding your insurance coverage or health plan, start with your insurance company or health benefits manager. If you do not have health coverage, we will try to help you and your family find financial help or make other arrangements. We need your help with collecting needed information and other requirements to obtain coverage or assistance.

While you are here, you will receive more detailed notices about some of the rights you have as a hospital patient and how to exercise them. We are always interested in improving. If you have questions, comments, or concerns, please contact *(name and number)*.

Modified from the American Hospital Association, 2003.

Pertinent Clinical Laboratory Tests

Laboratory tests are tools helpful in evaluating the health status of an individual. When gathering patient data before performing sonography, it is important to note any diagnostic tests the patient may have had. The following tests, arranged by organ/system, are most pertinent to general abdominal sonography and obstetric and gynecologic sonography.

HEMATOLOGY

Routine blood tests

Complete blood count (CBC): Routine screening of blood includes determinations of red blood cell (RBC) count, hematocrit (Hct), hemoglobin (Hgb), white blood cell (WBC) count, and differential WBC count (diff). An important additional observation is the sedimentation rate. Accurate hematologic diagnoses, as well as significant information about disease, can be gathered through the use of blood testing.

WBC: The number of white cells. High WBC can be a sign of infection. The WBC is also increased in certain types of leukemia. Low white counts can be a sign of bone marrow diseases or an enlarged spleen, viral infections, certain anemias, and diabetes. A low WBC (leukopenia) is also associated with HIV infection in some cases.

Total WBC count	Adults: 4000 to 11,000/mm^3
Differential count	Neutrophils 40% to 75%
	Eosinophils 1% to 6%
	Lymphocytes 20% to 45%
	Monocytes 2% to 10%
	Basophils 0% to 1%

Red blood cell (RBC): Red blood cells are the most common type of blood cell and are the vertebrate body's principal means of delivering oxygen to body tissues via the blood. RBCs are also known as *erythrocytes.*

Blood diseases involving RBCs include many kinds of anemias (sickle cell anemia, thalassemia, pernicious anemia, aplastic anemia). A surplus of RBCs occurs in a disease called *polycythemia vera.* Decreased RBCs are associated with Hodgkin disease, leukemia, and severe diarrhea.

Erythrocyte count: Male 4.5 to 6.5 million/mm^3; female 3.8 to 5.8 million/mm^3

Hemoglobin (Hgb): Hemoglobin is the amount of oxygen carrying protein contained within the RBCs. Low Hgb or hematocrit (Hct) suggests anemia. High Hgb can occur due to lung disease, living at high altitude, or excessive bone marrow production of blood cells.

Hgb: Male 13.5% to 17.5%; female 11.5% to 16.5%

Hct: The Hct or packed cell volume (PCV) is the proportion of blood that is occupied by RBCs. The packed cell volume can be determined by centrifuging the blood in a capillary tube (aka a hematocrit tube), which forces the cells to one end. The length of the tube containing blood cells divided by the length containing cells or plasma gives the PCV.

The Hct is not usually an important consideration when looking at a person's full blood count results, as most people are more concerned with the hemoglobin concentration and mean cell volume. However, the Hct gives an indication of how concentrated the red cells are in the blood and gives an indirect impression of whether the patient is dehydrated and how relevant the measured hemoglobin level is.

Hct (PCV): Male 40% to 54%; female 37% to 47%

Glucose: Glucose, a simple monosaccharide sugar, is one of the most important carbohydrates and is used as a source of energy. Carbohydrates are the human body's key source of energy. Glucose is absorbed into the bloodstream through the intestinal wall. Some of this glucose goes directly to fuel brain cells, while the rest makes its way to the liver and muscles, where it is stored as glycogen ("animal starch"), and to fat cells, where it is stored as fat. Glycogen is the body's auxiliary energy source, tapped and converted back into glucose when it needs more energy.

This test measures the sugar level in blood. High values are associated with eating before the test and diabetes.

Prothrombin time (PT): This test is used to determine the clotting tendency of blood, in the measure of warfarin dosage, liver damage, and vitamin K status.

PT: 7 to 10 sec

International normalized ratio (INR): 0.8 to 1.2

See also later section on digestive system tests.

Platelet (thrombocyte) count: Platelets are the smallest type of blood cell. They play a major role in blood clotting. When bleeding occurs, the platelets swell, clump together, and form a sticky plug that helps stop the bleeding. If there are too few platelets, uncontrolled bleeding may become a problem. If there are too many, the risk of a blood clot forming in a blood vessel is high. Platelets may also be involved in atherosclerosis (hardening of the arteries).

Normal values: 150,000 to 400,000/mm^3

DIGESTIVE SYSTEM TESTS

Bilirubin: Bilirubin is a waste product formed when hemoglobin breaks down. Insoluble in water, it is carried to the liver bound to albumin. Bilirubin is made water soluble in the liver by conjugation with glucuronic acid. As part of bile, the soluble bilirubin then passes through the common bile duct and is either temporarily stored in the gallbladder or passes right away into the gut. Some of the excreted bilirubin may be reabsorbed. Bacteria in the intestines modify bilirubin, causing the brown color of feces. The yellow color of urine is a result of products derived from bilirubin. The name of this metabolite is *urobilinogen*.

In diseases in which too much hemoglobin is broken down or the removal of bilirubin does not function properly, the accumulating bilirubin in the body causes jaundice. Low values are of no concern.

Bilirubin found unbound to albumin is referred to as "direct" bilirubin. When it is found soluble, or bound to albumin, it is referred to as "indirect" bilirubin. The terms "direct" and "indirect" refer to the fact that soluble bilirubin can be measured directly, whereas insoluble, or indirect, bilirubin must be solubilized before measurement.

Although both direct and indirect bilirubin can be measured separately, it is more common to just measure total bilirubin. Bilirubin is an excretion product, and the body does not control its levels. Bilirubin levels reflect the balance between production and excretion. Thus strictly speaking, there is not a normal level of bilirubin.

Bilirubin: Less than 1 mg/dl

PT and vitamin K administration test: PT is a liver enzyme that is part of the blood-clotting mechanism. The production of PT depends on adequate intake and utilization of vitamin K.

The increase of PT in liver disease may be the result of either malabsorption of the fat-soluble vitamin K or a deficiency in the formation of one of the clotting factors. Prolongation of PT manifests by bleeding tendencies. Persistently increased PT is associated with the presence of severe liver disease, with accompanying cellular damage (e.g., cirrhosis, metastatic disease).

A method of standardizing PT results, called the *INR system,* has been developed to compare PT results among laboratories using different test methods. Using the INR system, treatment to prevent blood clots (anticoagulant therapy) remains consistent even if a person has the test done at different laboratories. In some situations, only the INR is reported and the PT is not reported.

PT: Normal: 10 to 13 sec

INR: 1 to 1.4

The warfarin (Coumadin) dosage for people being treated to prevent the formation of blood clots is usually adjusted so that the PT is about 1.5 to 2.5 times the normal value (or INR values 2 to 3). PTs are also kept at higher levels for people with artificial heart valves, for the same reason.

Alanine transaminase (ALT): ALT is primarily a liver enzyme and is also called *serum glutamate pyruvate transaminase (SGPT)* or *alanine aminotransferase (ALAT).* This enzyme is released into the plasma by liver cell death, a normal event. However, when liver cell death increases, ALT levels rise above the normal range and the spillover of ALT is routinely measured as a marker of abnormal liver-cell damage. Alcoholic or viral hepatitis and severe congestive heart failure will increase ALT levels. An elevated ALT in the presence of normal levels of plasma alkaline phosphatase helps distinguish liver disease caused by liver-cell damage from diseases caused by problems in biliary ducts. The enzyme aspartate transaminase (AST) has a similar role, but because it tends to be found in other tissues such as the heart, it is not as specific to the liver.

ALT: Up to 40 U/L

Lactic acid dehydrogenase (LDH): LDH is present in nearly all metabolizing cells, with the highest concentrations in tissues of the kidneys, heart, skeletal muscle, brain, and liver, and in RBCs. Tissue damage causes this enzyme to be released into the bloodstream. Origin of the release cannot be determined by routine examination. Electrophoresis used to separate the isoenzymes of LDH, however, can determine the source of an elevation of this enzyme. Normal values may vary slightly from laboratory to laboratory.

LDH: 105 to 333 U/L

Although the LDH test is not specific for hepatic function, in combination with other diagnostic test results, its main use is to indicate the presence of myocardial and pulmonary infarction. Persistent, slightly increased LDH levels are associated with hepatitis, cirrhosis, and obstructive jaundice.

Aspartate transaminase (AST): Also called serum glutamic oxaloacetic transaminase (SGOT) or aspartate aminotransferase, AST is similar to ALT in that it is another enzyme associated with liver parenchymal cells. It is elevated in acute liver damage. It is also present in red cells and cardiac muscle.

AST: Up to 40 U/L

Alkaline phosphatase (ALP): An enzyme found primarily in the bones and liver. Expected values are higher for children and pregnant women, when damage to bones or liver has occurred, or when gallstones exist. Low values are probably not significant.

ALP: Adults 26 to 99 mu/ml

> NOTE: AST, ALT, and ALP are proteins found in muscles, the liver, and the heart, which help all the chemical activities within cells to occur. Injury to these cells releases the enzymes into the blood, resulting in high values.

Amylase: This digestive enzyme is mainly a constituent of pancreatic juice and saliva and is necessary for the breakdown of long-chain carbohydrates (such as starch) into smaller units.

Serum amylase: Up to 95 U/L

Lipase: A water-soluble enzyme. Human pancreatic lipase (HPL) is the main enzyme responsible for breaking down fats in the human digestive system; lipase converts triglyceride substrates found in oils from food to monoglycerides and free fatty acids.

Serum lipase: Less than 200 U/L

REPRODUCTIVE SYSTEM TESTS

Follicle stimulating hormone:

Female: Follicular phase 5 to 20 U/ml	Male: Not detectable to 20 U/ml
Luteal peak: 5 to 20 U/ml	Midcycle peak: 15 to 35 U/ml

Luteinizing hormone:

Female:

Postmenopausal: 5 to 20 U/ml	Postmenopausal: 40 to 200 U/ml
Ovulating females: Up to 8 U/ml	Male: Not detectable to 25 U/ml

Parathormone: A hormone synthesized and released into the bloodstream by the parathyroid glands. It regulates phosphorus and calcium in the body and functions in neuromuscular excitation and blood clotting.

Parathormone: Not detectable to 27 ng/dl

Serum alpha-fetoprotein (AFP): AFP is a substance naturally produced in the fetal liver that can appear in certain diseases of adults such as liver cancer. The amount of AFP in a pregnant woman's blood can help diagnose defects such as Down syndrome, spina bifida, anencephaly, chromosomal syndromes, and congenital defects. An AFP assay is a blood test performed to determine the level of AFP in a pregnant woman's blood. AFP is part of a specialized test, the triple screen.

Triple screen test: The maternal serum triple test is a screening test composed of three blood tests performed during pregnancy to assess the risk of birth defects in a fetus. Most accurate when performed between 16 to 18 weeks of pregnancy, each test measures the level of a particular substance in the maternal blood. Normal values for all three tests vary according to the age of the fetus. A high or low finding may mean that the fetal age has been miscalculated. Fetal ultrasound is done to determine fetal age more accurately. If the results of the triple screen are abnormal, the test is usually repeated. If the second test results are also abnormal, further testing is considered.

- **Maternal serum alpha-fetoprotein**
  Men and nonpregnant women: 0 to 6.4 U/ml
  Pregnant women: 0 to 20 U/ml
- **beta hCG (human chorionic gonadotropin):** Hormone secreted by the anterior pituitary gland and placenta; stimulates the gonads and controls reproductive activity. hCG is produced early in pregnancy, first by the embryo and then the placental trophoblasts, to cause progesterone secretions by the corpus luteum in order to prepare the endometrium for implantation. Detection of hCG in the urine and serum is the basis for one kind of pregnancy test.

  hCG may also be produced abnormally by certain tumors, especially germ cell tumors. Correspondingly, hCG testing is indicated in females with ovarian carcinoma or molar pregnancies. In men, hCG levels may be measured to determine the presence of testicular carcinoma.

  Beta hCG
  Non-pregnant: less than 10
  First month: 20 to 1000
  First trimester: 10,000 to 160,000
  Second trimester: 6000-30,000
- **Estriol:** A form of estrogen that increases during pregnancy, estriol is produced in large amounts by the placenta. Detection of estriol in the blood can be made as early as the ninth week of gestational age and continues to increase until delivery.

  Fasting blood sugar: For the fasting blood sugar test, the patient is NPO except for water 8 to 14 hours before testing. Fasting blood sugar levels higher than 126 mg/dl on more than two occasions in a pregnant patient are indicative of gestational diabetes.

  Fasting blood sugar: 80 to 120 mg/dl
  Postprandial blood sugar: up to 160 mg/dl

  Oral glucose tolerance test: A two-step oral glucose tolerance test is used to screen pregnant patients for gestational diabetes. In step 1, the blood is tested 1 hour after drinking 1.8 oz of a sweet liquid. If tests results reveal a glucose level greater than 140 mg/dl,* a second test is done. If that test reveals glucose levels greater than 130 mg/dl to 140 mg/dl, it indicates gestational diabetes.

  Hepatitis C virus (HCV): HCV causes a form of hepatitis (liver inflammation). Before this virus was discovered, in 1989, the syndrome was initially referred to as "non-A-non-B hepatitis."

*130 to 135 mg/dl is the value used in some laboratories.

Coinfection with HIV is common. Serologic tests are available to check for infection. The infection is spread by blood exchange and, less commonly, sexual contact. Before serologic tests became available, hepatitis C was often caused by the use of medical products derived from blood and by blood transfusion. Although hepatitis A, hepatitis B, and hepatitis C have similar names (because they all cause liver disease), the viruses themselves are quite different. Unlike hepatitis A and B, there is no vaccine for hepatitis C.

Pregnancy-associated plasma protein A (PAPP-A): A glycoprotein of placental origin that is used as a first-trimester screening test for chromosomal aneuploidies and an indicator of early pregnancy failure and pregnancy complications. The protein is normally present in high levels early in pregnancy and is thought to be crucial for normal fetal growth. Low levels have been linked with an increased risk for aneuploidy and with restricted fetal growth. PAPP-A also was reported to be depressed in established ectopic pregnancies.

The integrated PAPP-A test is performed in two stages:

- First stage: When the mother is approximately 12 weeks pregnant, a blood sample is taken from her to measure the concentration of serum PAPP-A. A nuchal scan is also carried out.
- Second stage: A second blood sample (at 15 or 16 weeks pregnant) is taken. Only after this second stage is a statistical result given. This blood sample measures four serum levels—AFP, unconjugated estriol (uE3), free beta hCG (free β-hCG), and inhibin-A (inhibin). The measurement of the total six markers, along with the mother's age, is used to estimate her chances of having a pregnancy with Down syndrome. Women with a chance greater than 1 in 100 are offered amniocentesis.

PAPP-A levels are elevated in hypercholesterolemic patients without clinical signs of atherosclerosis; therefore PAPP-A may serve as a marker of acute coronary syndromes.

CA-125: CA-125 is a substance produced by the fallopian tubes, the endometrium, and the lining of the abdominal cavity (peritoneum). CA-125 is used as a tumor marker—an indicator of some types of cancer, especially ovarian cancer. The amount of CA-125 in a woman's blood and body fluids often increases when cancer of the ovaries is present. However, it is important to know the following:

- Other conditions can also cause increased levels of CA-125 including menstruation, some nonovarian cancers, and some noncancerous disorders.
- CA-125 is also elevated during the first trimester of pregnancy and in women with pelvic inflammatory disease.
- CA-125 levels do not rise above the normal range in all women who have ovarian cancer.
- CA-125 levels often do not rise until the cancer is in an advanced stage.

Carbohydrate antigen 15-3 (CA 15-3): CA 15-3 is a tumor marker associated with breast cancer. It is most often used during treatment and remission.

Some research has shown that CA 15-3 is rarely elevated in early-stage breast cancer, while others show that it is. CA 15-3 may also be elevated, greater than 25 U/L in cancers of the pancreas, lung, ovary, and liver. Nonmalignant elevations may be seen in hepatitis and cirrhosis.

CA 15-3: 0.24 to 96.8 U/ml

Sexually transmitted diseases (STDs): Also known as sexually transmitted infections (STIs), these diseases are commonly transmitted between partners through some form of sexual activity, most commonly vaginal intercourse, oral sex, or anal sex. They were commonly known as venereal diseases (VDs) until around 1990. Bacteria, fungi, protozoa, or viruses are the causative agents.

> NOTE: The types of STDs on this list can be transmitted sexually. However, some of the diseases are commonly transmitted in other ways. For example, AIDS is also commonly transmitted through the sharing of infected needles by drug users, and candidiasis, which can be sexually transmitted, is very often not associated with sexual activity.

Bacterial
- Syphilis *(Treponema pallidum)*
- Gonorrhea *(Neisseria gonorrhoeae)*
- Chlamydia infection *(Chlamydia trachomatis)*
- Chancroid *(Haemophilus ducreyi)*
- Donovanosis (Granuloma inguinale or *Calymmatobacterium granulomatis*)
- Lymphogranuloma venereum (LGV) (*C. trachomatis* serotypes L1, L2, L3)
- Nongonococcal urethritis (NGU) *(Ureaplasma urealyticum* or *Mycoplasma hominis)*
  Viral
- Herpes/herpes simplex virus (HSV)
- HIV/AIDS
- Human papillomavirus (HPV)
  - Certain strains of HPV cause genital warts
  - Certain strains of HPV cause cervical dysplasias, which can lead to cervical cancer
- Cytomegalovirus
- Hepatitis (hepatitis A and hepatitis E are transmitted via the fecal-oral route, not sexually; hepatitis C is probably not sexually transmissable)
  - Hepatitis B
  - Hepatitis D
  Parasites
- Pubic lice *(Phthirus pubis)*
- Scabies *(Sarcoptes scabiei)*
  Fungal
- Candidiasis (thrush) *(Candida albicans)* is not strictly an STD but can be transmitted through sexual contact
  Protozoal
- Amebiasis *(Entamoeba histolytica)*
- Giardiasis *(Giardia lamblia)*
- Trichomoniasis *(Trichomonas vaginalis)*

Pap smear: A simple, effective test consisting of a cervical swab to collect a sampling of cells. The cells are checked for abnormalities in the laboratory. Approximately 5% to 7% of Pap smears produce abnormal results such as dysplasia, a possibly precancerous condition. Many of these abnormalities are NOT due to cervical cancer, but they are an indicator that increased vigilance is necessary.

Guidelines and screening programs vary; however, all sexually active women are urged to have an annual/biannual Pap smear and examination to detect any cancer early. If a smear is abnormal, depending on the nature of the abnormality, the test may need to be repeated in 3 to 12 months. If the abnormality requires scrutiny, the patient may be referred for a colposcopy.

URINARY SYSTEM TESTS

Blood urea nitrogen (BUN): A waste product produced in the liver and excreted by the kidneys. High values may indicate poor renal function. Heart failure, dehydration, high-protein diets, and strenuous exercise can result in increased levels of BUN. Liver disease or damage can result in decreased levels of BUN. Decreased levels of BUN can occur normally in the second and third trimesters of pregnancy.

BUN: 5 to 20 mg/dl
Blood urea: 15 to 50 mg/dl

Creatinine: A waste product largely from muscle breakdown. High values, especially with high BUN levels, may indicate renal problems.

Serum creatinine: 0.4 to 1.2 mg/dl
Creatine phosphokinase
Male: 16 to 110 U/L
Female: 16 to 94 U/L

Urinalysis: Urine tests are semiquantitative, and there is some variation from one sample to another on how the tests are scored.

Bilirubin: Normally there is no bilirubin or urobilinogen in the urine. These are pigments that are cleared by the liver. In liver or gallbladder disease, they may appear in the urine as well.

Blood: Normally there is no blood in urine. Blood can indicate an infection, kidney stones, trauma, or bleeding from a bladder or kidney tumor. Tests should indicate whether it is hemolyzed (dissolved blood) or nonhemolyzed (intact RBCs). Rarely, muscle injury can cause myoglobin to appear in the urine, which causes a false-positive result.

Glucose: Normally there is no glucose in urine. A positive glucose test occurs in diabetes. A small number of people with normal blood glucose levels have glucose in their urine. However, any glucose in the urine would raise the possibility of diabetes or glucose intolerance.

Leukocyte esterase: Normally negative. Leukocytes are WBCs (or pus cells). WBCs in the urine suggest a urinary tract infection.

Nitrate: Normally negative, this usually indicates a urinary tract infection.

pH: This is a measure of urine acidity.

Protein: Normally no protein is detectable. The presence of protein can indicate kidney damage, blood in the urine, or an infection. Certain diseases (e.g., diabetes) require the use of a special, more sensitive test for protein called a *microalbumin test,* which is useful in screening for early damage to the kidneys.

Sediment: A microscope examination of urine that has been spun in a centrifuge. Items such as mucous and squamous cells are commonly seen. Abnormal findings would include more than 0 to 2 RBCs, more than 0 to 2 WBCs, crystals, casts, renal tubular cells, or bacteria. (Bacteria can be present if there was contamination at the time of collection.)

Specific gravity (SG): Measures how dilute urine is. Water would have an SG of 1. Most urine is around 1.010 but can vary greatly depending on when the patient drank fluids last or if he or she is dehydrated.

SG: Normal 1.010

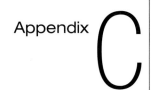

Common Medical Abbreviations

When beginning the clinical rotation phase of sonography training, a sonographer is expected to review patients' charts in order to correlate relevant clinical data. This information, along with the sonographic images recorded during the examination, is used to reach a sonographic diagnosis.

To streamline and expedite the reading and writing of chart data, common medical abbreviations have evolved. The following list contains terms that appear frequently on requisitions, charts, and reports. Although this is by no means a complete listing of medical abbreviations, it represents those a sonographer needs to know.

aa: Of each
AAA: Abdominal aortic aneurysm
Ab: Abortion
ac: Before meals
AFM: After fatty meal
AFP: Alpha-fetoprotein
ALL: Acute leukocytic leukemia
AML: Acute monocytic leukemia
Amnio: Amniocentesis
A-Mode: Amplitude modulation
AODM: Adult-onset diabetes mellitus
AP: Abdominal perimeter or anteroposterior
ASAP: As soon as possible
ATN: Acute tubular necrosis
BD: Binocular distance
BE: Barium enema
B-H: Braxton Hicks contraction
bid: Twice a day
B-Mode: Brightness modulation
BMR: Basal metabolic rate
BMT: Bone marrow transplantation
BP: Blood pressure
BPD: Biparietal diameter

BPH: Benign prostatic hypertrophy
BPM: Beats per minute
BPP: Biophysical profile
BSO: Bilateral salpingo-oophorectomy
BTD: Biliary tract disease
BUN: Blood urea nitrogen
Bx: Biopsy
C: Celsius (centigrade)
c: With
CBC: Complete blood count
CBD: Common bile duct
cubic centimeter: (write ml for milliliters)
CCA: Common carotid artery
CHD: Common hepatic duct
CHF: Congestive heart failure
CI: Cephalic index
CL: Corpus luteum
cm: Centimeter
CML: Chronic myeloid leukemia
CNS: Central nervous system
c/o: complains of
CD: Common duct
CPOD: Chronic obstructive pulmonary disease
Cr: Creatinine
CRL: Crown–rump length
CRT: Cathode-ray tube
CS: Cesarean section
CSF: Cerebrospinal fluid
CST: Contraction stress test
CT: Computed tomography
CVA: Cerebrovascular accident
CVS: Chorionic villus sampling
Cx: Cervix
db: Decibel
D&C: Dilatation and curettage
DGC: Depth-gain compensation
DM: Diabetes mellitus
dr: Dram
DTR: Deep tendon reflex
DTs: Delirium tremens
DVT: Deep venous thrombosis
Dx: Diagnosis
ECG: Echocardiogram
EDC: Estimated date of confinement
EEG: Electroencephalogram or echoencephalogram
EFW: Estimated fetal weight

EKG (ECG): Electrocardiogram
ERCP: Endoscopic retrograde cholangiopancreatography
ETOH: Ethanol (alcohol)
EUA: Examination under anesthesia
F: Fahrenheit
FDIU: Fetal death in utero
FH: Fundal height, fetal heart, or family history
FHT: Fetal heart tones
FSH: Follicle-stimulating hormone
FTT: Failure to thrive
F/U: Follow-up
FUO: Fever of unknown origin
Fx: Function, fracture
G: Gravida
GA: Gestational age
GB: Gallbladder
GI: Gastrointestinal
gm, g: Gram
gr: Grain
GS: Gestational sac
GTD: Gestational trophoblastic disease
gtt: drops
GU: Genitourinary
Gyn: Gynecology
HBP: High blood pressure
HC: Head circumference or hepatocellular
hCG: Human chorionic gonadotropin
HCT: Hematocrit
Hg: Mercury
Hgb, Hg: Hemoglobin
HIV: Human immunodeficiency virus
HLA: Human leukocyte antigen
HMG: Human menopausal gonadotropin
HP: Head perimeter
hs: At bedtime
HSM: Hepatosplenomegaly
Hx: History
Hydro: Hydrocephalus or hydronephrosis
IC: Iliac crest
IDDM: Insulin-dependent diabetes mellitus
IM: Intramuscular (use units)
IPPB: Intermittent positive pressure breathing
IUCD (IUD): Intrauterine contraceptive device
IUFD (IUD): Intrauterine fetal demise
IUGR: Intrauterine growth restriction
IUP: Intrauterine pregnancy

IV: Intravenous
IVC: Inferior vena cava
IVP: Intravenous pyelogram
IVS: Interventricular septum
JODM: Juvenile-onset diabetes mellitus
K: Potassium
Kg: kilogram
LCM: Left costal margin
LE: Lower extremity
LFT: Liver function tests (e.g., ALT, AST)
LH: Luteinizing hormone
LIF: Long internal focus (transducer)
LK: Left kidney
LLQ: Left lower quadrant
LMP: Last menstrual period
LNMP: Last normal menstrual period
LPO: Left posterior oblique
LSO: Left salpingo-oophorectomy
LSU: Left side up
LT: Ligamentum teres
Lt: Left
LUQ: Left upper quadrant
LV/HW: Lateral-ventricle/hemispheric width ratio
mEq: Milliequivalent
mg: Milligram
MHz: Megahertz
MI: Myocardial infarction
MIF: Medium internal focus (transducer)
ML: Midline
ml: milliliter (replaces cc)
mm: Millimeter
M-Mode: TM Motion modulation or time-motion modulation
MPV: Main portal vein
MRI: Magnetic resonance imaging
NGT: Nasogastric tube
NMR: Nuclear magnetic resonance (see MRI)
NPO: Nothing by mouth
NSS: Normal size and shape
NST: Nonstress test
NSVD: Normal spontaneous vaginal delivery
NTD: Neural tube defect
OA/OP: Occiput anterior/occiput posterior
Ob: Obstetrics
OC: Ocular diameter
OCG: Oral cholecystogram
OCT: Oxytocin challenge test

OFD: Occipital-frontal diameter
OR: Operating room
oz: Ounce
P: After
PA: Popliteal artery or popliteal aneurysm
Para: Number of full-term pregnancies, premature births, abortions, or living children
pc: After meals
PE: Pleural effusion or pulmonary embolus
PI: Pulsatility index
PID: Pelvic inflammatory disease
POC: Products of conception
POD #: Postop day (#_____)
Postop: After surgery
PP: Postpartum
PPD: Test for tuberculosis
Preop: Before surgery
PROM: Premature rupture of membranes
PSA: Prostate-specific antigen
PSI: Postsaline injection
PT: Pregnancy test
pt: Patient
PTA: Prior to admission
PTT: Prothrombin time
PV: Portal vein
qd: Every day
qh: Every hour
qid: Four times a day
qs: Sufficient quantity
RAS: Renal artery stenosis
RBC: Red blood cell
RCM: Right costal margin
Rh: Rhesus
RI: Resistive index
RIND: Reversible ischemic neurologic deficit
RK: Right kidney
RLL: Right lower lobe
RLQ: Right lower quadrant
R/O: Rule out
RPO: Right posterior oblique
RSO: Right salpingo-oophorectomy
RT: Real-time (dynamic imaging)
RUQ: Right upper quadrant
Rx: Treatment
s: Without
SAB: Spontaneous abortion
SBE: Subacute bacterial endocarditis

SD: Standard deviation
SIF: Short internal focus (transducer)
SMA: Superior mesenteric artery
SMV: Superior mesenteric vein
SP: Splenic vein or symphysis pubis
S/P: Status post
sp gr: Specific gravity
stat: Immediately
SVD: Spontaneous vaginal delivery
TAB: Therapeutic abortion
TAH: Total abdominal hysterectomy
TAS: Transabdominal scan
TCD: Transcranial Doppler
TCG, TGC: Time-compensated gain, time-gain compensation
TIA: Transient ischemic attack
tid: Three times a day
TIUV: Total intrauterine volume
tko: To keep open (re: intravenous line)
TOA: Tubo-ovarian abscess
Tr: Transverse
TURP: Transurethral resection of the prostate
TVH: Total vaginal hysterectomy
TVS: Transvaginal scan
Tx: Transplant or transducer
U: Umbilicus
UE: Upper extremity
UGI: Upper gastrointestinal series
UPJ: Ureteropelvic junction
URI: Upper respiratory tract infection
U/S: Ultrasound
UTI: Urinary tract infection
UVJ: Ureterovesical junction
VTX: Vertex presentation
w: Without
WBC: White blood cell
WES: Wall-echo shadow
XP: Xiphoid process

Medical Terminology

To master medical terminology, it is helpful to learn the root words and the prefixes and suffixes that commonly are incorporated into medical terms. The source or origin of a word is called a *root word*.

ROOT WORDS

angi- vessel
arth- joint
cardi- heart
cephal- head
cerebr- brain
chole-, chol- bile
chondri- cartilage
cost- rib
crani- skull
cyst- bladder
encephal- brain
enter- intestine
gastr- stomach
hem- blood
hepat- liver
hyster- uterus
leuk, leuc- white
lith- stone
nephr- kidney
oste- bone
phren- diaphragm
pneum- air
pyel- pelvis
viscer- organ

PREFIXES

a-, an- absent or deficient
ab- away from

adeno- glandular
an- absent or deficient
ante- front
anti- against
arthro- pertaining to joints
bi- two
brachio- arm
cardio- heart
co- together
colo- colon or large intestine
contra- against
cysto- bladder
dactyl- pertaining to fingers or toes
decub- side
dors- back
dys- difficult or painful
ecto- outside
encephalo- pertaining to brain
endo- within
entero- pertaining to the intestines
epi- upon
gastro- pertaining to the stomach
hema-, hemo- pertaining to blood
hemi- half
hepato- pertaining to liver
hydro- pertaining to water
hyper- above; a greater concentration
hypo- below; a lesser concentration
ileo- small intestine or ileum
infero- below
inter- between
intra- within
lipo- fat
mal- disorder
megalo- large
meningo- pertaining to membranes surrounding the brain
meno- pertaining to menstruation
meta- after or changing
myelo- spinal cord
myo- muscle
nephro- pertaining to the kidney
neuro- pertaining to nerve or nerves
olig-, oligo- too little or too few
oro- pertaining to the mouth
osteo- pertaining to bone
pan- all

para- beside or beyond
peri- around
phlebo- pertaining to vein or veins
pneumo- pertaining to air, lung, breathing
poly- many, too much
post- back, after
pre- before
psycho- mental
pulmo- lung
pyelo- pelvis (renal)
pyo- pus
retro- backward
sclero- hard
sub- under/below
super- over/above
trans- across
vent- front

SUFFIXES

-algia pain
-centesis puncture
-dia through
-dynia pain
-ectasis expansion
-ectomy surgical removal
-emia a condition of the blood
-genic origin
-glycemia pertaining to blood sugar levels
-iasis condition
-itis inflammation
-oid like
-oma tumor
-osis abnormal condition or process
-pathy abnormality
-phobia abnormal fear
-plasty surgical correction
-ptosis falling or drooping
-rhaphy suture
-scopy inspection
-tomy incision
-uria contained within the urine

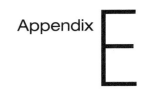

Abbreviated List of Helpful Spanish Phrases

GREETINGS AND INSTRUCTIONS

Hello, my name is _____. *Buenos dias, me llamo _____.*
I will be performing your ultrasound examination. *Voy a hacerle el ultrasonido.*
What is your name? *¿Cómo se llama?*
Please come with me. *Por favor, venga conmigo.*
Please remove all clothing and put on the gown. *Por favor quítese toda la ropa y póngase la bata.*
Please remove your clothing below the waist and put on the gown. *Por favor quítese la ropa de la cintura para abajo y póngase la bata.*
Please remove your clothing to/above the waist and put on the gown. *Por favor quítese la ropa de la cintura para abajo y póngase la bata.*
Are you too cold or too hot? *¿Tiene demasiado frío o demasiado calor?*

PATIENT PREPARATION

When was the last time you ate food or drank water? *¿Cuándo fue la última vez que comió o que tomó/bebió agua?*
How much water did you drink? *¿Qué cantidad de agua tomó?*

PATIENT HISTORY

What medicine are you taking? *¿Qué medicina toma?*
Are you in pain? *¿Tiene dolor?*
What kind of pain is it? *¿Qué tipo de dolor tiene?*
- dull/sharp? *¿sordo/agudo?*
- throbbing/constant? *¿punzante/constante?*
- on and off? *¿que va y viene?*
Where is your pain? *¿Dónde le duele?*

Are you pregnant? *¿Está embarazada?*

How many times have you been pregnant? *¿Cuántas veces ha estado embarazada?*

How many babies were born alive? *¿Cuántos bebés nacieron vivos?*

What was the date of your last menstrual period? *¿Cuándo tuvo la última regla/ menstruación?*

When are you due? *¿Para cuándo espera?*

What is your due date? *¿Cuál es la fecha del parto?*

Are you bleeding? *¿Tiene sangrado?* or *¿Está sangrando?*

There is an 85% chance of a boy/girl. *La probabilidad de que sea niño/niña es de 85 (ochenta y cinco) por ciento.*

POSITIONING AND SCANNING

Please lie down on the table. *Por favor, acuéstese en la camilla.*

Please turn over on your side. *Por favor, acuéstese de lado/sobre un lado.*

Breathe deeply. *Respire profundo.*

Lift your arms. *Levante los brazos.*

When I tell you, hold your breath. *Cuando le avise, aguante la respiración.*

Stop breathing. *Aguante la respiracion.*

You can breathe now. *Ya puede respirar ahora.*

Do not move. *No se mueva.*

ENDING THE EXAMINATION

I am finished. That is all. *Ya terminé. Es todo.*

I will return shortly. *Regresaré en seguida.*

Remain here. *Quédese aquí.*

Please sit here. *Siéntese aquí, por favor.*

Now you can get dressed. *Ya puede ponerse la ropa.*

Your doctor will tell you the results of this test. *Su médico le dirá los resultados de esta prueba.*

Thank you. Goodbye. *Gracias. Adios.*

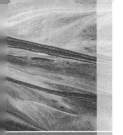

Illustration Credits

Chapter 1

Figures 1-1 **A** and **B,** 1-2, 1-3 **A** and **B,** 1-4, 1-5, 1-6, 1-7, 1-8, and 1-9 from Eastman Kodak Company.
Figure 1-10 **A** and **B** courtesy Joseph Woo, MD.
Figure 1-11 courtesy Terry J DuBose, RDMS.
Figure 1-12 courtesy Eric Blackwell, MD.
Figure 1-14 Courtesy Phillip J. Bendick, PhD, William Beaumont Hospital, Royal Oak, Mich.
Figure 1-15 from Rumack CM, Wilson SR, Charboneau JW: *Diagnostic ultrasound,* ed 3, St Louis, 2005, Mosby.
Figure 1-16 Courtesy SonoSite, Inc. Bothell, Wash.
Figure 1-17 courtesy GE Healthcare.

Chapter 4

Figures 4-1, 4-3, 4-4, and 4-5 courtesy Sound Ergonomics, Kenmore, Wash.

Chapter 5

Figures 5-4, and 5-8 from Perry AG, Potter PA: *Clinical nursing skills and techniques,* ed 5, St Louis, 2002, Mosby.
Figures 5-18, 5-19, and 5-20 from Ehrlich RA: *Patient care in radiography,* ed 6, St Louis, 2004, Mosby.

Chapter 7

Figure 7-1 from Society of Diagnostic Medical Sonography Educational Foundation, Plano, Tex, 1999-2005.

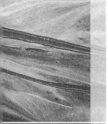

Glossary

The following list contains medical and technical words that are often used on patient charts and in sonography textbooks. It also contains definitions of the key terms listed at the beginning of each chapter.

This is by no means a complete listing of what a sonographer needs to know. For further study, the sonographer can consult any one of the many excellent medical dictionaries available in his or her school or hospital library.

A

abdomen: The large inferior cavity of the trunk, extending from the diaphragm to the brim of the pelvis. It is artificially divided into nine regions: right hypochondriac; epigastric; left hypochondriac; right lumbar; umbilical; left lumbar; right inguinal; hypogastric; and left inguinal regions.

abduction: Withdrawal of a part from the axis of the trunk or extremity.

aberrant: Varying/deviating from normal form, structure, or course.

abortion: The expulsion of the embryo or fetus from the uterus any time before week 28 of pregnancy, either by natural or by artificially induced means. When this occurs during the first 3 months, it is termed *abortion;* after 3 months time it becomes known as viability, *miscarriage;* and from the period of viability to full term, *premature delivery/birth.* Definitions of the types of abortions follow:
- Artificial abortion: intentional premature termination of pregnancy by medicinal/mechanical means.
- Complete abortion: the total expulsion of all products of conception from the uterus.
- Criminal abortion: the illegal interference with progress of pregnancy or illegal abortion.
- Habitual abortion: an accidental abortion recurring in successive pregnancies.
- Incomplete abortion: the partial expulsion of the products of conception.
- Inevitable abortion: an abortion that has advanced to a stage in which termination of pregnancy can no longer be prevented.
- Missed abortion: a condition in which the fetus has died but the products of conception are not expelled within 2 weeks.

- Partial abortion: the premature expulsion of one fetus in the presence of multiple gestation.
- Spontaneous abortion: the unexpected premature expulsion of the products of conception when no abortive agents have been applied.
- Therapeutic abortion: the termination of a pregnancy that poses a hazard to the life of the mother.
- Threatened abortion: the occurrence of signs/symptoms of impending loss of the embryo/fetus. May be prevented by treatment or may go on to inevitable abortion.
- Tubal abortion: the escape of the products of conception through the abdominal opening of the fallopian tube into the peritoneal cavity.

abruptio: A tearing away.

abruptio placentae: Premature separation of the placenta.

abscess: A pus-filled cavity that can develop anywhere, for example, on the skin or in any internal organ. Antibiotics may be helpful, but draining may be necessary to remove the pus.

accountability: Being required to answer for one's actions.

accreditation: The process that recognizes and authorizes a school or institution for demonstrated ability in a special area of practice or training. Currently, accreditation exists for diagnostic medical sonography programs, diagnostic ultrasound laboratories, and facilities.

acute: Describes sudden onset of relatively severe or sharp manifestations that run a short course. Acute problems may be mild or severe.

acute abdomen: An acute pathologic condition within the belly that requires prompt surgical intervention.

Addison disease: A disease resulting from decreased function of the adrenal glands.

adduction: Any movement of one part of a limb toward another or toward the midline of the body.

adhesion: Abnormal union of an organ or part to another by fibrous attachment.

adipose: Fatty, fatlike.

adnexa: Accessory parts or appendages of an organ.

adrenaline: Also known as epinephrine. A hormone produced by the adrenal glands. Available in drug form to improve breathing for persons with asthma, to treat severe allergic reactions, or to stimulate the heart in cardiac arrest.

advance directive: A legal document that helps ensure that your health care wishes will be respected if you become unable to speak or otherwise communicate.

aerobe: A microorganism that can only survive and replicate when free oxygen is present.

Agency for Healthcare Research and Quality (AHRQ): A government agency whose mission is to improve the quality, safety, efficiency, and effectiveness of health care for all Americans.

airway: A respiratory passage. Any of several devices used to maintain a clear and unobstructed respiratory passage.

albuminuria: Presence of protein or albumin in the urine.

Alpha-fetoprotein assay: AFP is a fetal protein, normally found in the maternal blood. Both increased or decreased AFP is associated with certain abnormalities. The test is usually performed at 16 weeks' gestation. AFP levels within normal range indicate low risk for fetal anomalies; higher AFP levels indicate an increased risk of neural tube defects, other fetal abnormalities, and threatened abortion; lower AFP levels indicate an increased risk of Trisomy 21, other rare genetic disorders, or impending fetal demise.

allergen: A substance that induces an allergic state or reaction.

ambulatory: Walking or able to walk; designating a patient not confined to bed.

amenorrhea: Absence of menses.

American Hospital Association(AHA): A nonprofit association of health care provider organizations that are committed to the health improvement of their communities.

amniography: Radiographic visualization of the fetus by injection of a dye through the abdominal wall and into the amniotic sac.

amniotic band syndrome: The firm attachment of adjacent serous membranes by bands or masses of fibrous connective tissue; caused by organization and scarring of exudates, resulting from infection or partial destruction of the surfaces.

amniotic fluid index (AFI): A method of estimating the volume of amniotic fluid present in second and third trimester pregnancies.

A-Mode: A one-dimensional representation of a reflected sound wave in a diagnostic scan. Also known as *Amplitude Modulation.*

analgesia: The absence of pain; usually denotes relief of pain without loss of consciousness.

analog scan converter: A device in which data are represented by continuously variable, measurable, physical quantities such as length, width, voltage or pressure.

anasarca: Massive generalized edema.

anastomosis: The joining of structures.

anechoic: Free from echoes, completely absorbing sound waves.

anemia: Low level of hemoglobin, the red blood cell chemical that carries oxygen to body tissues.

aneurysm: Weakening of a blood vessel because of disease, age, injury, or congenital defect. Rupture of the weakened wall is usually life threatening.

angina: Severe, often choking chest pain.

angiogram: Visualization of the blood vessels with x-ray examination.

angioplasty: Surgical opening of a clogged blood vessel by inflating a balloon and stretching the wall. Often performed after a heart attack, along with the administration of clot-dissolving medication.

anoxia: Lack of oxygen. Absence of oxygen in the tissues.

antibody: An immunoglobulin molecule that reacts specifically with a substance (antigen) that induced its synthesis or with a closely related antigen.

antigen: Any substance that induces the formation of antibodies with which it reacts specifically.

antiseptic: An agent that inhibits microorganisms.

anuria: Lack of urine production. The absence of excretion of urine from the body.

aorta: The main artery through which blood leaves the heart for distribution to the rest of the body.

aphasia: Defect or loss of power of expression in speech, writing, or signs or loss of comprehension of spoken or written language because of injury or disease of brain centers.

aplasia: Lack of development of an organ or tissue or of the cellular products from an organ or tissue.

apnea: Cessation of breathing for short periods of time (sleep apnea) or for prolonged and potentially life-threatening times (e.g., in premature babies).

artifact: A man-made artificial structure or changed appearance.

arrhythmia: Abnormality of heart rate or rhythm, or both.

arteriosclerosis: Hardening and loss of elasticity of the arterial wall. Common with aging and in certain diseases. Term often used interchangeably with atherosclerosis, a thickening of the inner wall of blood vessels from cholesterol deposits.

ascites: An abnormal collection of serous fluid in the peritoneal cavity.

aseptic/asepsis: Sterile, free of microorganisms.

assault: A threat to inflict physical injury on another person through force or violence. Included is the touching of another person without that person's consent, with intent to harm.

association: A connection in the mind between ideas, sensations, and memories.

asymptomatic: Showing or causing no symptoms.

ataxia: Failure of muscular coordination.

atherosclerosis: A form of arteriosclerosis.

atrophy: Diminution in the size of a cell, tissue, or organ.

attenuation: To weaken or lessen in intensity.

attitude: A manner of acting or thinking that shows one's disposition, opinions, and reactions.

auscultation: Listening for body sounds with the aid of a stethoscope.

autoclave: A device that sterilizes by steam under pressure.

autonomic nervous system: Part of the nervous system that regulates involuntary life-maintaining activities such as heart beat, respiration, and hormone secretion.

autonomy: The right to make our own decisions; to be independent and self-governing.

axillary: A small pyramidal space between the upper lateral part of the chest and medial side of the arm that includes the armpit, axillary vessels, brachial nerve plexus, and large numbers of lymph nodes.

azotemia: An excess of urea or other nitrogenous substances in the blood.

B

bacteria: Microbes or organisms, some of which cause disease and some of which live peacefully within the body, aiding such functions as digestion.

basal metabolism: The quantity of energy used by the body at rest. It is measured by the rate at which heat is given off.

battery: An assault in which any force, however slight, is applied to another (the assailant makes physical contact).

benign: Harmless; nonmalignant character of a neoplasm.

bilateral: Affecting both sides.

binder: An abdominal girdle or bandage used to support the abdominal walls (especially for postpartum patients).

biopsy: Removal of a small sample of tissue for microscopic examination.

bioethics: The study of moral values in health care and all biomedical sciences.

bi-stable: An electrical device or circuit that has two stable states at any given time, so it is possible to switch between them.

B-Mode: A two-dimensional presentation of echo-producing interfaces. Also known as *brightness modulation.*

bodily fluids: Consisting of cerebrospinal, synovial, pleural, peritoneal, pericardial, and amniotic fluids.

body language: Facial expressions, gestures, and body movements that send messages.

brachial: Region between the elbow and shoulder.

bradycardia: Abnormally slow pulse.

breach: The breaking of a promise or a pledge to perform an obligation under a precedent, either by commission or omission.

bronchi: Major air passageways in the lungs.

bronchoscopy: Direct examination of the bronchus.

bruit: A sound or murmur heard on auscultation.

burnout: A state of mental or physical exhaustion, or both, caused by excessive and prolonged stress.

C

calculus: A stonelike formation, usually composed of mineral salts.

caliper: A manual or electronic instrument used to measure thickness or diameter.

cannula: A small tube for insertion into a body cavity.

carcinogen: An environmental agent that can produce cancer.

carcinoma: Malignant neoplasm arising from certain tissues. Carcinoma in situ describes an early stage of cancer that is highly invasive.

cardiac arrest: The heart and breathing stop suddenly without warning.

cardiac output: The amount of blood—in liters per minute—flowing through the systemic circulation.

cardiology: Medical specialty that deals with disorders of the heart and cardiac vasculature.

cardiomegaly: Enlargement of the heart (cardiac hypertrophy).

cardiopulmonary resuscitation (CPR): Emergency techniques used on patients whose heart has stopped or who are not breathing, or both.

catheterize: The introduction of a hollow tube into a body cavity, such as the urinary bladder, to draw off fluid.

catheterization: Passing of a small tube through an opening into the body (e.g., blood vessel, urethra) to instill or remove fluid.

cavitation: The formation of cavities in a body tissue or an organ due to the sudden formation and collapse of low-pressure bubbles by means of mechanical forces.

cause: A reason, motive, or grounds for bringing a legal action, to be resolved by a court of law.

Centers for Medicare and Medicaid Services (CMS): Formerly know as the Health Care Financing Administration (HCFA). CMS is the federal agency within the Department of Health and Human Services that is responsible for the national administration of the Medicaid, Medicare, and State Children's Health Insurance Program (SCHIP).

cerebral vascular accident (CVA): Pathologic condition of a blood vessel in the brain, either rupture or occlusion, with formation of a blood clot.

certification: The process by which an individual institution or educational program is evaluated and recognized as meeting certain predetermined standards.

chemotherapy: Treatment of a disease by means of administering chemicals.

cholecystectomy: Surgical removal of the gallbladder.

cholecystitis: Infection of the gallbladder.

cholecystogram: An x-ray procedure used to visualize the gallbladder.

cholelithiasis: Gallstones.

chorionic villus sampling (CVS): The CVS test/procedure is a form of prenatal diagnosis to determine genetic abnormalities in the fetus in which a sample of the chorionic villi is obtained and tested. CVS is generally carried out on pregnant women older than age 35 and those who have a higher risk of Down syndrome and other chromosomal conditions. The advantage of CVS is that it can be performed at 10 to 12 weeks' gestation. This is earlier than amniocentesis (which is usually carried out at 15 to 18 weeks' gestation). However, CVS is riskier than amniocentesis.

chronic: Persisting over a long period; denoting a disease of slow progress and long continuance.

cirrhosis: Hardening of an organ.

civil law: All laws that affect the individual rather than the whole of society.

clustering: Gathering of things of the same sort.

code of conduct: The moral code, which guides the members of a profession in the proper conduct of their duties and obligations.

colostomy: Surgical procedure to form an artificial opening into the large bowel.

communication barriers: Fast talking, using slang or medical jargon, making it difficult for the listener to understand the message. Speaking a language foreign to the listener.

common law: Laws based on custom, usage, and the decisions of the court.

communication triads: A coalition formed by three people in a social situation, for exchanging information.

compassion fatigue: Lessening or loss of sympathy for the misfortune of others, caused by overwork and excessive emotional demands.

computerized axial tomography (CAT/CT scan): An x-ray imaging modality that produces detailed cross-sectional images of the soft tissue and bony structures.

conscious sedation: A type of sedation to induce an altered state of consciousness that minimizes pain and discomfort through the use of pain relievers and sedatives. Patients who receive conscious sedation usually are able to speak and respond to verbal cues throughout the procedure, communicating any discomfort they experience to the provider. A brief period of amnesia may erase any memory of the procedure.

congenital: Present at birth. Congenital problems can be inherited, the result of infection or drug use in the mother, or the effect of uterine abnormalities.

contamination: Soiling or making unclean by contact or the introduction of any organisms.

continuous subcutaneous infusion (CSQI): A useful method of drug administration for delivering a continuous subcutaneous infusion when other routes are inappropriate. Some of the more common drugs used are insulin, human growth hormone, and opioids. CSQI is indicated for patients who require the use of numerous drugs and those for whom the oral route is often no longer suitable. CSQI is used to ensure continued symptom control.

Using this method increases patient comfort, avoids the need for repeated injections, maintains constant plasma concentration levels of drugs, and maintains the patient's sense of independence.

convulsion: Violent, uncoordinated, involuntary contractions of the muscles.

coronal: A plane parallel to the long axis of the body.

cranial: Referring to the skull.

credential: An endorsement of confidence bestowed on a school or institution.

criminal law: Federal or state laws that affect the whole of society rather than the individual.

culdoscopy: Internal visual examination of the female reproductive organs through a small incision in the pouch of Douglas.

Current Procedural Terminology (CPT): A CPT code is a five-digit numeric code used to describe medical procedures performed by physicians and other health care providers. CPT codes were developed by HCFA to assist in the assignment of reimbursement amounts to providers by Medicare carriers. The American Medical Association (AMA) publishes the CPT codes.

cutaneous: Referring to the skin.

cyanosis: Bluish discoloration of the skin and mucous membranes caused by insufficient oxygen in the blood.

cyst: A sac or cavity filled with fluid or oily material; can form in any part of the body.

cystitis: Inflammation of the urinary bladder.

cystoscopy: Visual examination of the interior of the urinary bladder.

cytology: The study of cells.

D

dangling: A patient care technique that allows patients to sit on the edge of the bed and let their legs dangle loosely as a prelude to getting up and out of bed.

debride: To remove foreign material and contaminated or devitalized tissue by sharp dissection.

defamation: Any communication that holds a person up to contempt, hatred, ridicule, or scorn and lowers the reputation of the defamed person.

defecation: Elimination of wastes from the intestine.

dehumanization: To deprive of human qualities or attributes such as pity, kindness, and individuality.

dementia: Loss of mental posers due to organic disease.

deontology: The study of duty, moral obligation, and right action. Deontologists believe that one's duty is more important than bringing about good consequences; it is the motive or principle that determines right or wrong. One should do one's duty regardless of the consequences.

dependent position: The lowest area; hanging down (e.g., turning patients with gallbladder problems onto their right side so that any gallstones will layer to the dependent area).

diabetes insipidus: A disease caused by a deficiency of antidiuretic hormone (ADH).

diabetes mellitus: A metabolic disease in which carbohydrates are poorly oxidized.

diagnosis-related groups (DRGs): A classification of hospital case types into groups expected to have similar hospital resource use. The groupings are based on diagnoses (using International Classification of Diseases of the World Health Organization (ICD)), procedures, age, sex, and the presence of complications or comorbidities.

dialysis: Cleansing the blood by artificial means when kidneys have failed. Hemodialysis filters blood through a machine; peritoneal dialysis uses the peritoneal membrane that lines the abdomen to filter impurities.

diaphoresis: Excessive perspiration.

diastole: The relaxation of the heart between contractions. The dilation or enlargement of an opening or a hollow organ or tube.

didactic: Used or intended for teaching.

digital scan converter: Image processing device that uses a stable electronic circuit to store and manipulate ultrasonic images in memory. The device then reconstructs and displays these images simultaneously to create one single image.

disinfectant: An agent that kills some pathogens.

distal: Farther from the body or from the origin of a part.

diuresis: Increased urine production.

diuretic: A drug used to cause diuresis.

dobutamine: A potent cardiac stimulant used in stress echocardiography.

Doppler effect: Change in the observed frequency of a wave, occurring when the source and observer are in motion relative to each other. Frequency increases as the source and observer approach each other and decreases as they move apart. Any source motion causes a real shift in wave frequencies, while the observer motion produces only an apparent shift in frequency.

dorsal: The posterior aspect or back of the body or organ.

dorsiflexion: Flexion or bending of the foot toward the leg.

drawsheet: A drawsheet is an extra (short) sheet that is placed in the middle of the bed and under a patient who cannot move on his own. The patient can be rolled or moved from one area of the bed to another by two people on either side of the bed, using the drawsheet like a sling to move the patient.

dysfunction: Disturbed or abnormal function of an organ.

dysmenorrhea: Painful menstruation.

dysphagia: Difficulty in swallowing.

dysplasia: Abnormal change or growth; alteration in size, shape, and organization of differentiated cells.

dyspnea: Labored breathing.

dysrhythmia: Any disturbance in normal rhythm.

dystrophy: Faulty or defective nutrition.

dysuria: Painful or difficult urination.

E

ecchymosis: A bruise; a discoloration of the skin caused by the extravasation of blood.

echocardiogram: Sonographic examination of the heart.

ectopic: Out of place.

edema: Swelling caused by fluid retention; accumulation of abnormally large amounts of fluid in the interstitial spaces.

effusion: Escape of fluid into a space such as the pleural cavity.

elective: Not urgent. Elective surgery can be scheduled at the patient's convenience.

electric infusion devices (EIDs): Electronic infusion pumps are designed to ensure accurate administration of intravenous fluid volume (which may contain drugs) over a given period of time. Such devices, which include syringe drivers, are known as *volumetric pumps*, as they control and monitor volume, rather than drops per minute. The IVAC Model is an example of a volumetric pump that is in common use.

electrocardiogram: A graphic recording of the electrical current produced by the contraction of the heart.

electroencephalogram: A graphic recording of the electrical currents produced by brain action.

electrolyte: A solution, such as a salt solution, that can conduct electricity.

embolus: A mass of undissolved material traveling in the blood; it may be solid, liquid, or gaseous.

embryo: The fetus before the end of the eighth week of conception.

emesis: Vomitus.

empathy: Sharing another's emotion.

emphysema: A chronic lung disease usually characterized by greatly distended alveoli.

empyema: Pus in the pleural cavity.

endogenous: Originating within the body.

endoscope: An instrument used to inspect the interior of a body cavity.

endoscopic retrograde cholangiopancreatography (ERCP): An endoscopic x-ray procedure that permits visualization and biopsy of the biliary and pancreatic tissues.

endotracheal tube: A tube inserted into the trachea to provide a passageway for air. Also called *tracheal tube.*

endovaginal sonography(EVS): Also known as *transvaginal sonography (TVS).* EVS is an intracavitary ultrasound imaging technique employing the insertion of a specialized transducer into the vaginal canal.

enteral tube feeding: Feeding by way of or within the small intestine.

enterostomy: To provide with an opening, usually by surgical means.

enzyme: A protein that acts as a catalyst in biochemical reactions.

epidemiology: Study of the occurrence of a disease within a population.

epistaxis: Nosebleed.

ergonomics: The science of work. Ergonomics removes barriers to quality, productivity, and safe human performance by fitting products, tasks, and environments to people.

erosion: Wearing away of tissue.

erythema: An unusual redness of the skin.

esophagoscopy: Visual examination of the esophagus.

ethical decision making: Deals with concrete judgments in situations in which action must be taken despite uncertainty.

ethics: Systems of valued behaviors and beliefs that govern proper conduct to ensure protection of an individual's rights.

etiology: Study of the cause of a disease or condition.

eversion: Turning out or inside out.

evisceration: Protrusion of internal organs through a wound.

exacerbation: An increase in the severity or intensity of a disease and any of the symptoms.

excoriation: An area where the skin has been scraped away or chafed.

exogenous: Originating outside of the body.

extension: The increasing or straightening of the angle at a joint.

extrasystole: A premature contraction of the heart; a type of cardiac arrhythmia.

extravasation: An abnormality in flow that allows liquids (usually blood or IV fluid) to flow from a normal vessel into the surround body tissues.

exudate: A substance thrown out, such as pus or serous fluid.

F

fascia: A sheet of fibrous tissue that covers muscles and certain other organs.

feces: Excrement from the bowels.

fetal distress: Abnormal condition of the fetus characterized by irregular heart rhythm and meconium (fetal bowel movement) that discolors amniotic fluid. Turning the mother onto her side and administering oxygen often helps, but early delivery sometimes is necessary.

fetus: The unborn infant.

fibrillation: A type of cardiac arrhythmia.

fibrosis: The formation of fibrous tissue, usually as a reparative process.

filtration: The process by which water and dissolved substances are pushed through a permeable membrane from areas of high pressure to areas of lower pressure.

fissure: A cleft or groove.

fistula: Abnormal channel between two organs or an internal organ and the skin. A deep ulcer or abnormal passage often leading from a hollow organ to the body surface. Sometimes caused by congenital malformation or complications of surgery or childbirth.

flatus: Gas or air in the stomach or intestines.

flexion: Decreasing of the angle at a joint (e.g., the bending of the elbow).

flotation pads: Equipment designed solely for the use of people who are chronic invalids or have a physical disability. Example: alternating pressure pads and other flotation pads specially designed for the care and prevention of bed sores.

fluid volume deficit (FCD): The condition that results from excessive loss of water from a living organism.

fluid volume excess: A condition that results in excessive accumulation of fluid (e.g., polyhydramnios, ascites, edema).

fluoroscope: An x-ray machine used to allow visual examination of internal organs and to observe the movement and contour of the organs.

Foley catheter: A tube used for the continuous drainage of urine.

fossa: A shallow or hollow place in a bone.

fracture pan: A portable bedpan designed for users who are immobilized (e.g., because of fractures or hip operations). It is smaller and more compact than a standard bedpan and thus easier to position under this type of patient.

frontal: A plane that divides the body into front and back portions.

G

gastrectomy: Surgical removal of a part or all of the stomach.

gavage: Feeding by means of a stomach tube.

germicide: An agent that kills germs.

glutaraldehyde: A powerful solution used to disinfect transducers. Also known by trade names of Cidex, Metrex, and so on.

goiter: Enlargement of the thyroid gland.

granulation: Small, fleshy, beadlike protuberances consisting of outgrowths of new capillaries on the surface of a wound that is healing. Also called *granulation tissue.*

gray scale: A series of shades from white to black. The more shades or levels of gray, the more realistically an image can be recorded and displayed, especially a scanned photo.

grief: Intense emotional suffering usually caused by loss.

gynecology: Medical specialty that deals with the reproductive system of the nongravid female.

H

hallucination: Hearing, seeing, or feeling things that do not exist.

harmonic imaging: A quantitative method of characterizing and recognizing various tissue types, beyond what is visually possible from source images.

Health Insurance Portability and Accountability Act (HIPAA): Federal agency charged with overseeing many health care functions, the primary being patient confidentiality.

heart failure: The inability of the heart muscle to pump blood. Leads to fluid accumulation in the lungs, which makes breathing difficult and causes swelling of the legs, feet, liver, and other internal organs. Also known as *congestive heart failure.*

hematemesis: Bloody vomitus.

hematocrit: The percentage of the volume of a blood sample that contains erythrocytes.

hematology: The study of the blood.

hematoma: A localized mass of extravasated blood because of trauma. Usually clotted in an organ, space, or tissue.

hematuria: Blood in the urine.

hemiplegia: Paralysis of one side of the body.

hemodialysis: A procedure to remove waste or other toxic substances from the blood that cannot be eliminated by the kidney.

hemoglobin: Oxygen-carrying substance of the red blood cells.

hemolysis: Destruction of red blood cells.

hemoptysis: Bloody sputum.

hemostasis: Stopping the flow of blood.

hemostat: An instrument or clamp used to stop bleeding.

hemothorax: A collection of blood in the pleural cavity.

Hemovac drain: A Hemovac is a round drain with springs inside that must be compressed to establish proper suction.

Hepatic B virus (HBV:) A severe infectious liver virus. Classifications include hepatitis A, B, or C.

hernia: Protrusion of an organ or part of an organ through the muscular wall.

hierarchy: A group of things arranged in order of rank, grade or class.

hirsutism: Abnormal hairiness.

histology: The study of tissues.

Hodgkin disease: A malignant disease characterized by swelling of the lymph glands.

homeostasis: The maintenance of constant conditions in the internal environment. Environment of the body tends to return to normal whenever it is disturbed.

hormone replacement therapy (HRT): A combination of estrogen and progestin therapy used for relief of menopausal symptoms. Patients taking these drugs may present with increased endometrial thickening.

hydrogel: Hydrogel is a colloidal gel in which water is the dispersion medium. Hydrogels are superabsorbent (they can contain more than 90% water) natural or synthetic polymers. Most common uses in the health care environment are in disposable diapers to "capture" urine and in dressings for healing of burn or other hard-to-heal wounds.

hydrotherapy: The use of water in treating disease.

hyperemia: An excess of blood in any part of the body.

hyperglycemia: Excess sugar in the blood.

hyperplasia: An abnormal increase in the number of normal cells in a tissue or organ.

hypertension: A persistently high arterial blood pressure.

hypertrophy: An increase in the size of an organ or part because of an increase in the size of its constituent cells.

hypervolemia: An abnormal increase in the circulating blood volume.

hypoplasia: Underdevelopment of tissue or an organ usually caused by a decrease in the number of cells.

hypovolemic shock: Shock caused by a reduction in the volume of blood, as from hemorrhage.

hypoxia: Low oxygen content.

I

iatrogenic: Any adverse condition in a patient that results from treatment by a physician or surgeon (e.g., side effects of medication).

icterus: Jaundice.

idiopathic: Disease or condition whose cause is unknown.

ileostomy: An artificial opening into the ileum.

ileus: Obstruction of the bowel, usually because of the inhibition of nerve impulses necessary to the maintenance of normal peristalsis.

incident report: A form used in hospitals to document the possible injury of a patient or an employee or a visitor.

incontinence: Inability to hold urine or feces.

induration: Hardening.

infarct: An area of necrosis resulting from a lack of blood supply.

infection: Invasion of the body tissues by microorganisms, with multiplication of the microorganisms in the tissues.

inferior: Lower.

infiltration: The diffusion or accumulation in a tissue or cells, of substances not normal found there.

inflammation: A tissue response to injury. The signs are pain, heat, redness, and swelling.

informed consent: Permission obtained from a patient to have a test or procedure performed after the patient has been fully informed about the test or procedure. The consent may or may not be in writing, but a written consent provides better legal protection for the health care professional.

infusion pump: See **electronic infusion devices.**

intercostal: The space between the ribs.

interface: The boundary between two parts of matter.

interstitial: Lying between; the spaces between the cells; intercellular.

intravenous: Within a vein, often meaning an injection into a vein.

intubation: The insertion of a tube into a body opening.

invasive: Procedures that involve entering the body; tendency to spread to other parts of the body (e.g., tumors). Also known as *interventional procedures.*

involution: The return of an enlarged organ to its normal size.

irradiation: Exposure to any form of radiant energy, such as x-rays or radioisotopes.

ischemia: Decreased blood supply.

isolation: Separation from contact with others to prevent contracting or spreading disease.

J

jaundice: A yellow discoloration of the skin and eyes caused by excessive amounts of bile in the blood. May be normal in newborn infants. In adults it results from hepatitis, gallstones, or more serious liver problems.

Joint Commission of Accredited Health Organizations (JCAHO): An organization of health care institutions that is devoted to improving, regulating, and accrediting their member institutions, with the goal of providing safe and efficient patient care.

K

Kardex: Filing system for necessary information that can be located readily. Most often found at nurse's stations.

ketosis: Disturbance of the acid-base balance of the body.

L

laceration: A wound caused by tearing.

lateral: Toward the side.

latex allergy reactions: Allergic reactions to latex can include skin rash, itching, hives, swollen red skin, tears, itching or burning eyes, and swollen lips and tongue.

lavage: Irrigation or washing out of an organ or space.

law: Rules of conduct enforced by a controlling authority.

lesion: Any pathologic or traumatic change in a tissue.

leukocyte: White blood cell.

leukopenia: The reduction in the number of leukocytes in the blood (count of ≤5000).

licensure: Permission granted by a component authority or agency to an organization or individual, to engage in a practice that otherwise would be illegal.

ligation: The application of a tie around a vessel or hollow tube such as the fallopian tubes.

lipoma: Benign collection of fatty tissues.

lithiasis: Stone formation.

lithotomy: Surgical removal of a stone; also a common gynecologic position.

lithotripsy, litholapaxy: Use of sound waves to break up kidney stones or gallstones.

lumbar: Pertaining to the loin.

lumbar puncture: A procedure used to withdraw cerebrospinal fluid.

lumen: A cavity or channel within a tube.

lymph node: The primary infection fighters.

lymphocyte: A type of white blood cell.

M

magnetic resonance imaging (MRI): A diagnostic imaging technique that provides high-quality, cross-sectional images of the organs and bony structures of the body without the use of radiographs or radiation.

malabsorption: Impaired internal absorption of nutrients.

malaise: Weakness, lack of energy, and vague sense of bodily discomfort.

malignant: Tending to become progressively worse and to result in death; usually pertains to cancer or other life-threatening conditions.

mammary: Pertaining to the breasts.

mastectomy: The surgical removal of a breast.

medical malpractice: A dereliction from one's medical professional duty that results in injury, loss, or damage. A failure to exercise an accepted degree of medical professional skill/learning when rendering medical services.

memory: The process of calling to mind things remembered.

menarche: Onset of menstruation.

menopause: The cessation of menstruation at the end of the reproductive period of life.

menorrhagia: Profuse menstrual flow.

menstruation: The periodic discharge of blood and endometrial tissue from the uterus.

metabolism: The chemical processes of life.

metastasis: The transfer of a disease from one part of the body to another.

methicillin resistant *Staphylococcus Aureus* (MRSA): A specific strain of the Staphylococcus aureus bacterium that has developed antibiotic resistance.

metrorrhagia: Abnormal bleeding from the uterus during the intermenstrual period.

microorganism: A minute living organism.

micturition: The passing of urine.

midsagittal: A plane dividing the body or an organ into right and left halves.

M-Mode: Presentation of temporal changes in echoes, in which the depth of echo-producing interfaces is displayed along one axis, and time is displayed along a second axis. Also known as *motion modulation* or *time-motion mode.*

mnemonics: Techniques or systems for improving memory by the use of certain formulas.

modified Fowler position: The head of the patient's bed or table is elevated 18 to 20 inches above the level; the patient's knees are also elevated.

morals: Standards of right and wrong that are learned through socialization.

mucous membrane: A type of membrane that lines body cavities that open to the outside of the body.

mucus: A secretion produced by mucous membranes.

multiple sclerosis: A progressive disease of the nervous system.

muscular dystrophy: A progressive disease characterized by wasting of the voluntary muscles.

musculoskeletal injuries (MSIs): Injuries of the muscles, nerves, tendons, ligaments, joints, cartilage, and spinal disk due to physical work activities or workplace conditions. Also known as *musculoskeletal disorders (MSDs)* or *work-related musculoskeletal disorders (WRMSDs).*

myasthenia gravis: A disease characterized by progressive paralysis of muscles without any sensory disturbance.

myocardial infarction (MI): Heart attack.

myocardium: The heart muscle.

myoma: A muscle tumor.

myxedema: A disease caused by a deficiency of thyroid hormones.

N

Nasogastric tube (NG tube): A tube inserted through the nose and into the stomach or intestine.

National Patient Safety Goals (NPSG): Patient safety requirements developed by the Joint Commission for Accreditation of Healthcare Organizations (JCAHO) for all JCAHO-accredited institutions.

necrosis: The death or decay of one or more cells or a portion of tissue in which the growth is uncontrolled and progressive; usually results from an interruption of blood supply or injury.

negligence: The omission or commission of an act or action that a reasonably prudent sonographer would not have omitted or committed.

neoplasm: A mass of cells forming a new growth of tissue, such as a tumor, in which the growth is uncontrolled and progressive.

neovascularization: Proliferation of blood vessels in tissue not normally containing them. Proliferation of blood vessels of a different kind than usual in tissue.

nephrectomy: The surgical removal of a kidney.

nephritis: Inflammation of the kidney.

nephron: A microscopic functional unit in the cortex of the kidney.

nephroptosis: A downward displacement of the kidney.

nephrosis: A kidney disease.

nephrostomy: A surgical procedure involving placement of a tube into the renal pelvis of the kidney for drainage purposes.

neuropathy: Functional disturbances or pathologic changes in the peripheral nervous system.

neurosis: A psychic or mental illness usually characterized by anxiety and difficulties in adjusting to new or stressful situations.

nocturia: Excessive urination at night.

nonverbal communication: Communication that does not involve words (e.g., body language).

normal saline: A 0.9% solution of sodium chloride, frequently used for irrigations.

nosocomial infections: Infections acquired during a hospital stay.

nonsteroidal drugs (NSAIDs): Special class of drugs that reduce inflammation and relieve pain.

NPO: Nothing by mouth.

O

obesity: The condition of being excessively overweight.

objective: Having to do with a known or perceived object as distinguished from something existing only in the mind of the thinker.

obstetrics: Medical specialty that deals with pregnancy and childbirth.

occipital: Pertaining to the base of the skull.

occlusion: A blockage.

oliguria: Secretion of a diminished amount of urine.

oncology: The study of tumors.

oophorectomy: The surgical removal of an ovary.

ophthalmoscope: An instrument used to examine the interior of the eye.

organic: Pertaining to living matter.

orifice: The entrance or outlet of a body cavity.

orthopedics: A medical specialty dealing with disorder of the skeletal system.

orthopnea: Difficulty in breathing except in an upright position.

osseous: Pertaining to bony tissue.

ossification: Bone formation.

osteoarthritis: A chronic degenerative disease of the joints.

osteomyelitis: Infection of the bone.

osteoporosis: A disease in which there is a decrease in bone density.

ostomy: Any operation in which an artificial opening is formed between two hollow organs or between viscera and the abdominal wall.

ovulation: Release of a mature ovum from the ovary.

ovum: The mature female sex cell formed in the ovary.

oximetry: Determining the oxygen saturation of arterial blood.

oxygen saturation: In medicine, oxygen saturation (SaO_2) measures the percentage of hemoglobin binding sites in the bloodstream occupied by oxygen. An SaO_2 value below 90% is termed *hypoxia*.

P

palliative: Treatment that eliminates the symptoms but does not affect the cause of the symptoms.

palpation: Examination of the body by means of feeling with the hand.

palpitation: Rapid heart action felt by the patient.

papillae: Small nipple- or finger-shaped elevations.

papule: A small, raised lesion.

paracentesis: The removal of fluid from the peritoneal cavity.

paraphrasing: Restating the person's message in your own words.

paraplegia: Paralysis of the lower extremities.

parasympathetic: Pertaining to autonomic nerves that originate in the lower part of the brain and the sacral portion of the spinal cord.

parenchyma: The distinguishing or specific cells (functional elements) of a gland or organ as distinct from the connective tissue framework, or stroma.

parenteral: Piercing of mucous membranes or skin via needle sticks, cuts, abrasions, or bites.

paresis: Slight or incomplete paralysis.

parietal: Pertaining to the body wall; also the region of the head.

parity: A woman's reproductive history of viable/nonviable offspring. Also known as gravidity.

Parkinson disease: A progressive disease of the central nervous system characterized by stiffness; slowed movements; and rhythmic, fine tremors of resting muscles.

parturition: The birth of an infant.

patency: Being wide open.

pathogen: Anything that causes disease.

pathology: A branch of medicine concerned with structural and functional changes caused by disease.

patient care profiles (PCPs): A list of patient care plans, drugs, treatments, and so on.

Patient's Bill of Rights: Standards created by the American Hospital Association in 1993. Replaced by the Patient Care Partnership.

Patient Care Partnership: The new standard to replace the Patient's Bill of Rights, established by the American Hospital Association (see Appendix A).

pectoral: Pertaining to the breast or chest.

pediatrics: A medical specialty that deals with diseases of children.

pelvimetry: Radiographic measurement of the pregnant woman's pelvis to determine whether vaginal delivery is possible.

Penrose drain: A soft tube-shaped rubber or silicone drain, named for American gynecologist Charles Bingham Penrose (1862-1925). Frequently used in postsurgical patients.

percussion: A diagnostic procedure in which a part is struck with short, sharp blows to aid in determining the condition of the parts beneath by the sound obtained.

percutaneous: Performed through the skin.

percutaneous umbilical blood sampling (PUBS): PUBS, or fetal blood sampling, involves taking a small sample of blood from the fetal umbilical cord. PUBS are generally performed after the eighteenth week of pregnancy; however, the timing depends on the reason the test is being done (e.g., certain high-risk situations such as fetal blood type, fetal anemia, infection).

perfusion: A liquid pouring over or through something.

pericardium: The membranous sac that contains the heart.

perineum: The anatomic region at the lower end of the trunk between the thighs.

peripheral: Away from the center.

peristalsis: Contractions of smooth muscle, causing a wavelike motion.

peritoneum: A serous membrane that surrounds the abdominal organs and lines the abdominal cavity.

peritonitis: Inflammation of the peritoneum.

personality: The quality of personal identity: friendly, kind, humorous, and so on.

petechiae: Small hemorrhagic areas.

pH: The symbol relating to the hydrogen ion concentration or activity of a solution to that of a given standard solution.

phenotype: An organism's physical appearance.

phlebitis: Inflammation of veins.

phlebotomy: Insertion of needles into veins.

picture archiving and communication systems (PACS): Computer-assisted programs that allow the electronic storage, management, distribution, and viewing of images.

piezoelectric: The property of certain crystals that causes them to produce voltage when a mechanical pressure such as sound vibrations is applied to them.

piggyback infusion: An infusion system that provides both a primary line and a secondary line.

placebo: A substance with no pharmacologic action that is given to satisfy a patient's desire for drug treatment; also used in research to ensure that a medication rather than psychologic factors have caused a response.

placenta: The nutrient and excretory organ of the fetus.

plasma: The fluid portion of the circulating blood.

platelet: One of the formed particles of the blood that is important in clot formation.

pneumonectomy: The surgical removal of a lung.

pneumothorax: Air in the pleural cavity.

polyp: An abnormal growth from a mucous membrane.

polyuria: Greatly increased urinary output.

posterior: Situated behind or toward the rear.

pressure ulcer: Bed sore.

PRN: Latin term, pro re nata (as the situation demands; as needed).

proctoscopy: Visual inspection of the rectum.

prognosis: An opinion of the probable outcome of a disease or injury.

prolapse: Downward displacement of a tissue or organ outside of its normal position.

prophylaxis: The prevention of disease.

prosthesis: An artificial replacement for a part of the body that has been lost.

proximal: Closest to the point of attachment.

pruritus: Itching.

psychogenic: Caused by emotional factors.

psychosis: A severe form of mental illness in which the patient may have hallucinations and personality changes.

psychosomatic: A type of illness in which thought processes may disturb organic functions.

ptosis: A drooping or prolapse of an organ or part.

pulmonary: Pertaining to the lungs.

purulent: Containing pus.

pus: A product of inflammation consisting of fluid, white blood cells, and bacteria.

pustule: A small elevation filled with pus.

pyelonephrosis: Any disease of the kidney and its pelvis.

pyrexia: Fever.

pyuria: Pus in the urine.

Q

quadriplegia: Paralysis of all four extremities.

quality assurance (QA): A program that is intended, by its actions, to guarantee a standard level of quality and standard performance requirements.

R

radiation: The emission of radiant energy.

radioactivity: The spontaneous emission of alpha, beta, or gamma rays.

radioisotope: A radioactive element used as a tracer in the body because it can be detected and followed by its radioactive emissions.

radiology information systems (RIS): Computer programs designed to streamline scheduling/ordering of appointments, patient registration, work lists, billing, and medical and management reporting.

radiopaque: Not readily penetrated by radiographs.

rale: An abnormal respiratory sound usually associated with fluid in the air passages.

reflux: The backflow of material in the body.

registration: The process of placing one's name on a list of those eligible to practice a profession, by making an application in the prescribed way.

remission: Disappearance of the symptoms of a disease.

renal: Pertaining to the kidney.

repetitive strain injuries (RSIs): Tendon and nerve disorders resulting from many repeated, strong wrist motions. Also known as *repetitive motion injury (RMI), cumulative trauma disorders (CTDs),* or *overuse disorders.*

resection: Surgical removal of an organ or structure.

residual urine: Unexpelled urine.

respiratory arrest: Although breathing stops, the heart still pumps blood for several minutes.

restraint: A forceful confinement device.

resume: A summing up of a job applicant's previous employment, experience, and education.

resuscitation: Restoration to life or consciousness.

retroperitoneal: Behind the peritoneum.

rheumatoid arthritis: An inflammatory disease of the connective tissue characterized by remissions and exacerbation of pain and stiffness of the joints.

Rh factor: A substance in the red blood cells important in the typing of blood for transfusions and in obstetric care.

rights: Entitlements that one deserves according to just claims, legal guarantees, or moral principles. The categories of rights are freedom of choice, legal rights, and moral rights.

role-playing: Assuming a character or playing a part.

rugae: Folds inside some of the hollow organs (e.g., stomach, urinary bladder).

S

sagittal: Pertaining to a plane that divides the body into right and left portions.

salpingitis: Inflammation of the fallopian tubes.

sclerosis: Hardening.

seizure: Sudden, uncontrolled electrical activity in the brain that can cause reactions ranging from mild feelings of fear to loss of consciousness and generalized twitching (convulsions).

self-esteem: Belief in oneself; self-respect.

self-actualization: Experiencing one's potential. Full development of one's abilities, ambitions, and so on.

sepsis: Poisoning by bacteria.

septicemia: Bacteria (circulating in the blood) that multiply and produce toxins; blood poisoning.

serology: The study of antigen-antibody reactions in vitro.

serosanguineous: Pertaining to or containing both serum and blood.

serum: The fluid portion of the blood obtained after removal of the fibrin clot and blood cells.

sharps containers: Rigid containers for the safe disposal of needles and other sharp items.

sign: An objective manifestation of disease.

social conversation: The type of communication people use out of habit; superficial chitchat.

spastic: Involuntary muscle spasms.

sperm: The mature male sex cell formed in the testes.

sphincter: A muscle that closes an orifice.

sphygmomanometer: An instrument used to measure blood pressure.

standard precautions: Suggested program to provide safety to both patient and caregiver from blood or airborne infections. The Centers for Disease Control and other federal agencies have compiled these recommendations.

stasis: A stoppage of the flow of any body fluid.

statutory law: Laws established and enforced by federal or state legislators in response to perceived needs for social regulation.

stenosis: Narrowing of a passage.

stent: A device used to provide support for tubular structures that are being attached within the body.

sterilization: A process by which materials are made free of microorganisms; a procedure that makes an individual incapable of reproduction.

stethoscope: An instrument used to listen to sounds produced within the body.

stricture: A narrowing of a passageway.

subcutaneous: Beneath the skin.

subjective: Affected or produced by the mind, or a particular state of mind, resulting from the person thinking.

sublingual: Beneath the tongue.

supine: Lying on the back, face upward.

subpoena: A court document that requires a witness to appear and testify or to produce documents or papers pertinent to a pending controversy.

supportive communication: Goal oriented and information bearing.

suture: Surgical stitch or the material used to make the stitch.

sympathetic nerves: Fibers of the autonomic nervous system that originate in the thoracic and lumbar regions of the spinal cord.

symphysis pubis: The place where the pubic bones join; common landmark for pelvic scanning.

symptom: Subjective evidence of disease.

syncope: Fainting.

syndrome: A set of signs and symptoms.

systole: The contraction of the heart.

T

tachycardia: An abnormally fast heart rate. Can be caused by heart problems, fever, an overactive thyroid, or drugs.

tamoxifen: An estrogen antagonist used to treat breast cancer. Female patients may present with endometrial thickening.

teleology: The use of ultimate purpose or design as a means of explaining phenomena. Teleologists believe that an act is right if it results in a good outcome.

T-Tube: During liver-transplant surgery, a small tube called a *T-tube* is placed into the bile duct to allow bile to drain out of the patient's body into a small pouch, known as a bile bag. The T-tube is attached to the skin with a stitch. The dressing around the tube should be changed at least once daily, and more often if it becomes moist. Knowing how to change the dressing without pulling out the T-tube is important.

temporal: Pertaining to the region of the body anterior to the ear; the temple.

tetany: Muscle twitching and cramps caused by hypocalcemia.

therapeutic ultrasound: Sound at a controlled high-level dose that is used to selectively break down diseased or damaged tissues.

therapy: Treatment.

thoracentesis: A procedure used to remove fluid from the pleural cavity.

thorax: Pertaining to the chest.

thrombosis: Formation of a stationary clots (thrombus) inside a blood vessel.

torsion: Twisting; any organ that moves freely can become twisted. Surgical correction required to deter organ death from lack of blood supply.

tort: A wrongful act resulting in injury to another's person, property, or reputation—independent of a contract—for which the injured party is entitled to seek compensation.

toxemia:
A general intoxication resulting from the absorption of bacterial products; also may occur in pregnancy for reasons not completely understood.

toxin: A poison.

transcutaneous electrical nerve stimulation (TENS): A technique used to relieve pain in an injured or diseased part of the body in which electrodes applied to the skin deliver intermittent stimulation to surface nerves, blocking the transmission of pain signals.

transesophageal echocardiography (TEE): A two-dimensional, real-time imaging of the heart employing the placement of a specialized transducer within the esophagus.

transthoracic echocardiography (TTE): A noninvasive, two-dimensional, real-time imaging technique used to evaluate cardiac structure and function through the chest wall.

transvaginal sonography (TVS): The ultrasonic examination the vagina, uterus, fallopian tubes, ovaries, and bladder achieved by inserting a specialized transducer into the vagina. Also called endovaginal ultrasound.

trauma: Any type of injury.

tremor: Involuntary shaking or trembling.

Trendelenburg position: The head of the patient's table or bed is tilted downward 30 to 40 degrees, and the table or bed also is angled beneath the knees.

tumor: Any swelling or new growth.

U

ulcer: An open lesion.

ultrasound: Sound with frequencies above the upper limits of the human ear (2 to 20 mHz).

unilateral: Occurring on only one side of the body.

urea: A nitrogenous substance that is one of the end products of protein digestion.

uremia: A condition in which there is an excess accumulation of waste products in the bloodstream.

ureter: The tube leading from the kidney to the urinary bladder.

urethra: The tube leading from the urinary bladder to the outside of the body.

urinalysis: Laboratory examination of urine.

urology: A medical specialty that deals with disorders of the urinary system.

V

vaccine: A preparation made from a killed or weakened pathogen.

values: Concepts, goals, and ideals that provide a framework for one's decisions and actions and give meaning to one's life.

Valsalva maneuver: An expiratory effort against a closed glottis, which increases pressure within the thoracic cavity and thereby impedes venous return of blood to the heart.

vancomycin-resistant enterococcus (VRE): Virus commonly found in hospital patients.

varices: Enlarged and tortuous veins.

vasoconstriction: A decreased in blood vessel diameter, which leads to decreased blood flow.

vasodilatation: An increase in blood vessel diameter, particularly the peripheral arterioles.

vasomotor: Presiding over the expansion or contraction of blood vessels.

ventilation: Exchange of air (breathing).

ventral: Pertaining to the anterior surface.

verbal communication: Communication that uses written or spoken words.

vertigo: Extreme dizziness.

vesicle: A blister.

viable: Capable of living.

virus: A small disease-causing particle too tiny to be seen by conventional microscopes. Most viral infections are untreatable until the patient's own immune defenses eliminate the virus.

viscera: Internal organs of the body (particular within the abdominal and thoracic cavities).

visualization: Envisioning or forming a mental image of something not present to the sight. Also known as an *abstraction*.

vital capacity: The amount of air that can forcibly be expelled after the largest possible inhalation.

vital signs: Temperature, pulse, respirations, and blood pressure.

Z

zygote: The fertilized ovum.

Index